Medical Theory and Practice in Early Modern Italy

Medical Theory and Practice in Early Modern Italy

Edited by
Sandra Cavallo
and John Henderson

HARVEY MILLER PUBLISHERS

HARVEY MILLER PUBLISHERS
An Imprint of Brepols Publishers
LONDON TURNHOUT

British Library Cataloguing in Publication Data
A catalog record for this book
is available from the British Library

ISBN 978-1-915487-65-0

D/2025/0095/127

Printed in the EU on acid-free paper

List of Contents

Hospitals and Public Health

Abbreviations

AAV: Archivio Apostolico Vaticano.
ACUd: Archivio Capitolare di Udine.
Adel: Adelsarchiv.
AG: Archivio Gonzaga, in Archivio di Stato di Mantova.
AHK: Alte Hofkammer.
APCFi: Archivio Provinciale dei Cappuccini, Montughi, Firenze.
ASFi: Archivio di Stato di Firenze
ASDP: Archivio Storico Diocesano di Pisa
ASLi: Archivio di Stato di Livorno.
ASMi: Archivio di Stato di Milano.
ASMn: Archivio di Stato di Mantova.
ASPi: Archivio di Stato di Pisa.
ASRo: Archivio di Stato di Roma.
ASVe: Archivio di Stato di Venezia.
AT-OeStA: Österreichisches Staatsarchiv, Wien.
AVA: Allgemeines Verwaltungsarchiv, in Österreichisches Staatsarchiv.
BAV: Biblioteca Apostolica Vaticana.
BCRo: Biblioteca Civica di Rovereto.
BNCF: Biblioteca Nazionale Centrale di Firenze
BNCR: Biblioteca Nazionale Centrale, Roma
BNMVe: Biblioteca Nazionale Marciana, Venezia.
BR: Biblioteca Riccardiana
BTMi: Biblioteca Trivulziana, Milano.
BUBo: Biblioteca Universitaria di Bologna.
BUW: Biblioteka Uniwersytecka we Wrocławiu.
CORRERVe: Biblioteca del Museo Correr, Venezia.
FHKA: Finanz- und Hofkammerarchiv, in Österreichisches Staatsarchiv.
FSV: Fondo Spada Veralli, in Archivio di Stato di Roma.
HA: Hofarchive.
HAN: Sammlung von Handschriften und alten Drucken, in Österreichische Nationalbibliothek, Wien.
HAUSA: Habsburgisch-Lothringische Hausarchive, Hausarchive.
HHSTA: Haus-, Hof-, und Staatsarchiv, in Österreichisches Staatsarchiv.
KONVOLUT: Konvolut zu den Medici und Physici.
MdP: Mediceo del Principato.
NÖHA: Niederösterreichische Herrschaftsakten.
OHMA: Obersthofmeisteramt (13. Jh.-1921), Obersthofmeisteramt (1650-1921).
ÖNB: Österreichische Nationalbibliothek, Wien.
OSMN: Ospedale di Santa Maria Nuova.
RAA: Reichsadelsakten.
SR: Sonderreihe.

Illustrations

23b. Tariff (Taxa) for 1672. ACUd, Ospedale di S. Maria della Misericordia, b. 1064. (Courtesy of the Historical Archives of the Archdiocese of Udine).

23c. and d. Covers of the 1671 and 1682 Tariffs. ACUd, Ospedale di S. Maria della Misericordia, b. 1064. (Courtesy of the Historical Archives of the Archdiocese of Udine).

24a and b. *Taxa anni MDCLX seu Pretia Veneta rerum medicinalium tum simplicium tum compositarum [...] anno praescripto observanda* (Venice: Typographia ducali Pinelliana, 1660), pp. 15-16. ACUd, Ospedale di S. Maria della Misericordia, b. 1064. (Courtesy of the Historical Archives of the Archdiocese of Udine).

25. Order of the Avogadori di Comun, March 1617. ASVe, *Giustizia Vecchia*, b. 211. (Courtesy of the ASVe).

26. Page from [Dionisio Andrea Sancassani], *Dilucidazioni fisico-mediche tendenti a richiamare la medicina pratica alla preziosa purità in cui ce la lasciò il grande Ippocrate*, 1731. (Wellcome Collection. Creative Commons - Public Domain Mark).

27. Frontispiece of Lodovico Settala, *Hippocrates: Ludovici Septalii Mediolanensis medici in librum Hippocratis Coi De aeribus, aquis, locis commentarii V* (Cologne: Ciotti, 1590). (München, Bayerische Staatsbibliothek Public Domain Mark CC 0 1.0 No Copyright). https://www.digitale-sammlungen.de/de/view/bsb10147904?page=1

28. Giuseppe Ceredi, *Tre discorsi sul modo d'alzare l'acque da' luoghi bassi* (Parma: Seth Viotti, 1567), p. 69. (ETH-Bibliothek Zürich, Rar 1335, Public Domain Mark: PDM 1.0 DEED Public Domain Mark 1.0 Universal).

Introduction

Sandra Cavallo and John Henderson

Traditionally, the history of medicine in early modern Italy was a field divided between the study of theory and the study of practice, yet not only was this separation not historically justified, but the attention paid to these two elements was not equal. Whereas the intellectual foundations of the discipline were given significant consideration from the outset, there was comparatively little focus on how and when this body of knowledge was translated into practical expressions, such as diagnoses, cures, recipes, and public health measures. This was underlined as long ago as 1990 by Nancy Siraisi in her magisterial survey of the field. She commented that while much work had been done on the more theoretical learned medicine, 'At present, however, modern studies of medieval and Renaissance medical practice based on local studies are still few and scattered.'[1]

Furthermore, the ways in which medical practice influenced theory were largely overlooked. Correctives to these imbalances have emerged in recent years, thanks especially to the expansion of scholarly interests in bedside medical practice, i.e. in the medical treatment implemented by both formal and informal practitioners, as well as in domestic healthcare and in self-treatment.[2]

Attention has also shifted to how different types of healers understood the way in which medicaments worked and indeed what they understood to be medicaments. Furthermore, there is now much greater interest in understanding how a wide range of agents, from ordinary people to the authorities, sought to preserve health.[3] These new approaches have begun to highlight the ways in which the conceptual underpinnings of practice interacted with everyday medical experience.

The field has thus moved on considerably from the time Nancy Siraisi wrote her survey in 1990. Even so, there still does remain a gap between studies of medical theory and studies of medical practice in Renaissance and early modern Italy. This book, by building on recent studies, contributes to redress this imbalance by bringing together scholars at the forefront of these new approaches to take forward this fascinating field.[4] The chapters in this volume reveal the entangled inter-relationship between these two realms in a period that was characterized by the rise of empirical approaches and experimentation, as well as the growing need to incorporate novel drugs and unfamiliar diseases into the classic paradigms of professional medicine. In order to achieve these aims, we have divided the book into four sections: Bodies and Diseases, Medical Treatment, Pharmacy, Public Health, and Hospitals. The following pages first outline the themes discussed and the basic arguments developed by each chapter, emphasizing their different perspectives in relation to their sources. We then go on to examine the chapters in relation to one

1. Siraisi, *Medieval and Early Renaissance Medicine*, pp. xi-xii.
2. These include: Park, *Secrets of Women*; Pomata, 'Sharing Cases'; Nicoud, 'Salute, malattia e guarigione'; Stolberg, *Experiencing Illness; Pathology in Practice*; Quaranta, 'The Consilia'; Stolberg, 'Examining the Body; Strocchia, *Forgotten Healers.*
3. These include: Henderson, *The Renaissance Hospital*, ch. 8; Nicoud, *Les régimes de santé*; Cavallo and Storey, *Healthy Living*; Donato, *Sudden Death*; Minuzzi, *Sul filo dei segreti*; Wallis, 'Medicine and the Senses'; *Conserving Health*; Stevens Crawshaw, *Cleaning up Renaissance Italy.*
4. This volume stems from the conference 'Medicine in Early Modern Italy: Between Theory and Practice, 1500–1700', which took place at The Medici Archive Project in Florence on Friday, 19 November 2021. The event was organized by Sheila Barker, Rose Byfleet, and John Henderson. We extend our sincere thanks to MAP's director Alessio Assonitis and Elisa Paoli for their support.

another, highlighting how, collectively, they advance our understanding of the relationship between theory and practice. In this way, we shall underline the original contribution to the field of not just each author but of the volume as a whole.

THEMES AND SOURCES

In the first section, 'Bodies and Diseases', Michael Stolberg challenges the standard scholarly narrative according to which early modern doctors saw disease as generated by an 'imbalance of humors'. Drawing on a variety of medical writings (*observationes, curationes, collegia*, students' notebooks, and *consilia*) by physicians who taught or studied at Italian universities, he shows how simplistic this account is. Through a detailed analysis of these sources, the chapter aims to provide a more accurate and complex description of the medical theory that underpinned the understanding of pathological mechanisms and informed diagnosis and treatment. The aim of medical practitioners was not to balance the humors but to rid the body of morbid matter, which accumulated in certain organs and led to putrefaction, causing swellings, tumors and obstruction of organs. Morbid matter also produced vapors which rose to the head, causing catarrh and even melancholy.

Many of the arguments proposed by Stolberg are corroborated by other chapters in the volume: in particular, the notion that pathologies were typically perceived as localized rather than deriving from an imbalance affecting the whole body; and the view that, for early modern people, recovery from disease could only be attained through the expulsion of the morbid matter that caused the pathology. More open to debate and rather different from the picture emerging from other chapters is Stolberg's view that such noxious matter was thought to be out of place and of foreign, preternatural origin, rather than the product of an internal degeneration of undigested bodily residues, with the implication that early modern doctors were closer to an ontological concept of disease.

A different approach is adopted in the chapter by Alessandra Quaranta, who examines the medical practice of Italian doctors at the Habsburg Court in the second half of the sixteenth century. Her study encompasses not just the attitude of learned physicians to medical theory and practice, but also the interaction between physician and patient during the medical encounter, and how this affected the relationship between the written medical tradition and empirical practice. Indeed, her analysis emphasizes the centrality of the link between the socio-professional context and the extent to which practice diverged from theory. Quaranta reveals the extent to which medical practitioners were influenced by their patients' expectations, alongside the clinical observation conducted at the bedside. Furthermore, she shows that some physicians accepted empirics' views and treatment, reflecting a much more flexible approach in practice and in the interpretation of theory than often presented in historical studies.

In the second section of the book, 'Medical Treatment,' Sandra Cavallo's chapter, based on a close reading of the seventeenth-century correspondence of the noble Roman family of the Spadas, examines the practical use of drugs. In this way, she moves us beyond the study of printed recipe collections, which has hitherto tended to dominate the field, to an analysis of actual practice. It is clearly shown that the basic ideas of humoral medicine remained central to treatment, contrary to the frequent assumption of a shift in early modern medical treatment away from the Galenic paradigm to a world where drugs alone could heal diseases. These findings are also confirmed over the same period by two popular vernacular medical treatises, which underscore the centrality of time-honored methods of purging, evacuation, and venesection, with medicines used to aid the process rather than as ends in themselves. However, both types of sources also reveal an increased emphasis on gentler treatments and the role of the six non-naturals, an integral component of Hippocratic and Galenic thought, in promoting health and combatting disease. The impact of the relationship between patients and practitioners upon cures is further highlighted in this chapter: it is suggested that it was perhaps the influence of medically knowledgeable patients that accounts for the discrepancy between the new medical theories found in the Latinate treatises and the more conservative healing practices, also reflected in the highly popular vernacular texts.

Lucia Dacome shifts the focus to a more public context, the study of the treatment of galley slaves in early modern Livorno, a rarely analyzed site of health management. The extensive walled area in the town center known as the Bagno, which was used to house Christian and Turkish slaves, included shops, dormitories, mosques, and churches, as well, as health facilities. If treatises and decrees emphasized the economic necessity to provide good treatment to restore galley slaves to health, especially to ensure reciprocity of treatment for Christan slaves held by Turkish powers, the reality of medical practice was not always as humane as presented by the authorities. The large Bagno hospital was at the same time a center of surveillance and control, but also of medical treatment and innovation. Indeed, it was characterized by the enforcement of contemporary notions of cleanliness of air and environment and became an important center for the observation of the sick body, also through the systematic practice of morbid anatomy. Another significant finding is that the Bagno also became a center of innovation by adopting cures derived from vernacular practice, as illustrated by the case of two of its medical practitioners, the galley physician Giovanni Cosimo Bonomo and the apothecary Diacinto Cestoni, who promoted external medical treatment of scabies rather than the traditional internal treatment.

The chapters in the following section, on Pharmacy, engage with a range of sources which prompt us to explore the actual nature, dissemination, production, and sale of drugs within different contexts. Elisa Andretta examines the career of the papal physician, Michele Mercati, in the second half of the sixteenth century. Mercati also held important posts as head of the botanical garden in the Vatican and of the museum of medicine and minerals. These roles, as well as his active engagement with collecting and studying plants and minerals, have in the past often been examined separately. It is through these multifarious activities, combined with the application of his treatises on medicine, and above all on minerals and stones, that Mercati exemplifies the relationship between theory and practice. Indeed, the results of his major work, the *Metallotheca*, were reflected both in the physical layout of the museum collection and in the way individual ingredients were used in his therapeutic practice, as in the case of the Bezoar stone. Mercati's influence also spread beyond the Vatican, affecting papal public health policy through the implementation of the advice found in his treatises on plague and poison, as part of the drive to promote the health of the inhabitants of Rome. This chapter, then, extends the remit of our enquiry by examining theory and practice through not just written evidence, but also through botanical and mineral collections and the practical use of their components.

Sharon Strocchia's chapter shares a theme which has emerged from Andretta's study and in many of the other chapters, the broader shift in the sixteenth century towards increased observation and experiment. Strocchia takes Indies balsam as a case study to ask wider questions about reactions to New World drugs in early modern Italy, demonstrating the importance of not just medical, but also commercial interests, as merchants promoted its introduction and use, thereby gaining handsome profits from its sale. However, as she shows, vested interests were suspicious of this new drug, especially as this imported variety was much cheaper than the balsam already available in the Mediterranean. This suspicion led to investigation by medical authorities of its properties and effects in sixteenth-century Tuscany, where the medical college was reluctant to accept it as part of the official pharmacopeia. The trials set in motion provide a fascinating window into the relationship between theory and practice. Initially they adopted the traditional approach of sensory information to assess the balsam's humoral qualities, though complicated by the fact that balsam had not been mentioned by classical medical authorities. They rapidly adopted experimental methods, observing the effects of balsam both on the patients at the major medical hospital of Santa Maria Nuova and on deliberately poisoned dogs, usually with negative effects. After initial reluctance, eventually the medical establishment did accept this new version of balsam, especially following the publication of the book promoting new world drugs by the well-known Spanish physician Monardes. It was included in the city's *Ricettario* in 1657, following also demand from apothecaries. This chapter, by examining a range of sources, foregrounds the importance in sixteenth-century Italy of the combination of sensory approaches with new methods for determining the empirical effects of drugs through trials and experimentation.

Gaston Javier Basile also examines early modern Tuscany, and in particular the role of medicinal and cosmetic waters, a curiously under-studied topic, despite their central role in Renaissance medicine. He addresses the differences between the importance ascribed to manufactured waters in official pharmacopeia and in vernacular collections, and how this changed over time. In the more restrictive nature of official *Ricettari,* recipes tended to be more conservative, reflecting the beliefs of members of the College of Physicians, who were naturally disposed to be suspicious of the preparation of waters often associated with empirics. In contrast, it is shown that an ever-increasing number of manufactured waters were included in the recipes of a range of vernacular manuscripts in Florentine libraries. While one major collection belonged to the hospital of Santa Maria Nuova and others were associated with the Medici court, the vast majority were anonymous. However, they all had in common an openness to experimentation. They recorded the effects of medicinal waters on patients and drew as much on the practice of empirics as on officially registered practitioners, more broadly reflecting vernacular methods of recording and transmitting medical knowledge. In this chapter, then, Basile draws out the importance of the vernacular medical tradition, showing that over time, even the official *Ricettari* began to include more theoretical discussions of manufactured waters, reflecting also the increased emphasis on alchemical experimentation within the ducal court.

Sabrina Minuzzi's chapter shifts the focus to early modern Venice and its territory and the production and selling of pharmaceutical products. Venice was a special case since, in contrast to Florence and many other major cities, the College of Physicians did not produce an official pharmacopeia. Instead, thanks to the influence of their organization—the Capitular, which dated back to the thirteenth century—apothecaries had surprising independence from the College's control, which led to a much greater flexibility in the sale of medications in terms of both outlets and prices. Indeed, this chapter demonstrates the general acceptance that a wide range of individuals and institutions prepared and sold medicines. While many studies have documented the granting of licenses to empirics and charlatans to sell their secret remedies, this chapter takes us into a novel area of research, the analysis of pharmacies of friaries, particularly those of the Franciscans and Dominicans. A detailed discussion reveals that they provided recipes to a wide range of customers outside their institutions, from artisans to the wealthier. Furthermore, through a comparison with an important, but little-known source, official tariffs of the amounts to be charged for medicines, it is shown that the friars often asked no more than the cost price for their recipes, leading inhabitants, and especially poorer ones, to frequent conventual rather than commercial pharmacies. In this way, Minuzzi has been able to demonstrate how far practice departed from theory, not just in terms of which medicines were actually prescribed, but also in terms of the actual amounts charged.

The two chapters in the final section, Public Health and Hospitals, develop themes raised by previous contributors, but take them in new directions. Maria Pia Donato examines the controversies surrounding the theory, practice, and effectiveness of the treatment of wounds and ulcers in eighteenth-century Italy within the context of the hospital in Florence, Santa Maria Nuova, which also provide evidence for the studies of Strocchia and Basile. Here debates between practitioners were quickly made public, for they had implications for practice well outside the institutional environment. Donato examines an important controversy over the treatment of wounds, and the challenge to the common, complex, and repeated method of medication by a new simpler method, the 'rare' medication, which no longer understood suppurating wounds as a sign of healing. This was part of a wider challenge to Galenic physiology resulting from developments in anatomy and physical observation, prompting some practitioners to reframe the rationale behind treatments. This new approach was championed by Angelo Nannoni, master surgeon at Santa Maria Nuova, in his 1761 treatise on surgery, relying on reason and experiment rather than ancient authors. At the same time Donato finds a new reliance on broader empirical evidence to support observations backed up by the outcome of patients' cures, analyzed through statistics and the comparison of case histories. Giuseppe Cavallini's treatise, for example, based on his continued observation of patients between 1762 and 1779, represented a synthesis of qualitative information. This study underlines the importance of hospitals in encouraging debate, with practitioners' treatises boosting the reputation of their treatment and of the hospital for which they worked, which in turn helped to justify the enormous expense of running these substantial institutions.

The last chapter, by Lavinia Maddaluno, broadens still further our exploration of the key themes of this volume by shifting attention to public health and focusing on the long-standing disputes in the Milanese territory over the status of rice fields. While there was a clear case for the economic importance of paddy fields in, for example, feeding the army, dependence on stagnant water led many to criticize them as the source of corrupt air, disease and depopulation. Central to the criticism of rice production were the arguments in the Hippocratic *Airs, Waters and Places* on the relationship between health, disease and the environment, backed up by the political discourse of the public good that stressed the necessity to protect the population, their territories, and activities. These theoretical positions were reflected in a very concrete way through the employment of engineers and doctors to advise the public health boards concerning the salubriousness of rice fields in the Milanese state and the best way to maintain the region economically productive while safeguarding the health of its inhabitants. This study thus speaks to the themes of this volume, demonstrating how medical and political theories were marshalled to support the divergent policies of different professional groups, institutional bodies and economic interests.

NEW PERSPECTIVES ON MEDICAL THEORY AND PRACTICE

Up to this point, our aim has been to briefly outline the main contributions of each chapter. In the following section, we take a more selective approach to highlight how, taken together, the findings of these chapters help identify common trends and form a picture of the relationship between theory and practice—one that is innovative in many ways.

Stolberg seeks to reconstruct the theory of disease that informed the reading of the sick body in the sixteenth and seventeenth centuries; he aims, in other words, to define the common ground and shared assumptions that guided physicians' practice in this period. Quaranta, working on the same period, stresses instead that diagnoses were often contentious and provides therefore a less solid and more uncertain and negotiated image of early modern theories of disease. While for Stolberg, physicians' medical practice and the medical theory underpinning it are one and the same, other contributions in the volume provide instances of a significant gap between the two. They suggest that trust in the codified ways of reading and treating illness derived from the classical tradition was challenged in what could be labeled as 'the century of empiricism' through careful observation of the pathology and the outcome of cures (Quaranta, Andretta, Dacome, Donato).

Indeed, it is well known that the tendency to infer the nature of the disease and potential solutions, in contrast to conventional ones, from the attentive observation of the sick body, intensified in the late sixteenth and early seventeenth centuries. Alongside the development of autoptic practices, which have already attracted considerable scholarly attention, our essays underscore the importance of the clinical method first introduced at the university of Padua, and its emphasis on sensory observation in achieving these results. Furthermore, they highlight the role of hospital medical practice, which offered physicians numerous cases to examine and compare (Dacome, Donato).

This opportunity grows especially in the following period, studied by Donato. With the expansion and bureaucratization of hospitals, also brought about by the handover of these institutions to the state in the eighteenth century, empirical observation took a leap forward. It was no longer based simply on the in-depth examination of individual cases but had access to a mass of data (relating to the personal details of patients, the treatment they had received and its outcome) and to new statistical methods capable of highlighting the benefits of different healing practices.

However, as indicated by Andretta and Strocchia, the refinement of therapeutics did not only concern the human body but also inanimate things. The new method of inquiry extended to the study of nature in the sixteenth century, as the assessment of the medicinal virtues of a natural element now required clinical proof. It was no longer acceptable to simply rely on ancient doctrine, especially since the natural elements under scrutiny were often new specimens unknown to the traditional pharmacopeia. Based on their physical characteristics, response to experiment, and the results of dissections—which made it possible to retrospectively assess the validity of diagnoses and treatments–, doctors like Mercati expanded pharmacological knowledge and promoted new remedies (especially, mineral ones), not only systematizing the wisdom of the ancients but correcting and extending it.

Observation and experimentation also extended to vernacular healing practices, even to those in use among the largely non-Christian, enslaved population serving the grand duke of Tuscany (Dacome). The open-minded, inquiring approach of the doctors in charge of the health of these captives led them to modify their way of treating scabies, replacing the internal remedies prescribed by Galenic medicine with the topical ones used by the slaves. In this case, the successful trial of a new cure prompted a re-conceptualization of the nature of the disease, now related to the presence of small parasites in the body detectable under the microscope, and no longer seen as caused by an excess of black bile or degenerated blood. The new theory of scabies emerged in this case from below, from lay medical practice and experience, reflecting the openness of established physicians to learning from empirical traditions.

Quaranta, however, highlights the potential conflict between the expected conformity to the written medical tradition and the new value attributed to empiricism, and thus the difficulty for early modern medical practitioners to entirely divorce themselves from time-honored knowledge. Not only had humanist thought made it imperative to show constant reverence for the ancient texts, but the confidence in long-established ideas and practices, in a delicate matter such as health management, was a powerful inhibitor of innovation. As Strocchia and Dacome underline, 'the test of time' was a recurring preoccupation. Thus, even an enlightened figure like the well-known papal physician Giovanni Maria Lancisi dismissed the new treatment of scabies, arguing that its apparent, recent success could not invalidate 'the experience of many centuries.' Therefore, as exemplified by Quaranta, introducing novelties into medical practice required stratagems, such as searching for contradictory passages or omissions in ancient texts, to avoid openly clashing with tradition.

However, some of the essays caution us against establishing a simplistic opposition between 'traditional' humoral theory and 'new' medical views and therapeutic approaches. In the period examined, the Galenic paradigm was not static but subject to modest shifts, which nevertheless made a significant difference to the patients' experience. Both Cavallo and Dacome suggest, for example, that attention to the effects of environmental factors and lifestyles, the non-naturals, became increasingly important in both the prevention and treatment of disease in the seventeenth century. In the medical treatment of the Roman nobility as in the health management of the enslaved galley-rowers, factors like diet, good air, rest, exercise, hygiene, and the soothing of emotions, acquire a greater role in the healing process, at the expense of an over-reliance on drugs and violent purging and bloodletting.

The introduction of milder forms of treatment is also signaled by Donato in relation to the medication of surgical cases. Elements of change therefore are detectable but, as this author explains, we cannot expect dramatic interpretive shifts and major breakthroughs in the therapies adopted, only small yet significant adjustments within a general trend of continuity of the humoral paradigm. Focusing on the eighteenth century, Donato shows how slow the emergence of a new way of treating wounds was, where rare medication of the affected part replaced the traditional habit of over-medication. Moreover, as for the new therapy against scabies, the application of 'rare' medication only concerned certain hospitals or hospital wards. Therapeutic practice, in other words, seems particularly resistant to change; at the turn of the seventeenth century, it failed to adapt to the new ways of conceptualizing physiology, such as blood circulation and a corpuscular understanding of the body and medicinal substances. Hence, as noted by Cavallo, the cures prescribed by Girolamo Brasavola, a physician considered an innovator in medical theory based on his academic writings, are not so different from those adopted a few decades earlier by Fonseca, a far more traditional doctor, marginal to new trends of thought and ongoing scientific debates.

But how helpful is the conservative/innovative binary division that we have just employed and that often characterizes discussions about change in medical theory and practice? Usually, the theoretical stance of a physician is deduced from his professional writings, including treatises, letters, *consilia*, etc., and his attitude towards tradition and innovation is assessed from there. Quaranta, however, warns us that the content of these texts cannot be taken at face value, as a reflection of the physician's thought. She shows that, depending on the circumstances, the same person may express opinions that appear to us progressive or regressive depending on the context in which they were expressed and their intended and unintended recipients. In general, she shows that it was easier to deviate from doctrine at the patient's bedside than in writing. In talking to colleagues and patients, doctors could take unconventional positions in diagnosing disease and deciding on cures; in writing, adopting an heterodox position more easily exposed the doctor to the criticism of competitors. Even letters were not immune to this risk since they were public, were often shown to others, circulated widely, and could provoke condemnations negatively affecting a practitioner's reputation.

As already noted, patients also had agency and influenced diagnosis and treatment, but not all of them commanded the same authority. On the basis of the examples collected in this volume, it seems that therapeutic innovations were more likely to be applied to the poor seeking medical care in hospitals, and to prisoners, i.e. to categories with limited power to influence the cures they received, rather than to the more vocal, paying sick.

Our essays also illustrate the massive assimilation of new medicinal substances (mineral, animal, exotic and chemical) into Western therapeutic practice, offering further evidence of the capacity for renewal of the humoral paradigm. But how did this inclusion come about? How were the medical authorities and consumers themselves persuaded of the value of these new products? Several chapters draw attention to the role of printed texts in the vernacular, aimed at a wide audience as formidable 'promotional vehicles,' to use Strocchia's words, for new cures and new drugs. Alongside published works, Andretta also highlights the influence and didactic role played by 'museums of medicine,' such as Mercati's, which displayed little-known minerals, stones, and metals to visitors, illustrating their medicinal properties and thus promoting their use.

Focusing on the case of Indies balsam, Strocchia explores the passages that led many new products to be included in Western medical treatment from many new angles. On the one hand, she illustrates the process of Europeanization of these medicinal substances, i.e., their justification in terms of humoral qualities and a familiar pharmaceutical nomenclature. But she also highlights the sophisticated promotional strategies employed, such as the collection of eyewitness testimonies and practitioners' reports on the efficacy of the drug. Moreover, she shows how large institutions, like hospitals or monasteries, were deliberately persuaded to use the drug to provide the public with reassuring evidence of its validity. In other words, she reveals the often-forgotten role of market dynamics and marketing stratagems in a process that was not only of an intellectual nature, but was also driven by economic considerations, i.e., the quest for profit and the need to meet demand. Although much has been written in recent years on the testing of new drugs as a purely intellectual pursuit, things were more complex. Strocchia points out that these clinical trials were often inconclusive and therefore decisions were ultimately made regardless of the drug's poor proof of efficacy.

Strocchia also shows how the thoroughness of the tests and the caution with which new drugs were accepted into medical practice varied from country to country, Spain being much more casual in promoting the commercialization of drugs about which little was known, and Tuscan authorities, doctors and pharmacists adopting much more scrupulous procedures to ascertain the validity of the product. This comparison invites us to avoid the easy generalization of results obtained from the study of a single region or country. The importance of paying attention to differences between places is also noted by Minuzzi, who shows how Venice stands out for being particularly liberal in granting patents and privileges to new drugs, and never produced an official pharmacopoeia, which in other areas, such as Tuscany, was intended to act as a barrier to the spread of new medicines.

Even when they existed, however, pharmacopoeias were still largely ignored in practice, as demonstrated by Basile's comparison between the contents of the *Ricettario Fiorentino*, in its various editions, and numerous manuscript recipe books. While the former long resisted the inclusion of medicines produced by distillation and other chemical procedures, he finds that chemical remedies were already frequently mentioned in recipe books compiled as early as the fifteenth century. Pharmacopoeias thus hardly reflected the actual medicinal treatment adopted in society. To illustrate everyday practice, we must turn to other sources: in addition to the manuscript collections of recipes studied by Basile, the tariff books analyzed by Minuzzi offer a more accurate picture of the type of drugs sold in pharmacies. Undoubtedly, as these two essays demonstrate, the evolution of pharmaceutical theory was stimulated by extensive independent practice and by experimentation from below. This is shown clearly by Minuzzi in relation to monastic pharmacies, which supposedly just made medicines for friars but in practice served numerous external customers, largely outside the control of the authorities. Not only was access to medicines far more extensive than previously assumed, but far more unregulated.

A rarely asked question about medicinal remedies concerns the role they played in cures. Undoubtedly their availability and use increased significantly during this period, as suggested by many of the chapters in this volume. But is this sufficient to justify the assumption that they were now used independently, on the ground of their direct therapeutic efficacy, and supplanted time-honored evacuative cures, based on purgation and bloodletting, as well as dietetic measures? Cavallo demonstrates the importance of addressing these questions through sources that document actual practice, like family letters. The evidence from letters, backed by vernacular medical texts, suggests that medicinal remedies were just one component of more complex treatments, consisting of a combination of dietary, pharmaceutical, and evacuative procedures. Drugs were thought to play an ancillary role: they were used to encourage and facilitate the expulsion of the noxious matter responsible for the pathology but were not seen as capable of curing directly; this epochal change was still to come.

So far, we have discussed the relationship between medical theory and practice limited to the treatment of individual patients and the effects of remedies. Lavinia Maddaluno broadens this question to the field of public health, thus extending the implications of other chapters, such as that by Andretta on Rome and Donato on Florence. Moreover, while the other essays consider medical theory in isolation from other traditions of thought, Maddaluno's reminds us that medical views coexisted with often competing bodies of ideas about health, not only of an economic nature, as Strocchia and Minuzzi have also shown, but also, for example, of a political and religious nature. In this particular case, physicians' views about the impact of rice fields on health were at odds with economic considerations supported by the state, which favored this type of cultivation over other, more salubrious functions of the marshes. Conversely, medical perspectives were more aligned with the position of advocates of the *ragion di stato*, who, aware of the impact of increased morbidity and death, encouraged a policy of re-population of the area, and with religious authorities, preoccupied by the inability of those employed in paddy fields to perform their religious duties. This case thus illustrates how medical theory sometimes converged, other times collided, but always needed to negotiate its practical applications with different bodies of thought.

WORKS CITED

Cavallo, Sandra and Storey, Tessa, *Healthy Living in Late Renaissance Italy* (Oxford: Oxford University Press, 2013).

Conserving Health in Early Modern Culture. Bodies and Environments in Italy and England, ed. by Sandra Cavallo and Tessa Storey (Manchester: Manchester University Press, 2017).

Donato, Maria Pia, *Sudden Death: Medicine and Religion in Eighteenth-Century Rome* (Farnham: Ashgate, 2014).

Henderson, John, *The Renaissance Hospital: Healing the Body and Healing the Soul* (New Haven and London: Yale University Press, 2006).

Minuzzi, Sabrina, *Sul filo dei segreti: Farmacopea, libri e pratiche terapeutiche a Venezia in età moderna* (Milan: Unicopli, 2016).

Nicoud, Marylin, *Les régimes de santé au Moyen Âge. Naissance et diffusion d'une écriture médicale en Italie et en France (XIIIe-XVe siècle)* (Rome: Ecole Française de Rome, 2007).

Nicoud, Marylin, 'Salute, malattia e guarigione. Concezioni dei medici e punti di vista dei pazienti', *Quaderni storici* 46 (2011), 47–74.

Park, Katharine, *Secrets of Women: Gender, Generation, and the Origins of Human Dissection* (New York: Zone Books, 2006).

Pathology in Practice: Diseases and Dissections in Early Modern Europe, ed. by Silvia De Renzi, Marco Bresadola, Maria Conforti (Routledge: London, 2017).

Pomata, Gianna, 'Sharing Cases: The *Observationes* in Early Modern Medicine', *Early Science and Medicine*, 15 (2010), 193–236.

Quaranta, Alessandra, 'The Consilia by Learned Physicians Pietro Andrea Mattioli and Francesco Partini. Dialectic Relations between Doctrine, Empirical Knowledge and Use of the Senses in Sixteenth-Century Europe', *Social History of Medicine*, 35:1 (2022), 20–48.

Siraisi, Nancy, *Medieval and Early Renaissance Medicine. An Introduction to Knowledge and Practice* (Chicago—London: Chicago University Press, 1990).

Stevens Crawshaw, Jane, *Cleaning up Renaissance Italy. Environmental Ideals and Urban Practice in Genoa and Venice* (Oxford: Oxford University Press, 2023).

Strocchia, Sharon, *Forgotten Healers. Women and the Pursuit of Health in Late Renaissance Italy* (Cambridge, Mass.: Harvard University Press, 2019).

Stolberg, Michael, 'Examining the Body, c.1500–1750', in *The Routledge History of Sex and the Body*, ed. by Sarah Toulalan and Kate Fisher, (London-New York: Routledge, 2013), pp. 91–105.

Stolberg, Michael, *Experiencing Illness and the Sick Body in Early Modern Europe* (Basingstoke-New York: Palgrave Macmillan, 2011).

Wallis, Faith, 'Medicine and the Senses: Feeling the Pulse, Smelling the Plague, and Listening for the Cure', in *A Cultural History of the Senses in the Middle Ages*, ed. by Richard G. Newhauser (London: Bloomsbury Academic, 2016), pp. 133–52.

1
The Myth of Humoral Imbalance.
How Renaissance Physicians Explained and Treated the Diseases of Their Patients

Michael Stolberg

According to the standard historical narrative, the principles of early modern humoral pathology were remarkably simple: health rested on the balanced mixture of the four natural humors in the body (yellow and black bile, blood, and phlegm) and on the balance of the four primary qualities (cold, hot, dry, and moist) which were associated with these four natural humors in pairs: yellow bile was hot and dry, black bile cold and dry, phlegm cold and moist, and blood hot and moist. Diseases were due to *intemperies* or *dyscrasia,* that is, to an imbalance of the four primary qualities and/or the four natural humors in the body. 'For most people', Mary Lindemann has summarized this view, 'disease arose from humoral imbalance, that is, from a general state of disequilibrium that the environment could affect or influence.'[1] According to Ian Maclean, one of the leading experts on sixteenth-century medical theory, physicians ascribed diseases to 'asymmetric or unbalanced states of the body'.[2] Although some authors, most notably Andrew Wear and recently Evan Ragland,[3] have offered a different, more nuanced picture, this has been well-established textbook account of early modern Galenic medicine for decades and it continues to be widely taken for granted in scholarly writing as well as in books, articles, radio programs, and documentaries for the general public.

As I will argue in this chapter, there is a fundamental problem with this narrative, however: the idea that early modern Galenist physicians explained diseases as resulting from an imbalance of the primary qualities or the four natural humors in the body does not correspond to the medical theory as it was taught in Padua, Bologna, and other leading universities at the time. And, more importantly even, it is very much at odds with what we know about the ways in which physicians actually diagnosed, explained, and treated the overwhelming majority of cases of disease in their everyday practice.

The misconception results to a considerable degree from a confusion of the early modern understanding of the healthy body with that of the sick body and from a lack of awareness of the prominent place of localized pathology in early modern medicine. The temperament or *krasis,* the specific, quite literally idiosyncratic mix of humors in the body, did play a key role in early modern Galenic medicine. Medical students already learnt how to assess a patient's temperament, from the color of the hair and the skin and from the 'character' of a person. Letters from patients requesting an epistolary consultation show that lay people often had quite firm ideas about their own bodily temperament. They knew whether their body was dominated, for example, by yellow bile or rather by phlegm.[4]

While a certain temperament might predispose an individual to certain diseases, it was not considered a disease in itself. It was the natural physical constitution of that person, which could change with age and under the influence of environmental conditions. Dietetic recommendations for the choice of the right food and drink, appropriate physical exercise, place of living in sickness and

1. Lindemann, *Medicine and Society*, p. 13.
2. Maclean, *Logic, Signs and Nature*, p. 260.
3. Wear, *Knowledge & Practice*; Ragland, *Making Physicians.*
4. Stolberg, *Experiencing Illness*, pp. 86-87.

in health, and the prescription of medicines, had to take the patient's temperament into account. A patient with a hot and dry temperament, for example, had to be particularly careful with consuming hot food and drink. When it came to explaining diseases, however, learned physicians relied on a fundamentally different explanatory model, one which was already present to some degree in the writings of Hippocrates and Galen. They attributed virtually all diseases, with very few exceptions, to some kind of foreign, impure, preternatural, morbific, 'peccant' matter in the body. The specific nature of this matter and its location in the body—and not some humoral imbalance—explained the symptoms and sequels of most diseases.

SOURCES

This explanatory model is ubiquitous in the rich but under-exploited body of sources on how physicians in the sixteenth and early seventeenth centuries, the heyday of Galenic humoral medicine, were taught to understand and explain diseases and on how they diagnosed and treated them. These sources are crucial, if we want to assess the importance and impact of the general medical theories we find in contemporary textbooks on actual practice. In fact, as the late Iain Lonie rightly remarked, 'without some kind of access to practical medicine and its teaching, we are in danger of ending with a history of medicine which includes everything except the craft of medicine itself.'[5] Printed collections of *curationes* and *observationes*, a very popular genre from the 1550s onwards, offer thousands of case histories on the diagnosis and treatment of individual patients.[6] Many *observationes* were moreover followed by a learned *scholion*, which put the case history into a theoretical context. In countless medical *consilia*, physicians responded to patients' and colleagues' requests for epistolary advice, often with a quite extensive discussion of the presumable nature and causes of the patient's disease, on which they based their therapeutic recommendations.[7] In places like Ferrara, Padua, and Bologna, the students also accompanied their professors on patient visits, in local hospitals or in the patients' private homes, witnessing and documenting how the professor explained the patient's disease and justified his choice of treatment. In Padua, moreover, students could attend public presentations and discussions of individual cases, the so-called *collegia* for which the university was famous. In a *collegium*, the case of patient was presented, based on a written *historia morbi* or orally by one of the professors. Then, one professor after the other expressed his opinion about the cause and the nature of the disease in question and its treatment. Student notes on dozens of such patient visits and *collegia* were published in print, while others have survived in manuscript form.[8] Practice journals, personal notebooks of physicians, and similar sources documenting the daily practice of medicine outside academia have rarely been preserved from this period, though there are notable exceptions.[9] One of the most significant among them is the richest known source on the everyday medical practice of sixteenth-century Galenic physicians. The little-known Bohemian physician Georg Handsch, first as a student in Italy and later as a practicing doctor, compiled several notebooks containing over 4,000 pages of notes. These detailed his observations of patients seen alongside his professors and, later, with other physicians in Prague and Innsbruck. Among his colleagues were Andrea Gallo from Trento and the renowned botanist Pietro Andrea Mattioli from Siena.[10]

MORBID MATTER

There is thus a wealth of sources that demonstrate in great detail how Galenist physicians in the sixteenth and early seventeenth century explained and treated their patients' diseases. Yet it is very difficult—and indeed virtually impossible—to find in these sources cases in which

5. Lonie, 'The "Paris Hippocratics"', p. 157.
6. Particularly successful and widely quoted examples are Amatus Lusitanus, *Curationum medicinalium*; Foreest, *Observationum et curationum medicinalium*—Foreest eventually published almost forty books of medical and surgical observations; Schenck von Grafenberg, *Observationum medicarum*; on the genre, see Stolberg, 'Formen'; Pomata, 'Observation Rising'.
7. e.g., Monte, *Consultationum medicarum*; Trincavelli, *Consilia medica*.
8. Cf. Stolberg, 'Bedside Teaching'; ibid., 'Kasuistischer medizinischer Unterricht'.
9. See the contributions to Dinges et al., *Medical Practice*, which all draw primarily on physicians' practice journals. The most extensive practice journal that has so far been found for a *doctor medicinae* in the sixteenth and early seventeenth century is that of the Zwickau town physician Hiob Finzel. It documents more than two decades of his medical practice, with almost 10,000 consultations, in three heavy folio volumes (Ratsbibliothek Zwickau, MS. QQQQ 1, MS. QQQQ 1a und MS. QQQQ 1b).
10. In particular, ÖNB, Cod. 11183, Cod. 11205, Cod. 11206, and Cod. 11207

physicians attributed the disease of an individual patient to an imbalance of the humors or primary qualities in her or his body. The physicians routinely assessed the patient's temperament but their diagnosis of the actual disease did not refer to some imbalance of humors or qualities in the body. Their diagnostic method—and their choice of suitable treatment—required first and foremost that they establish the cause of the disease. This involved identifying the nature of the preternatural morbific matter in question, its primary location in the body, and the source or origin of the pathological processes that generated this morbid or 'peccant' matter or promoted its accumulation in the body or specific parts of it.

As the above-mentioned sources show, physicians were familiar with a range of reasons why preternatural, morbid matter was generated and/or accumulated in the body. To some degree, the generation of preternatural matter was inevitable. After all, the body was constantly ingesting foreign, impure substances with the food. According to contemporary Galenic theory, this incoming foreign matter had to be quite literally 'concocted' in several steps by the body's vital heat: first in the stomach, where the useful parts of the food were turned into chyme, then in the liver which produced nutritious blood from the chyme, and finally in the individual parts of the body which the blood nourished.[11]

Due to its crucial place in the first step of concoction the stomach played a particularly significant role in this explanatory model. In the vast majority of cases, it was thought to be involved, even though often further organs such as the liver, spleen, intestine, lung, and brain might be taken to play their part as well. A weak stomach that did not have 'its natural digestion,' as the physicians explained to their patients,[12] could not properly concoct the raw, foreign matter that humans constantly ingested with food and drink. And even a strong stomach could be overtaxed by excessive amounts of raw, cold food. In both cases, raw, sticky, slimy matter would accumulate in the stomach. 'A foul mucus is lying in his stomach,' Handsch declared in such cases.[13] This 'foul' mucus or slime must not be confused with the phlegm that was considered one of four natural humors. It originated from the raw food in the stomach, the same way in which rotting vegetables turned slimy. When cold, raw, slimy, foul matter accumulated in the stomach and stuck to its walls, a vicious circle was initiated. The ability of the stomach to concoct the incoming food was further compromised and more and more preternatural matter would fill the stomach and counteract the efforts of the vital heat to concoct the food.

When the concoction of the incoming food and drink by the stomach was imperfect, the resulting chyme that arrived from the stomach to the liver was also inevitably insufficiently concocted, raw, or even slimy. The liver could not produce good blood from it but only imperfect, somewhat raw, and impure blood, or at least blood that was mixed with insufficiently concocted, raw matter. One result was that the various parts of the body were deprived of their proper nutrition. 'The stomach does not do a natural digestion,' Handsch and his colleagues found in such cases: 'most of that which should give nourishment to the body turns into slime.'[14] Moreover, the raw, insufficiently concocted matter could putrefy or become more harmful in other ways. The body therefore needed to get rid of it. As Thomas Erastus explained to a patient with a smelly urinary flux along these lines, for example, parts of his blood were insufficiently concocted. Some of this raw blood oozed from the veins into the surrounding flesh and slowly putrefied. The patient's urinary flux resulted from his body's attempt to evacuate the bad, evil matter, which, in patients who suffered from gout, migrated to the extremities, and formed calcareous deposits.[15]

Insufficient concoction and the slimy, viscous blood often resulting from it were also believed to affect the physical quality of the blood and particularly its mobility. Here, we encounter another explanatory element that has so far been insufficiently appreciated in standard accounts of early modern humoral pathology. Renaissance physicians also widely relied on mechanistic, hydraulic explanations—something medical historians have traditionally described only for the iatromechanical theories of the seventeenth and early eighteenth centuries. When the blood was insufficiently concocted and slimy or mixed with mucilaginous, preternatural matter, the physicians believed, it moved more slowly. The matter

11. On the disease concepts that informed sixteenth-century learned medical practice, see also Stolberg, *Learned Physicians*, esp. pp. 121-145.
12. ÖNB, Cod. 11206, fol. 126^{v}.
13. Ibid., fol. 23^{v}.
14. Ibid., fol. 20^{v}.
15. Staatsbibliothek Berlin, Depot Breslau 10, Nr. 9, *consilium* for Lazarus von Schwendi, Basel, 15 March 1581 (detailed summary by Ulrich Schlegelmilch in the Würzburg database on Early Modern Physicians' Letters, www.aerztebriefe.de/id/00003394).

stuck to the walls of the vessels and clogged them, and, in the worst case, disrupted the movement of the blood altogether: 'the blood cannot move freely, it is all pain and narrowness', the physician might say in such cases.[16] Or he might explain in somewhat more elaborate terms: 'The blood is soiled, spoiled, filled with mucus and clogged; it lacks its natural flow, gets stuck and is constricted in the veins like water in the pipes.'[17] Sometimes the physicians compared this process more specifically to the effects of dirt or lime scale that slowed down or indeed blocked the flow of water.[18]

Even when the concoction in the stomach, the liver, and, at a later stage, in the individual parts of the body was sufficiently strong, the concoction and assimilation inevitably left behind some impure residual matter, which the body could not use for nutrition, and which had to be excreted. Early modern medical writers discussed a full range of excretions, from earwax, tears, and hemorrhoidal bleeding to fingernails, toenails, and hair. Four major excretory pathways stood out, however, for their sheer volume and their sensory qualities: feces, urine, sweat, and, in women, menstruation. When one of these excretions was diminished or, even worse, entirely 'suppressed,' excremental matter would accumulate in the body and could seriously jeopardize health. Thus, when a noblewoman developed fever and pain in the uterus and the flanks after having given birth, Benedetto Vittori in Bologna immediately concluded that she suffered from a retention of the 'purgationes' and 'menstruum'; her postpartum flux had only lasted for six days.[19]

When the sick body made every possible effort to rid itself of the preternatural morbid matter, some of this matter would also also mingle with the natural excretions, changing the color, consistency, and smell of the feces or the menstrual blood, for example, or swimming or forming a sediment in the urine flask. For good reasons, physicians, far into the eighteenth century, routinely resorted to uroscopy to diagnose diseases.[20] Sometimes, the careful examination of other excretions could also provide valuable diagnostic clues. In the case just cited, Brasavola asked the patient to collect his sputum in a vessel and examined it afterwards together with his students.[21]

When the blood was insufficiently concocted or mixed with morbid, peccant matter it could undergo further pathogical changes or indeed putrefy inside or outside the vessels, and even well-concocted, healthy blood, semen, and other natural fluids in the body could spoil and become corrupted, when they remained stagnant for a longer period of time in certain parts of the body. Humors and fluids could also become sharp and acrid when they were burnt by some pathological heat. In this sense, Giovanni Battista da Monte in one of the Paduan collegia, attributed the disfiguring impetigo of a female patient to evil, adust humors which moved towards the skin of her face. Her very hot liver, he believed, had literally burnt these humors.[22]

Drawing on this complex but coherent explanatory model, the physicians resorted to a wide range of medicines when they treated their patients. As the 'servants of Nature,' they used above all medicines and other forms of treatment such as cupping and bloodletting that supported the body in its evacuative efforts. In addition, they prescribed medicines that acted against the further generation and accumulation of morbid matter in the body. Some medicines were also taken to change the nature of the morbid matter itself, to make it less harmful and/or more suitable for excretion, for example, by softening and mobilizing morbid matter that had accumulated and hardened in certain parts of the body. Other medicines, again, served to strengthen individual organs, such as the heart or the stomach.

In the seventeenth and eighteenth centuries, a range of new and often contradictory medical theories were put forward, ranging from iatrochemistry, Helmontianism and mechanistic accounts to Stahlianism and vitalism. They were meant to take the place of the traditional explanatory model I just sketched out. Among patients and in the lay medical culture in general the attribution of diseases to morbid, 'foreign' matter of which the body had to be cleansed, prevailed far into the nineteenth century, however.

16. ÖNB, Cod. 11206, fol. 24^{r}.
17. Ibid., fol. 15^{r}.
18. Ibid., fol. 121^{v}.
19. Biblioteca comunale, Forlì, MS. III, 94 (notes by an unidentified student on patients he saw with his professors in Bologna), fol. 6^{v}, 1 February 1540.
20. Stolberg, *Uroscopy*.
21. Biblioteca comunale Ariostea, Ferrara, MS. Antonelli, 531, fol. 17^{r}.
22. Wellcome Collection, London, Western Manuscripts 567, fols 18^{r}-20^{v}.

Ordinary people continued to consider drastic laxatives and emetics, with bloodletting and cupping and other evacuative means, as indispensable for successful treatment. As a physician who worked in mid-nineteenth century rural Bavaria summarized his experience: 'People expect quick and tangible results from the medicine, especially much sweating and copious evacuations, which they consider desirable results. [...] The more drastic and quicker [the effects], the more confidence-inspiring the medicine.'[23]

ORGANIC 'INTEMPERIES'

It is virtually impossible to find any cases in the abundant casuistic medical writings of the period in which physicians declared an imbalance of the primary qualities in the whole body to be the cause of the disease. Fevers might seem to be the most obvious counterexample because they were often associated with heat. However, physicians and laypeople also knew 'cold' fevers, characterized by shivering. More importantly, the feverish heat itself was considered pathological. It was a *calor extraneus*, a foreign heat, which was inflamed in the heart, according to Avicenna's often-quoted definition in his *Canon medicinae,* which remained the foundational text of learned fever theory far into the seventeenth century.[24]

One specific point—and a possible objection against my account—still needs to be discussed, namely the notion of an *intemperies*, of an imbalance of the primary qualities of individual organs. This notion did play a considerable role in sixteenth- and seventeenth-century Galenic medicine. Galenic theory saw the workings of body, from the concoction and assimilation of food to memory and reason, as resulting from specific powers or 'faculties'. Ultimately these faculties were attributes of the soul, but they needed bodily 'organs,' i.e. literally 'instruments' or 'tools', to take effect. Different faculties had their seat in different organs, and they depended on the healthy constitution of these specific organs. A pathological *intemperies* of an organ therefore could affect the faculties that depended on that organ as its tool.

Renaissance physicians were well-aware of the prominent place the *intemperies* of individual organs held in Galen's writings. Organic *intemperies* ranked among the standard topics of the medical theory teaching. Around 1550, Bassiano Landi in Padua, for instance, in his lectures on Galen's *Ars medica*, extensively and systematically discussed the different forms and signs of *intemperies* that could be identified in individual organs, from the brain to the genitals. He elaborated in great detail, for example, on how an excessively hot, cold, dry, or moist liver could impair the functions—or more precisely, the *facultates*—of that organ, and what the typical consequences and symptoms would be. The range of possible diverse types of organic *intemperies* was considerable. After all, each of the major organs could be too cold, hot, moist, or dry, or it could be too cold and moist, too cold and dry, too warm and moist, or too warm and dry at the same time. Georg Handsch's manuscript notes on Landi's lectures run over more than two hundred pages.[25]

As I have found in my extensive survey of early modern medical *consilia*, case histories and physicians' practice notes, most varieties of *intemperies* that Landi listed were largely irrelevant in everyday practice. Only a handful were quite frequently diagnosed. The most important among them were an excessively cold stomach, which could not concoct the incoming food sufficiently and produced raw, slimy matter, and an excessively hot liver which burnt the blood and other humors, making them sharp, acrid, or biting. An excessively cold stomach and an excessively hot liver also frequently came together. Handsch and his Italy-trained colleagues in Prague often diagnosed both in the same patient, sometimes explicitly suggesting a causal connection: the crude, poorly concocted, slimy, viscous chyme the cold stomach sent to the liver caused an obstruction in the liver. The ensuing stagnation and accumulation of blood and humors in the liver resulted in corruption and putrefaction, generating excessive heat.

In this sense then we do find an *intemperies* explaining certain diseases, but it was not an *intemperies* of the whole body. In fact, the frequent simultaneous diagnosis of a cold *intemperies* of the stomach and a hot *intemperies* of the liver illustrates that opposing types of *intemperies* could coexist in the same patient. Moreover, strictly speaking, the pathological consequences of an *intemperies* in a specific organ did not result from an 'imbalance.'

23. Bayerische Staatsbibliothek, Munich, manuscript collection, Cgm 6874-111, medical topography and ethnography of the district of Mindelheim, 1861.
24. Avicenna, *Canon medicinae*, lib. 4, fen 1, tr. 1.
25. ÖNB, Cod. 11224, *Dictata in artem parvam Galeni.*

When the liver was too hot, for example, this was not in comparison with the three other primary qualities. The heat as such was excessive and acted like a fire, burning, or even charring fluid and solid matter.

LOCAL PATHOLOGY

The peccant, preternatural matter that was at the core of the disease process could spread throughout the body or settle in a specific area. When it mingled with the blood in vessels or 'infected' it, as this was commonly termed,[26] the whole body was affected. This was the principal explanation for fevers. In many cases, some of the morbid matter that 'infected' the blood was moreover taken to move through the walls of the veins and to accumulate in the flesh around them. This helped explain a certain periodicity which physicians and patients often thought they could discern in fevers: depending on its nature, the peccant matter, they believed, could be mobilized, and hence moved back into the veins at regular intervals. In quartan fevers, patients got worse or had 'attacks' of fever every third day, in tertian fevers every second day and in semi-tertian fevers every day, because the preternatural matter, depending on its nature, periodically reentered the vessels at certain times every third or second day or indeed daily.[27]

In most diseases, the morbid, peccant matter was taken to settle in specific parts of the body, however, causing local symptoms. Sometimes such local accumulations of morbid matter could be seen from the outside, as local swellings of limbs and joints, for example, or as apostemes, boils, or pustules in the skin or as the typical 'tophi' on the big toe in gout. In other cases, the body evacuated some of this morbid matter, bringing it quite literally to the surface, as when patients had slimy or purulent expectoration or when boils burst and released a smelly, unappetizing fluid. A nobleman at the court of Schwerin, for example, suffered for years from a painful affection of the skin, with boils that sometimes released stinking pus. Consulted about the case, Dr Johann Kuhn and the Nuremberg collegium medicum had no doubts that the boils originated from impure, infected and salty phlegmatic blood and from adust melancholic blood, which the body sought to expel through the skin.[28]

The dangers to the patient's health and life were even greater and potentially more lasting when the morbid matter, due to its often viscous, slimy consistence, accumulated in a certain organ and 'obstructed' it. Organ obstructions were feared by physicians and laypeople alike, and they ranked among the most common diagnoses. The liver, the spleen, and the uterus were taken to be at particular risk. In the worst case,obstructions directly affected the excretion of impure excremental matter. In this sense, an obstruction of the uterus was feared as the major reason for a 'suppressed' menstruation and the many diseases that were believed to follow from it. When the monthly 'cleansing' or 'benefit of nature', as it was sometimes called, was diminished or totally obstructed, the harmful, impure menstrual matter would accumulate in the body. Morefore, excremental matter that accumulated and stagnated in and around the uterus as or in another organ was particularly prone to putrefy and to become even more harmful

When morbid matter accumulated in one of the abdominal organs it sometimes could even be felt from the outside as a swelling or 'tumor'. For this reason, medical students already learned how to explore a patient's body, and particularly the abdomen, through manual palpation. Some of the earliest evidence for this practice comes from student notes on the bedside-teaching of Antonio Musa Brasavola in early sixteenth-century Ferrara. In the case of a fever patient with copious expectoration, for example, Brasavola palpated the abdomen and the chest and pressed down with his hands to identify the site of the disease. He felt a hardening in the area of the spleen and the liver but the patient's pain was most acute when he touched the lowest parts of the thorax on the back. Brasavola concluded that pus had accumulated in this area and affected the diaphragm.[29]

26. Temkin, 'An Historical Analysis'; cf. e.g., ÖNB, Cod. 11183, fol. 209^{r}, on a 'contagion' that 'infected' ('inficit') the gums and the teeth of a patient, and ibid., fol. 204^{r}, on Andrea Gallo's comparison of morbid matter which 'infected' the blood with the color change of milk to which minuscule amounts of red paint were added.
27. ÖNB, Cod. 11238, fol. 105^{r} and Cod. 11240, fol. 4^{r}, student notes on the teaching of fever theory in 1550s-Padua.
28. Landeshauptarchiv Schwerin, 11.1 (Historische Handschriften and Drucksachen), Vol. XXIV, Fasc. 2, *consilium*, Nürnberg, 5 June 1599.
29. Biblioteca comunale Ariostea, Ferrara, MS. Antonelli, 531, fol. 17^{r}; in another case, Brasavola found some hardness and a swelling in the hypochondriac area of a young man (ibid., fol. 34^{v}). On the practice of manual palpation in the sixteenth century, see also Stolberg, 'Examining the Body'.

As people knew from the fumes that ascended from dung heaps in the morning, impure, excremental matter could set free vapors and fumes. Accordingly, physicians and patients alike believed that fluid morbid matter that accumulated in the abdomen or one of its organs could also produce vapors or fumes which ascended to the head were the skull cap prevented them from leaving the body.[30] In the head and brain, the fumes or vapors could cause dizziness, headaches or indeed hallucinations. This notion of 'vapors' could conveniently be combined with a range of other concepts. In a detailed consilium for the Elector Friedrich III of the Palatinate, for example, Thomas Erastus concluded that Friedrich's unhealthy eating habits resulted in large amounts of undigested matter which the liver could not convert into good, nutritious blood. Some of the fluid was turned into slimy, phlegmatic blood, which among others made it difficult to pass urine. Other fluid parts were burnt by the liver and became pungent, salty, and acrid. Some of these morbid fluids moved towards the stomach, the chest, and the mouth, causing a foul-smelling breath, and they also 'fell' into his limbs and his tendons, making them rigid. The head was affected as well, by slimy blood and salty phlegm which accumulated there and by vapors that ascended from the hot liver like the smoke from a fire, which explained the dizziness and the Elector's eye problems and also caused the red marks and the scales in his face.[31]

When the hot ascending vapors arrived at the relatively cool brain, they were prone to condense back to water in turn. This was a widely accepted cause of 'fluxes' or 'catarrhs', two very common diagnoses at the time—the terms were largely synonymous. 'Catarrh'—the term is derived from the Greek word for 'flowing down'—referred not only to colds in the modern sense but to all kinds of diseases that were attributed to the flow and local accumulation of morbid matter that originated from the head. A 'catarrh' could also 'fall' into the joints, for example, or settle in the lungs or in other parts and patients and physicians alike feared 'catarrhs' as a major cause of tooth-ache.[32]

To sum up: the physician who wanted to arrive at a precise diagnosis and devise a causal treatment based on it needed to identify the localization of the underlying pathological process and the place(s) where the the resulting preternatural matter morbid settled and accumulated. The importance physicians attributed to localized pathology also throws some light on one of the mysteries of early modern medicine. It is well known that a major reason why hundreds if not thousands of medical students and future medical practitioners from all over Europe came to Ferrara, Padua, Bologna, and other Northern Italian universities in the sixteenth and early seventeenth centuries, was that anatomical teaching in Italy was far superior to what they could obtain at home. In Italy, they could witness public and private anatomical demonstrations and could learn from some of the leading anatomists of the time. If diseases had been attributed primarily to an intemperies or a humoral imbalance in the body, anatomical knowledge would have been quite useless, however. By contrast, to the degree diseases were seen as localized phenomena or at least attributed to a local accumulation or stagnation of impure, peccant matter, anatomical knowledge gained crucial importance and with it pathological anatomy, autopsies on patients, that is, who had succumbed to a certain disease. Post-mortems revealed 'obstructions' of individual organs, like the liver or the intestines, swellings and tumors, which could be attributed to a local accumulation of preternatural matter, kidney-, bladder-, and biliary stones which were considered to result from a hardening or burning of morbid matter, and other macroscopic pathological changes. Already around 1500, Antonio Benivieni connected a number of case histories with the relevant post-mortem findings, such as a total obstruction of the small intestines by a tumor.[33] By the late sixteenth century, we have already scores of post-mortem reports.[34] Even minor town physicians now came forth with collections of medical case histories that included their findings in the post-mortem.[35] For good reasons, anatomists like the famous Gabrielle Falloppia in Padua also frequently alluded to post-mortem findings in their anatomical lectures and demonstrations, as surviving student notes show.[36] The notion that the pathological changes and

30. Stolberg, *Learned Physicians*, pp. 138–40.
31. Universitätsbibliothek Heidelberg, Cod. Pal. Germ. 239, copy of a *consilium* which Erastus probably wrote in 1563.
32. ÖNB, Cod. 11183, fol. 364^r, Cod. 11207, fol. 203^r, and Cod. 11251, fol. 115^v, on different patients who came forward with this explanation.
33. Benivieni, *De abditis*.
34. Stolberg, 'Post-Mortems'.
35. Chifflet, *Singulares tam ex curationibus, quam ex cadaverum sectionibus observationes*.
36. Stolberg, *Gabrielle Falloppia*, pp. 36-37.

processes were often located in specific sites and could affect or indeed spread into the surrounding organs and structures, depending on the spatial relationship and on vessels and other anatomical connections, added greatly to the relevance of anatomical knowledge—and their own expertise—also for medical practice.

MELANCHOLIA

It should be clear at this point that the dominant explanatory model of sixteenth- and early seventeenth-century Galenism, with its focus on preternatural, morbid humors and local pathology differed fundamentally from the idea that diseases resulted from an 'imbalance' of the primary qualities or the four natural humors in the body. In what follows, I would like to illustrate these findings by sketching the sixteenth- and seventeenth-century understanding of a disease that has widely been taken for a prime example of a disease from 'humoral imbalance': melancholy or *melancholia*. According to countless scholars, early moderns explained *melancholia* as resulting from an excess of natural black bile in the body. There is a crucial difference, however, between a 'melancholic' temperament and the disease 'melancholia.' The melancholic temperament attracted considerable attention at the time, especially in the wake of Marsilio Ficino's work.[37] People with a melancholic temperament—like Ficino himself—were believed to have more natural black bile in the body than others but they were not sick. On the contrary, drawing on the (Pseudo-)Aristotelian *Problemata,*[38] Ficino and others after him described a melancholic temperament as a token of genius. This is the tradition in which Albrecht Dürer's famous *Melencolia I* stands (fig. 1).[39]

The disease *melancholia* was quite a different matter. Those diagnosed with *melancholia* in the Middle Ages and in the early modern period often exhibited dramatic symptoms, such as delusions, hallucinations, weird, or aggressive behavior, massive fears, or severe despondency. It was the standard term for all kinds of lunacy.[40] In a certain sense, the disease *melancholia* was also associated with black bile. It was not the natural black bile, however, that was believed to be at work here but some kind of preternatural blackish bilious matter. This preternatural 'atrabiliary' matter—derived from the Latin term 'ater,' meaning dark or blackish—was thought to sometimes originate from natural black bile but could also come from yellow bile or blood. Its black color was not a natural characteristic but resulted from the humor being burned to the point of turning black. In this sense, Jakob Horst attributed the *melancholia hypochondriaca* of a court official to his hot liver which burnt the blood and produced lots of ashes. The result was a 'melancholic' blood ('gebluett'), which obstructed the spleen and resulted in a range of other ailments.[41] Similarly, he attributed the *melancholia hypochondriaca* of a pregnant woman to a 'burning of the warm blood by the hotter liver.'[42]

The excessive heating and burning also was taken to be responsible for a peculiar characteristic of this 'atrabiliary matter': it was biting, sharp, acrid. Accordingly, it not only caused the disease *melancholia* but could also destroy flesh and skin, as in the case of ulcers. Thus, when 51-years old Marx Gropp was suspected of suffering from leprosy, the Augsburg town physicians could diagnose a 'biting melancholic mange' instead.[43]

Moreover, blackish, dark fumes were believed to frequently rise from melancholic matter in the abdominal area to the heart and lungs, and from there to the brain. These dark, atrabiliary fumes were thought to be primarily responsible for affecting the power of imagination, leading to hallucinations and delusions. In this sense, Horst and his colleague Johannes Neefe explained the *melancholia* of Caspar von Rechenberg, for example, as resulting from his atrabiliary, burnt blood and to harmful vapors or fumes that ascended to the head, weakening the brain and making him sad, fearful, and faint-hearted.[44] Martin Luther described *melancholia*

37. Ficino, *Three Books on Life*.
38. Pseudo-Aristotle, *Problemata*, ch. 30,1.
39. See the classic survey by Klibansky/Panofsky/Saxl, *Saturn und Melancholie.*
40. Jackson, *Melancholia and Depression.*
41. Staats- und Universitätsbibliothek Göttingen, MS. Meibom 146, pp. 160-167, *consilium* for Melchior Richardus, Helmstedt, 10 May 1585.
42. Ibid., notes preceding a *consilium* for the wife of Ascha von Mohrenfeld (*c.* 1585).
43. Stadtarchiv Augsburg, Collegium medicum XXVI, 120, medical certificate for Marx Gropp, Augsburg, 24 April 1603; cf. www.aerztebriefe.de/id/00019129, summary by Simone Herde.
44. Ibid., pp. 222–228, letter to Caspar von Rechenberg, February 1569.

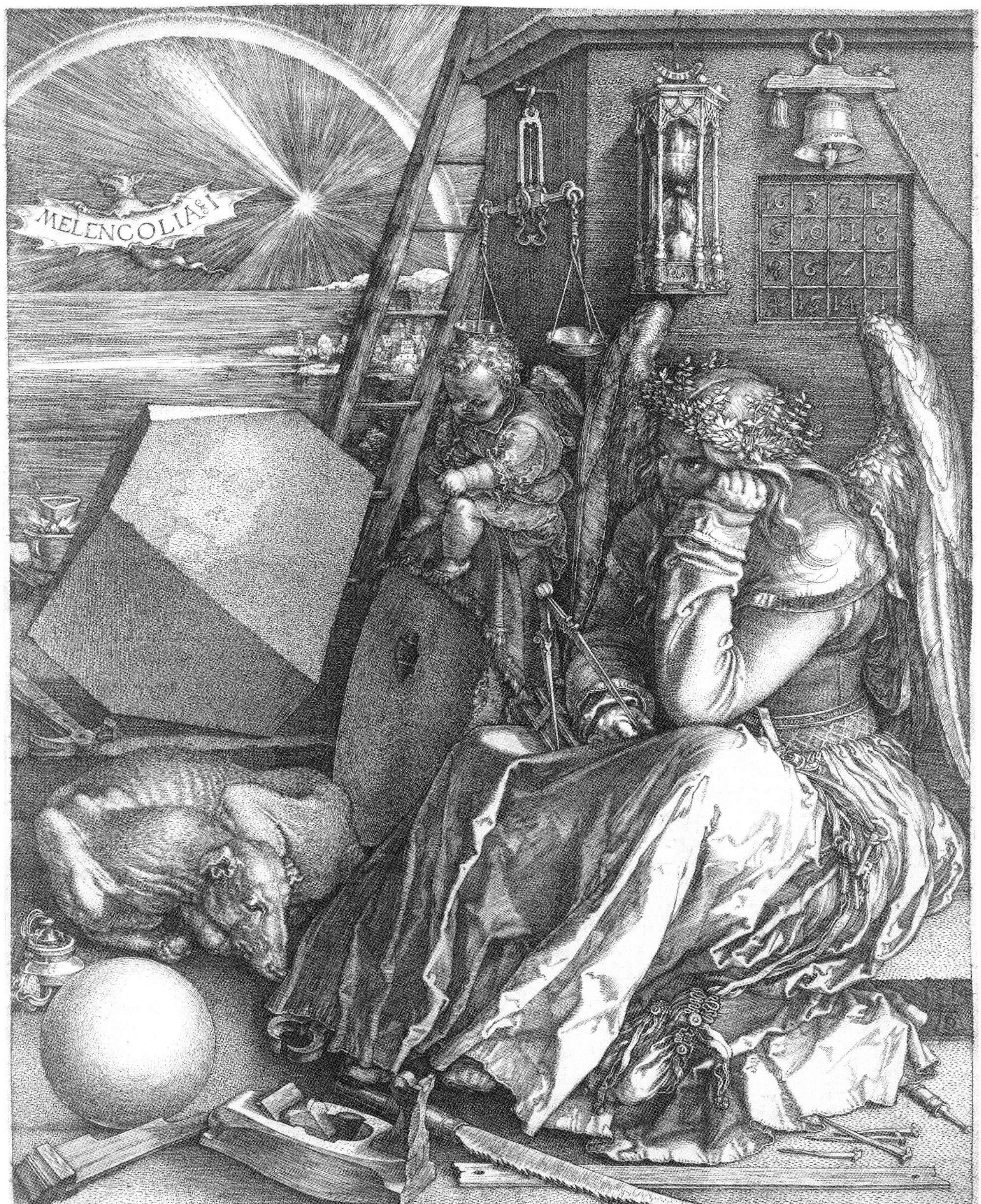

1. Albrecht Dürer, Melencolia I (1514).

as a 'devil's bath' in fact, because the devil—whose powers were limited to an artful manipulation of natural objects and powers—could easily manipulate the power of imagination through atrabiliary fumes, sometimes even making them take on specific shapes, so that his victims would sincerely believe that they saw demons and witches or even had sexual intercourse with the devil himself. As I have argued elsewhere,[45] it was this new understanding of *melancholia* as a disease—rather than the melancholic temperament, as in Dürer—which Lukas Cranach represented in his famous *Melancholia*-paintings. The surviving versions differ in the details but in addition to the figure of *Melancholia*, who is sitting peacefully in a room and in some versions carving a stick, they have a striking characteristic feature in common which is missing in Dürer: a dark cloud with demonic figures, such as witches riding backwards on animals. In the 1533 version (fig. 2), this cloud, populated with various demonic figures, is particularly prominent, filling the entire upper space. Notably, a face on the right side appears to either speak or blow the word 'melancholia' toward the figure's head.

It is here, in the head, I would argue, that Cranach wants us to locate the cloud, using an artistic device like the thought bubbles in modern comics. Since the demonic action is only happening in the head of the figure, the children or putti who are playing around her in some of the versions remain blissfully ignorant of the ominous demonic figures. Cranach's message seems clear: the demonic figures in the cloud are a mere figment of the imagination. They are caused by the dark vapors or fumes that rise to the head and assemble under the skull, affecting the power of imagination or indeed condensing like clouds into the shape of demonic figures. So strong is her conviction that these figures and creatures are real rather than just figments of her imagination that she is carving a stick which will serve her to join the witches' Sabbath.[46] In sum, with his visual representation of the contemporary attribution of the disease *melancholia* to some preternatural atrabiliary matter and the fumes that ascended from it, Cranach set a very negative, distinctly Lutheran understanding of pathological *melancholia*, which could easily be exploited by the devil, against Dürer's much more positive, Neoplatonist representation of a melancholic temperament.

CONCLUSION

The central argument of this chapter has been that sixteenth- and early seventeenth-century learned medicine did not attribute diseases to an imbalance of the humors or the primary qualities in the body as numerous accounts of early modern medicine have claimed. Instead, the medical beliefs of learned physicians, just like those, for all we know, of the patients and their families, were grounded in the conviction that pathological processes in the sick body were, in most cases, caused by a more a less specific impure, foreign morbific matter. This matter, accumulated in the body due to an insufficient concoction of food, the (further) corruption of matter inside the body, or a decrease or total suppression of natural evacuations. Sometimes an *intemperies*, an imbalance of the primary qualities in a specific organ, might affect the 'faculties' and functions of that organ, which then changed bodily humors into preternatural, morbid ones or made the morbid matter even more harmful. The disease *melancholia,* which historians have often attributed to a dominance of natural black bile in the body, confusing it with a mere melancholic temperament, is an illustrative example. Often natural black bile was not even involved at all because the pathological 'melancholic' matter resulted from a burning of blood or yellow bile. Even in fevers, it was not a humoral imbalance in the body as such which was taken to cause the disease but some morbid matter or at least a 'foreign' heat, a *calor extraneus*. Accordingly, the treatment of diseases did not aim at reestablishing humoral balance in the body but at getting rid of the preternatural, foreign matter.

These findings also have wide-reaching implications for our more general, theoretical understanding of early modern disease concepts. Medical theorists and medical historians with them have traditionally distinguished between 'physiological' and 'ontological' disease concepts and they have, more specifically, attributed the rise of 'ontological' disease concepts in Western medicine to Thomas Sydenham in the seventeenth century. In 'physiological' concepts, disease is defined as a deviation by degrees from a normal or ideal state. The interpretation of illness as resulting from of a humoral imbalance or *intemperies* in the body would offer a prime example of such a physiological understanding. By contrast,

45. Stolberg, 'Lukas Cranachs "Melancholia"-Darstellungen'.
46. Klibansky/Panofsky/Saxl, *Saturn und Melancholie*, p. 567 (newly added appendix by Raymond Klibansky).

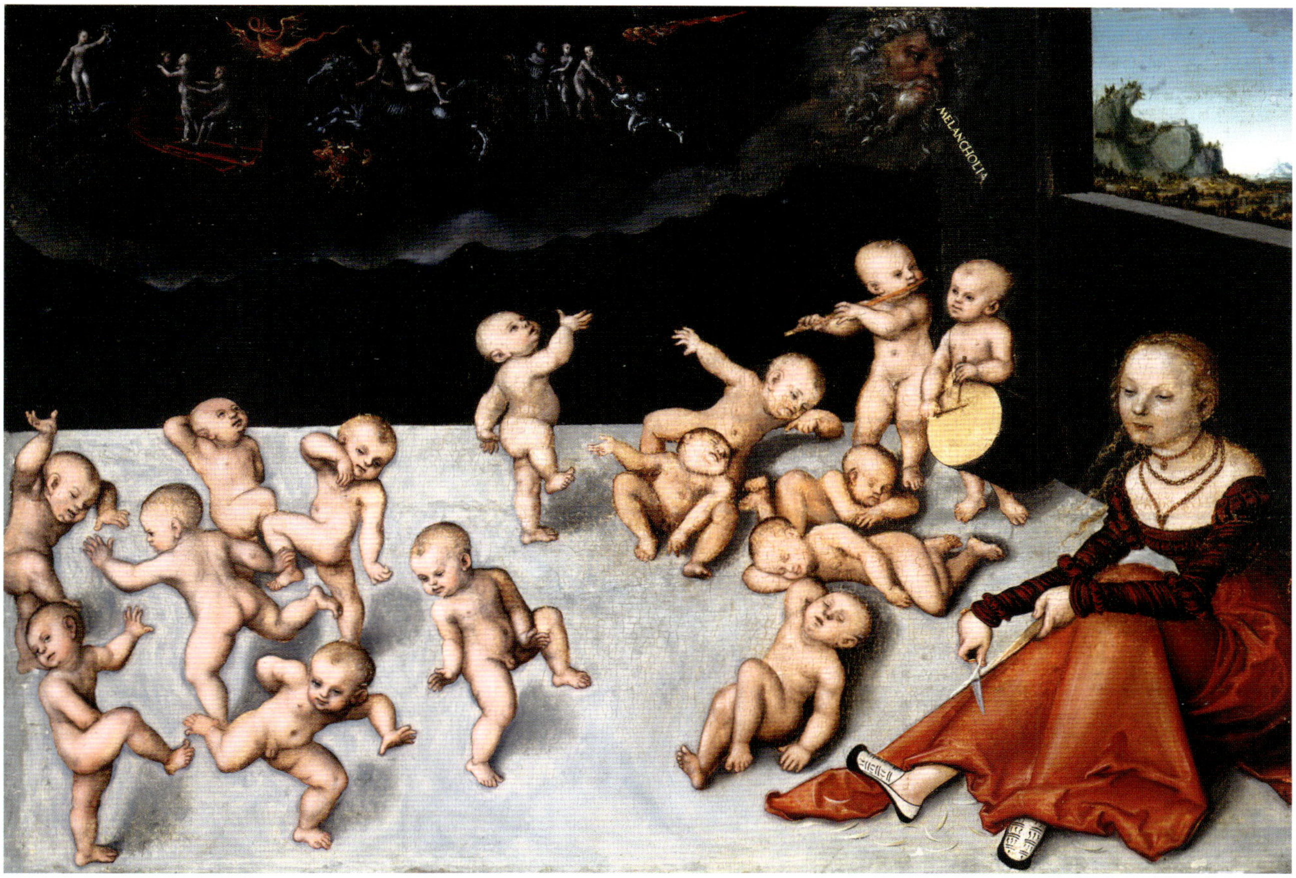

2. Lukas Cranach, Melancholia (around 1533).

'ontological' theories describe diseases as an entity apart rather than as a qualitative variation or deviation from a normal, healthy state.[47]

In the sixteenth and early seventeen centuries, learned physicians did not categorize diseases like plants, as Sydenham and the eighteenth-century nosologists later did.[48] The dominant medical paradigm I have described in this chapter entailed to a large degree an 'ontological' understanding of disease, however, or was at least much closer to such an 'ontological' understanding than to a 'physiological' one. Diseases were not a deviation from an ideal, balanced state but in most cases ultimately due to some morbid, 'peccant' matter,' which was quite literally 'matter out of place', to quote Mary Douglas's famous definition of 'dirt' or 'impurity'.[49] It was 'foreign'. Like an enemy that entered a city or a whole country, it had to be repelled, driven out beyond city walls or the borders, if the disease was to be overcome.[50] This was what the body sought to achieve, especially by means of the natural evacuations and sometimes by opening additional pathways, such as pustules or oozing ulcers and it was the physician's task to support it in this struggle. When they succeeded, when the 'foreign' enemy had been defeated, a 'radical' cure had been achieved and the patients regained their health.

This 'ontological' understanding of diseases as entities found its telling expression in one of the major innovations in early modern medical practice. From the sixteenth century onwards, physicians increasingly resorted to 'empirical' remedies, i.e. medicines that were chosen not because of their *complexio*, the relative intensity of the primary qualities in them, but because in their own

47. Henríquez Garrido, 'The Ontological Concept'; Pagel, 'Paracelsus, Virchow'.
48. Boissier de Sauvages, *Nosologia methodica*; Alibert, *Nosologie naturelle*.
49. Douglas, *Purity and Danger*.
50. On the metaphorical understanding of diseases as enemies, see Rather/Frerichs, 'On the Use of Military Metaphor'.

experience, or that of others, these medicines had proved beneficial in the treatment of certain types of disease.[51] The underlying assumption was that there were different types of diseases and that, in this sense, diseases were entities that could be distinguished from each other. At closer analysis, the same idea was also already at the heart of the range of disease names that structured medieval and early modern textbooks and lectures on medical practice, and which were also frequently used in the communication between physicians and patients: people suffered from one disease rather than another, and not from a quite literally 'idiosyncratic' imbalance of natural humors or/and primary qualities in the body.

My account contradicts the well-established standard narrative which, to this day, is taught to students, presented in major textbooks, and taken for granted in the media and in popular writing. Some readers will understandably remain skeptical. They may suspect a selective reading of the sources on my part. Or they might argue that my sources, which come primarily from Italy and Germany, may not be representative of the medicine in other parts of Europe, even though Latin as the *lingua franca* and a lively international market for medical books (in Latin) created a pan-European republic of letters. There is a pretty straightforward test, however, that allows us to settle the debate: I would quite simply ask anyone who continues to support and teach the traditional narrative to disprove my account by pointing out sources that document a substantial number of concrete individual cases in which sixteenth- and early seventeenth-century physicians, in actual practice, did attribute the diseases of their patients to an imbalance of the humors or of the primary qualities in the whole body which had to be corrected. If such sources cannot be found, however, something clearly is deeply wrong with the traditional standard account: it is a myth.

WORKS CITED

Printed Primary Sources

Alibert, Jean-Louis, *Nosologie naturelle ou les maladies du corps humain distribuées par familles* (Paris: chez Caille et Ravier, 1817).

Amatus Lusitanus, *Curationum medicinalium centuria prima, multiplici variaque rerum cognitione referta* (Florence: Torrentinus, 1551).

Avicenna, *Canon medicinae* (Basel: Hervagios, 1556, repr. Teheran 1976).

Benivieni, Antonio, *De abditis non nullis ac mirandis morborum et sanationum causis.* With an English translation by Charles Singer (Springfield, Ill.: Charles C. Thomas, 1954; first publ. in Florence, 1507).

Boissier de Sauvages, François, *Nosologia methodica sistens morborum classes juxta Sydenhami mentem et botanicorum ordinem*, 2 vols (Venice: apud Franciscum ex Nicolao Pezzana, 1773).

Chifflet, Jean, *Singulares tam ex curationibus, quam ex cadaverum sectionibus observationes* (Paris: Richer, 1612).

Ficino, Marsilio, *Three Books on Life. A Critical Edition and Translation with Introduction and Notes*, ed. by Carol V. Kaske and John R. Clark (Binghamton, New York: Medieval & Renaissance Texts & Studies, 1989).

Foreest, Pieter van: *Observationum et curationum medicinalium libri tres [...] in quibus eorum caussa, signa, prognoses, curatio graphice depinguntur. Etiam adiectis scholiis* (Leiden: Plantin, 1590).

Monte, Giovanni Battista da, *Consultationum medicarum opus absolutissimum*, ed. by Johannes Crato (Basel: Petri and Perna, 1565).

Pseudo-Aristotle, *Problemata Aristotelis, ac philosophorum medicorumque complurium* (sine loco, 1558).

Schenck von Grafenberg, Johannes, *Observationum medicarum, rararum, novarum, admirabilium, et monstrosarum tomus unus* (Frankfurt Rhodius, 1600).

Stocker, Johannes, *Empirica: sive medicamenta varia, experientia diuturna comprobata et stabilita, contra plerosque omnes corporis humani morbos tam internos quam externos*, ed. by Tobias Dornkrell von Eberhertz (Frankfurt: Bassaeus, 1601).

Trincavelli, Vettore, *Consilia medica* (Basel: Waldkirch, 1587).

Vittori, Benedetto, *Medicatio empirica singulorum morborum* (Paris: Foucher, 1551)

Secondary Sources

Dinges, Martin, and others (eds), *Medical Practice, 1600-1900. Physicians and Their Patients* (Leiden: Brill, 2016).

Douglas, Mary, *Purity and Danger. An Analysis of Concepts of Pollution and Taboo* (London: Routledge & Kegan, 1966).

Henríquez Garrido, Rui J.: 'The Ontological Concept of Disease and the Clinical Empiricism of Thomas Sydenham', *Sciendo*, 22 (2019), 10.2478/kjps-2019–0013.

Jackson, Stanley W., *Melancholia and Depression. From Hippocratic Times to Modern Times* (New Haven and London: Yale Universty Press, 1986).

Klibansky, Raymond, Erwin Panofsky, and Fritz Saxl, *Saturn und Melancholie. Studien zur Geschichte der Naturphilosophie und*

51. For example, Vittori, *Medicatio empirica*; Stocker, *Empirica*.

Medizin, der Religion und der Kunst (Frankfurt: Suhrkamp, 1992).

Lindemann, Mary, *Medicine and Society in Early Modern Europe*. 2nd edn (Cambridge: Cambridge University Press, 2010).

Lonie, Iain M., 'The 'Paris Hippocratics'. Teaching and Research in Paris in the Second Half of the Sixteenth Century', in *The Medical Renaissance of the Sixteenth Century*, ed. by Andrew Wear, Roger K. French and Iain M. Lonie (Cambridge: Cambridge University Press, 1985), pp. 155–74.

Maclean, Ian, *Logic, Signs and Nature in the Renaissance. The Case of Learned Medicine* (Cambridge: Cambridge University Press, 2002).

Pagel, Walter, 'Paracelsus, Virchow und die Wandlungen im ontologischen Krankheitsbegriff', *Virchows Archiv A*, 363 (1974), 183–211.

Pomata, Gianna, 'Observation Rising. Birth of an Epistemic Genre, 1500-1600', in *Histories of Scientific Observation*, ed. by Lorraine Daston and Elizabeth Lunbeck (Chicago and London: University of Chicago Press, 2011), pp. 45–80.

Ragland, Evan R., *Making Physicians. Tradition, Teaching, and Trials at Leiden University, 1575-1639*. Vol. 1 (Leiden/Boston: Brill, 2022).

Rather, L.J. and J. B. Frerichs, 'On the Use of Military Metaphor in Western Medical Literature: The *Bellum contram morbum* of Thomas Campanella (1568-1639)', *Clio medica*, 7 (1972), 201–08.

Stolberg, Michael, 'Bedside Teaching and the Acquisition of Practical Skills in Mid-Sixteenth-Century Padua', *Journal of the History of Medicine and Allied Sciences*, 69 (2014), 633–61.

Stolberg, Michael, 'Examining the body (c. 1500-1750)', in *The Routledge History of Sex and the Body, 1500 to the Present*, ed. by Sarah Toulalan, and Kate Fisher (Oxford: Routledge, 2013), pp. 91–105.

Stolberg, Michael, *Experiencing Illness and the Sick Body in Early Modern Europe* (London: Palgrave, 2011).

Stolberg, Michael, 'Formen und Funktionen ärztlicher Fallberichte in der Frühen Neuzeit (1500-1800)', in *Fallstudien: Theorie—Geschichte—Methode*, ed. by Johannes Süßmann, Susanne Scholz, and Gisela Engel (Berlin: trafo, 2007), pp. 81–95.

Stolberg, Michael, *Gabrielle Falloppia, 1522/23-1562. The Life and Work of a Renaissance Anatomist* (London: Routledge, 2023)

Stolberg, Michael, 'Kasuistischer medizinischer Unterricht im 16. Jahrhundert: die paduanischen *collegia*' in *Anfänge—Umbrüche—Wendungen*, ed. by Marina Hilber, Elena Taddei and Alois Unterkircher (Innsbruck: Innsbruck University Press, 2025), pp. 43–46.

Stolberg, Michael, *Learned Physicians and Everyday Medical Practice in the Renaissance* (Berlin: De Gruyter 2022), pp. 121–45.

Stolberg, Michael, 'Lukas Cranachs "Melancholia"-Darstellungen und die zeitgenössische Medizin', in *Medizin und Sozialwesen in Mitteldeutschland in der Reformationszeit*, ed. by Stefan Oehmig (Leipzig: Evangelische Verlagsanstalt, 2007), pp. 249–71.

Stolberg, Michael, 'Post-Mortems, Anatomical Dissections and Humoural Pathology in the Sixteenth and Early Seventeenth Centuries', in *Pathology in Practice. Diseases and Dissections in Early Modern Europe*, ed. by Silvia De Renzi, Marco Bresadola, and Maria Conforti (New York and London: Routledge, 2017), pp. 79–95.

Stolberg, Michael, *Uroscopy in Early Modern Europe* (Farnham: Ashgate, 2015).

Temkin, Oswei, 'An Historical Analysis of the Concept of Infection', in idem, *The Double Face of Janus, and Other Essays in the History of Medicine* (Baltimore: Johns Hopkins University Press, 1977), pp. 456–71.

Wear, Andrew, *Knowledge & Practice in English Medicine, 1550-1680* (Cambridge: Cambridge University Press: 2000).

2

Italian Medical Practice at the Habsburg Courts (1550–1600).

Encounters and Exchanges between Learned Physicians, Empirics, and Patients

Alessandra Quaranta

Early modern European courts represented sought-after workplaces for university-trained physicians, who aspired to acquire professional prestige and social acknowledgement. They also provided a safe harbor from the academic context, often characterized by intellectual constraints and torn by internecine conflicts.[1] In some cases, princely courts played a key role in encouraging physicians to cultivate their scientific interests. Archduke Ferdinand II of Tyrol (1529–95), for instance, actively promoted the descriptions of naturalia made by his personal physician Pietro Andrea Mattioli from Siena (1500–77).[2] Ferdinand also helped Mattioli obtain illustrations for the German and Czech editions of his *Discorsi*, based on the work of the Greek naturalist Dioscorides (first edition: Venice, 1544).[3]

This article will explore the role of Italian learned physicians who served the imperial Habsburg family at the courts of Vienna, Prague, Innsbruck, and Graz in the second half of the sixteenth century. In particular, I will investigate these physicians' attitudes to medical theory and practice within both scholarly debates and medical encounters. On the one hand, the Hippocratic-Galenic and Arabic-medieval tradition represented the cornerstones of their academic education, and the works belonging to these traditions were increasingly interpreted, commented on, and even criticized by medical scholars from a humanist philological perspective over the course of the sixteenth century.[4] The medical classics were thus essential sources of knowledge within academic dissertations, learned medical writings, and doctrinal discussions. On the other hand, learned physicians relied on empirical practices to verify and extend their knowledge in the field of anatomy, pathology, and therapeutics, and to examine and treat patients.

The sixteenth-century learned physician Ulrich Lehner from Prague, in his correspondence with Pietro Andrea Mattioli, stated that doctors must support their assertions with both 'reason and experience.'[5] But what happened in practice? Were learned physicians consistently respectful of the medical literature or did they diverge from it and why? And how large was their room for maneuver in this respect? How did they react when the outcomes of empirical practice did not conform to the medical tradition, or even contradicted it? The answers to these questions vary according to the circumstances, physicians' aims, and their interlocutors. As we will see, the doctors' relationship with theory and practice was influenced by the socio-professional contexts in which they acted, i.e., in written medical correspondence, and at the patient's bedside.

---

1. The present research was funded by the Austrian Science Fund (FWF), project number: M 2709-G. Sincere thanks go to Sandra Cavallo and John Henderson, for their valuable comments and for their linguistic revision of the essay. I am also grateful to Michael Stolberg for his useful remarks.
   On court medicine cf. at least Amsler, 'The Work of Many Bodies', 391–406; *Medicine at the Courts*, ed. by Nutton; *Patronage and Institutions*, ed. by Moran; Nolte, 'Der kranke Fürst'; Nolte, '*Zu fürsterlicher Körperlichkeit*'; Cavallo, *Artisans of the Body*; De Renzi, 'Medical Competence'; *Être médecin*, ed. by Andretta and Nicoud; Nicoud, *Le prince et les médecins*; Herrmann, *Tomaso Rangone*; Herrmann, 'Ärzte am Hof von Mantua'.
2. Moran, 'Patronage', p. 174.
3. Vlachová, 'Known and Unknown Creators', p. 159.
4. Siraisi, 'Giovanni Argenterio', pp. 162–63.
5. Ulrich Lehner to Pietro Andrea Mattioli, without date, in Matthiolus, *Epistolarum medicinalium*, p. 220: 'ratio' and 'experientia'.

A second aspect to be considered is the interaction with non-university-trained medical practitioners, who were often called upon by the Habsburg family. These included female healers, who were called in for medical consultations. Working side by side, the medical perspectives of non-learned practitioners and Italian physicians interacted in unexpected ways, and this could have an impact on how the latter conceived the relationship between theory and practice. Finally, we will analyze how the interests of physician and patient during the medical encounter balanced the relationship between the written medical tradition and empirical practice.

A considerable number of Italian physicians (thirty-five) were employed at the Habsburg political centers between the 1540s and the 1620s. They regularly attended to the health of the imperial family and were involved in numerous medical discussions within and outside the court. In this professional context, Italian imperial and court physicians produced a significant body of documents that can attest to the physicians' relationship with theory and practice: medical consultation papers, reports of patient visits, letters concerning medical issues, descriptions of autoptic examinations, and reports of meetings (*collegia*), during which physicians discussed clinical cases together.

Italian physicians moved to imperial political hubs to find better job opportunities. To secure court positions, they relied on their networks of social contacts, as exemplified by the case of physicians from the Prince-bishopric of Trento. The lack of both a university and a *Collegium medicum* penalized local learned physicians in professional and economic terms,[6] and led several to seek service with the imperial family. The Habsburgs were closely connected to the Prince-bishopric through numerous political, administrative and military bonds making it easier for physicians to find intermediaries to help them reach the imperial courts. For instance, imperial physician Francesco Partini from Rovereto (1500–69) was recommended to Ferdinand, King of Bohemia and Hungary, by a trusted collaborator in 1538.[7] This intermediary was probably a member of the Madruzzo family, political ally of the House of Austria. In fact, in the 1530s, Partini provided medical assistance to Cristoforo Madruzzo, prince-bishop of Trento, and his elder brother Nicolò, commander of the imperial troops.[8] Other physicians profited from the recommendations by influential personalities close to the Habsburgs. Cristoforo Guarinoni-Fontana from Verona (1540–1604) became personal physician to Rudolf II in 1590, thanks to the support of the Gonzaga family, to whom the Habsburgs were connected through marriage.[9]

Recommendations counted even more than medical experience, as the case of Giovanni Merenda from Brescia (1510–67) shows. He became personal physician to the Archduke Ferdinand's sons at the court of Innsbruck in 1542, although the government of that region preferred another physician, Johann Mörl. The latter had practiced medicine for twenty-six years, extensively proving his expertise in the field.[10] In contrast, Merenda had little practical experience at the time, although he had attained a medical degree at the University of Padua in 1538.[11] His father-in-law, Giovanni Cazzani from Schwaz, who had practiced medicine at the court of Innsbruck from the 1530s, suggested that the Archduke employ Merenda.[12]

Kinship bonds with court officers were also crucial, as in the case of Giulio Alessandrini (1506–90). His father, Pietro Alessandrini, was imperial ambassador in Trento as well as personal counselor of Emperors Maximilian I and Charles V in the first decade of the sixteenth century. As his father had already rendered excellent service to the imperial crown and won its trust, in 1553 Giulio was appointed personal physician to Emperor Ferdinand I at the Viennese court.[13]

Only in two cases did recommendation play a minor role in the recruitment process, whereas scholarship and specialized competences counted more. By virtue of his 'considerable medical erudition', Girolamo Mercuriale (1530–1606) was called to treat Emperor Maximilian II.[14]

6. Garbellotti, 'Al servizio della comunità', pp. 139–40; Garbellotti, 'Confini giurisdizionali', pp. 273–74; Garbellotti, *Le risorse dei poveri*, pp. 74–81.
7. AT-OeStA, AVA, Adel, RAA 307.49, 8 February 1538, fol. 2^{r}; AT-OeStA, AVA, Adel, RAA, 307.50, 9 September 1561, fol. 3^{v}.
8. Cf. Partini's medical consultation papers in BCRo, MS 24, fol. 29^{r-v}, 49^{r-v}; 50^{r}–54^{r}; 55^{r}–58^{v}; 59^{r-v}; 61^{v}–63^{r}.
9. Guidobono Guidoboni to Vincenzo I Gonzaga, 23 June 1590, in ASMn, AG, Corte Cesarea, 464–V, fol. 474^{r}.
10. Bachmann, 'Dr. Johann Peter Merenda', pp. 5–6.
11. *Acta graduum academicorum ab anno 1538 ad annum 1550*, ed. by Martellozzo Forin, p. 228.
12. Bachmann, 'Dr. Johann Peter Merenda', p. 7.
13. AT-OeStA, AVA, Adel, RAA 5.15, 1 May 1573, fol. 2^{v}.
14. AT-OeStA, AVA, Adel, RAA 272.53, 10 October 1573, fol. 1^{v}: 'praeclara in re Medica scientia'; Emperor Maximilian II to Girolamo Mercuriale, 4 August 1573, in AT-OeStA, HHStA, Große Korrespondenz 25.30, fol. 269^{r}.

He stayed at the Viennese court from August to October 1573.[15] Likewise, Mattioli was appointed to the court of Prague after Emperor Ferdinand I had learned of his fame as a botanist.[16] He was also chosen because of his excellent surgical skills.[17]

MEDICAL DEBATES AT COURT: THE AMBIVALENT ROLE OF THE WRITTEN MEDICAL TRADITION

This section will explore how the relationship between medical theory and practice was conceived in the medical debates that took place at court. These discussions either took the form of written medical correspondence between court physicians or occurred in the context of their medical practice. In the latter case, they were mainly concerned with individual patients, their specific disorders, and related treatments. When examining patients, Italian physicians adopted the clinical method promoted by Giovanni Battista da Monte (1489–1551), professor of medicine in Padua. This method was based on the direct observation of both the symptoms and the objective signs perceived by the physician.[18]

Let us start by analyzing how the relationship between theory and practice was addressed in the correspondence, both printed and manuscript, between physicians. I will consider four examples: the first three are from a printed collection of letters, the last from manuscript correspondence.

In one of these letters, Pietro Andrea Mattioli and Stephan Laureus from Amersfoort (fl. 1556–64), both personal physicians to Archduke Ferdinand II at the court of Prague, discuss the properties of *terra sigillata*. The latter was a red healing clay, sold in small medallions or troches stamped with a seal, an image of Diana, which served to authenticate its purity.[19] In agreement with the opinions of Alexander of Tralles and Mesue, who listed *terra sigillata* among lethal medicaments, Mattioli held that it should not be administered to children affected by epilepsy. When Laureus reported that the Spanish learned physician Andrés Laguna (1499–1559) from Segovia, had successfully cured children with a scruple of *terra sigillata*, Mattioli did not change his mind. He stated that the opinions of ancient authors on this topic were 'unquestionable'.[20] Mattioli based his opinion on theory; in fact, he disregarded Laureus's report on Laguna's experiments, or the outcomes of Laguna's therapy.

An emphasis on theory also emerges from the correspondence between Mattioli and Iacobus Camenicenus (Jakub Kamenický) from Žatec (in Bohemia), an ecclesiastic with a medical education, who moved to Prague in 1554 to practice medicine.[21] In an undated letter to Mattioli, Camenicenus recounted that, according to some of his colleagues, it was almost impossible to find an abnormal quantity of water under the peritoneum (the membrane that envelops the intestines) in men suffering from dropsy. In his response to Camenicenus, Mattioli remarked that, in *De locis affectis*, Galen had argued that a lot of water could collect under the peritoneum in men affected by dropsy. Galen had also added that similar cases were not isolated and, according to Mattioli, there was no reason to question Galen's statements.[22]

The third example is taken from the letters between Mattioli and Ulrich Lehner, focusing on the following Hippocratic aphorism: 'It was the raw body matters, not the cooked ones, which needed to be treated.' It referred to the process of *coctio* that took place in the stomach, where food was cooked as if in an oven and transformed. If this process was correctly completed, cooked matter was generated that could feed the body. In the opposite case, raw and crude matter was produced that was harmful to the body and had to be treated with purgative medicines and expelled. There was a danger, however, that evacuative remedies would have affected not only the crude matters but also those which should remain within the body and nourish it. When Lehner asked Mattioli for his opinion on the subject, he drew a distinction between powerful

15. Girolamo Mercuriale to Crato von Craftheim, 4 November 1579, in *Girolamo Mercuriale*, ed. by Agasse and Pennuto, p. 182.
16. Findlen, 'The Formation of a Scientific Community', p. 377.
17. Bachmann, 'Dr. Johann Peter Merenda', p. 7.
18. Bylebyl, 'The Manifest'; Pomata, '*Praxis historialis*', pp. 128–29.
19. Stephan Laureus is mentioned in the imperial account book of 1563 as court physician with a salary of 50 golden florins per month: AT-OeStA, HHStA, HA, OHMA, SR, 183.45, 1563, fol. 5^{v}. On *terra sigillata* cf. Dannenfeldt, 'The Introduction', and Rankin, *The Poison Trials*, pp. 163–65.
20. Pietro Andrea Mattioli to Stephan Laureus, without date, in Matthiolus, *Epistolarum medicinalium*, pp. 275–76.
21. Wernisch, 'Der Adiaphoristische Streit', pp. 427–28.
22. Pietro Andrea Mattioli to Iacobus Camenicenus, without date, in Matthiolus, *Epistolarum medicinalium*, p. 324.

purgative syrups and mild ones; the former had to be avoided and the latter had to be administered with caution. With these words, Mattioli provided a more nuanced interpretation of the general Hippocratic prescription, but he did not contradict it.[23]

The last example concerns the letters exchanged between Bartolomeo Guarinoni from Trento, personal physician to Emperor Maximilian II from 1572 to 1618, and Crato von Craftheim.[24] To treat oedema of the feet, Crato intended to prepare a 'healing water' by himself. In contrast, assuming a more cautious position, Guarinoni suggested a remedy recommended by Galen in the second chapter of his *De arte curativa ad Glauconem*, i.e., oxicraton. It was a mixture of vinegar and water applied to the skin with bandages to pulverize stagnant liquids.[25]

The fact that Mattioli and Guarinoni argued in favor of the medical classics can be explained by the context in which their opinions were expressed: in all the cases examined, this was an epistolary exchange between colleagues. In the first three, the letters belong to the printed collection of medical correspondence which Mattioli published in 1561. These types of collections were addressed to the entire community of medical writers and students and were often presented as the summa of the knowledge on a certain medical theme. The public nature of the printed letters made them vulnerable to criticism. Mattioli noted the harshness of these critiques, particularly regarding his unconventional views on purgative syrups for the stomach, which caused him considerable distress and fear of 'the bites of his adversaries.' This pattern persisted as his letters continued to be reprinted.[26]

While the letter Bartolomeo Guarinoni wrote to Crato von Craftheim was not conceived for publication, handwritten letters, too, were not read only by the sender and the recipient, but often by their closest friends and colleagues. Within the Habsburg courts, the letters of Italian imperial physicians to colleagues were also read by court officers for various purposes, including obtaining information about their travels and to ascertain their Catholic orthodoxy.[27] Thus, to preserve their scientific reputation, physicians tended to express more 'conservative' opinions in their correspondence. While they shared original hypotheses, they were careful not to lend themselves to criticism from competitors, even if this meant compromising the exploration of new avenues, as in the case of *terra sigillata*.

In their practice, however, physicians were less likely to follow the written medical tradition. For instance, Andrea Camuzzi from Lugano (1512–87), personal physician to Emperor Maximilian II, diverged from Galen's standpoint, when, in July 1576, he examined the case of a noblewoman named Aloysia. Camuzzi discussed this case in person with Giulio Alessandrini. Alessandrini assumed that the woman's life was at risk, as she was affected by a general form of pleurisy, bolstering his diagnoses with a reference to a passage from Galen. According to the Greek physician, a general form of pleurisy usually degenerated into empyema (i.e., a purulent sore in the pleural space), and all those who suffered from empyema died. Camuzzi disagreed, basing his conviction on a different interpretation of the same passage. He held that Galen meant that they would only die if they made mistakes either in their lifestyles or in their medications. But this did not hold true in the case of Aloysia.[28]

Camuzzi obviously deviated from Galen, and his 'daring' choice depended on the context of the patient's examination, where, in contrast to the more 'public' nature of correspondence, only a small number of physicians was present. This encouraged more spontaneous exchanges and informal face-to-face discussions. However, in Camuzzi's case, we must also consider the professional rivalries that permeated the court environment. These rivalries often led physicians to emphasize their own value in the eyes of the prince and thus to express even more daring opinions. We cannot therefore exclude that, in refuting Alessandrini's opinion, Camuzzi was also

23. Pietro Andrea Mattioli to Ulrich Lehner, without date, in Matthiolus, *Epistolarum medicinalium*, pp. 221–22. The mentioned Hippocratic aphorism is: 'concocta medicari atque non cruda'.
24. On the year of Guarinoni's employment cf. Divišová, 'Ärzte', p. 91; on his departure from the imperial court of Prague cf. AT-OeStA, FHKA, AHK, NÖHA, W 61/A/22, KONVOLUT, 20 March 1618, fol. 24^{r}.
25. Bartolomeo Guarinoni to Giulio Alessandrini, 7 July 1579, in BUW, MS Rehdiger 248, no. 49, fol. 73^{r}.
26. Pietro Andrea Mattioli to Ulrich Lehner, without date, in Matthiolus, *Epistolarum medicinalium*, p. 221: 'constitui [...] adversariorum morsus pertimescere'.
27. Bartolomeo Guarinoni to Martin Weinrich, 31 October 1588, in Weinrich, *Fama posthuma*, fol. 4^{v}.
28. Camutius, *Brevis excussio*, pp. 48–50 and 55.

attempting to win the goodwill of the high-ranking patient at the expense of his colleague.

The fierce rivalries between court physicians were not the only reason why they often diverged from the classical medical sources, during the patient's examination. Physicians relied on the clinical method, which enabled them to gather a sizable amount of information about the patient's health from their appearance, bodily signs, symptoms, and excrements. Accurate empirical knowledge was considered extremely important in formulating a diagnosis and could not be easily ignored, even when it contradicted medical theory.

Italian physicians at the imperial courts encountered contradictions between theory and practice when diagnosing symptoms. For example, in Francesco Partini's medical consultation, he failed to find a correspondence between what he had observed in his clinical examination and the terms used by ancient authorities. In his diagnosis of Count Bernardino Thun, who was passing only a few drops of urine, and was experiencing a sharp burning sensation when urinating, Partini realized that the terms used by Galen to describe the disorders of the urinary tract did not accurately reflect his analysis of the symptoms. In fact, Galen used both 'strangury' and 'dysuria', but these terms did not indicate precise symptoms, allowing for misunderstanding.[29] Partini decided to use only those terms that he believed corresponded to the tangible symptoms he had personally ascertained: 'burning sensation while urinating' and 'difficult discharge of urine'.[30]

The second example concerns Giovanni Planerio from Brescia (1509–1600), personal physician to Maximilian II from 1557.[31] He made a diagnosis of a count affected by fever based on medical classics, but then rectified it after analyzing the body's excretions. Initially, by considering the signs described in Galen's *De arte curativa ad Glauconem*—'thirst, vomit, sweat, and bilious matter'—, Planerio assumed that the count was afflicted by a simple tertian fever, which occurred every three days. However, by examining the patient's excrements, Planerio was able to correct his diagnosis. By observing that the count's urine was red, and his feces were 'compact,' 'cooked' and 'burnt,' Planerio inferred that the patient had been suffering from a continuous tertian fever. In his opinion, this was mainly due to pituitary matter, mixed with some bilious humors. Planerio's interpretation of the symptoms differed in part from Galen's in his *De arte curativa*. While both considered red urine to be a distinguishing symptom of a continuous tertian fever, Galen also stated that coarse, uncooked feces—not compact and cooked ones—generally accompanied this kind of fever.[32]

Like Partini, Planerio was not afraid to attribute greater importance to the empirical information derived from his clinical analysis. What mattered most to physicians was not so much their adherence to theory, but the patients' recovery, and thus they relied on all the knowledge at their disposal, whether theoretical or empirical.

In medical practice, physicians provided further arguments to back up opinions that differed from the written medical tradition. To this end, they used at least two strategies. First, they searched in the medical literature for other passages that might support their hypothesis, as when Planerio formulated a diagnosis that contradicted that of his colleagues who followed Galen. After examining a noblewoman who presented a severely swollen abdomen, these physicians assumed that the woman had a lesion in her uterus, caused by the 'flatulence' accumulated in her womb. They believed that the menstrual flow was not 'in the right quantity' and the fact that she had still not become pregnant was unequivocal proof of a womb lesion.[33] This opinion was based on Greek medical thought, according to which a small amount of menses was a sign of serious disease.[34] Planerio expressed a completely different opinion. He touched the woman's belly and relied on the patient's reaction to this palpation to identify the seat of the disease: since the pain was perceived by the woman in a region of the abdomen far away from the uterus, Planerio excluded that this organ was responsible for the belly's swelling and instead suggested that the

29. BCRo, MS 24, fol. 11^{r}: 'stranguria' and 'dysuria'.
30. Ibid.: 'mordicatio or punctio urinae', and 'difficultas urinae'.
31. Brumana, '*Si serviendum est*', p. 42.
32. Planerius, *Dubitationum*, fols 47^{v}–48^{r}. Planerio adopted the terms 'egestiones compactas, et concoctas' and 'humores adusti'. On the Galenic description of tertian fevers cf. Leonicenus, ed., *De arte curativa*, 20.
33. Planerius, *Dubitationum*, fol. 45^{v}. Planerio respectively used the terms 'ventositas', and 'in debita quantitate'.
34. Bonnard, 'Male and female bodies', p. 9.

peritoneum had ruptured, and the intestines had been pushed out.[35]

Planerio supported his hypothesis by referring to ancient medical *auctoritates*, suggesting that the woman's failure to engender an embryo could be due to flawed male seed, as attested in both Aristotle's *De generatione animalium* and Galen's *De femine*. Finally, Planerio argued that neither a lack of pregnancy nor a small quantity of menstruation were undisputable signs of a uterine lesion; the former could simply depend on narrow uterine canals.[36] Planerio thus mentioned passages from the classical medical sources to make his diagnosis more acceptable to his colleagues.

The second strategy for validating an opinion that was not in line with the written medical tradition was to demonstrate that this divergence was not based on fact and its absence did not imply that ancient authors had ignored a symptom or disorder. This is reflected in the discussion between Pietro Andrea Mattioli and Jakob Camenicenus. The latter recounted that, during the dissection of a corpse, he had found stones in its liver, which had not been mentioned by Galen. Mattioli replied that stones could certainly develop in the liver when rough and viscous humors accumulated in it, were hardened by the heat of the liver itself, and were transformed into stones, and Galen had simply not discussed them.[37] This way, Mattioli showed that his opinion did not actually diverge from Galen's texts, which remained essential to assess the validity of medical hypotheses.

THE COURT: A MEETING PLACE FOR DIFFERENT HEALING PRACTICES

In early modern Europe political power was a birthright, and the health of a sovereign and his family was central to political and religious affairs, and was tied to international politics, affecting both dynastic interests and the stability of a state.[38] When a prince fell ill, the court sought the best way to present the situation to both political partners and subjects without undermining the ruler's reputation and honor.[39]

The vital importance of the health of the Habsburg monarch was the reason the roles and tasks of court physicians began to be defined more clearly, and their numbers were increased, especially in the second half of the sixteenth century.[40] This trend was perceived as a threat by the established physicians. Gilberto Vosso, active at the court of Graz, was the personal physician to Maria Anna (1551–1608), the wife of Charles II, Archduke of Innerösterreich-Steiermark, who in April 1608 employed five other medical practitioners. In his medical report on Maria Anna's disease, Vosso stated that, since he had carefully and diligently treated her, further medical consultations were not necessary, underlining that he feared being replaced.[41]

The increase in the number of court physicians was also necessitated by Rudolf II's poor health. It also reflected his multifarious cultural and scientific interests, which ranged from the natural sciences to medicine and alchemy, to mathematics and astronomy. Furthermore, the court was characterized by conflicting factions, thus courtiers often interpreted the physicians' behaviors instrumentally, to favor one doctor to the detriment of another. For example, as I have demonstrated elsewhere, the emperor's entourage compelled Andrea Camuzzi to leave the court in 1576.[42]

Despite professional rivalries, the court could potentially be an ideal breeding ground for discussions about causes of disease and therapeutic approaches, as those concerning Emperor Maximilian. From 1552, he had repeatedly suffered from episodes of shortness of breath, heavy sweating, pain, and accelerated heartbeat. These symptoms bespoke serious cardiac diseases.[43] The 'long-lasting heart palpitation' still afflicted the emperor shortly before his death, as the imperial *Secretum Consilium* recorded on the day he died.[44] Maximilian was also affected

35. Planerius, *Dubitationum*, fols 45^{v} –46^{r}.
36. Ibid., fol. 46^{r}.
37. Pietro Andrea Mattioli to Iacobus Camenicenus, without date, in Matthiolus, *Epistolarum medicinalium*, pp. 323–24.
38. Stolberg, *Gelehrte Medizin*, p. 415; Strocchia, *Forgotten Healers*, p. 15; Andretta, 'Les multiples visages', p. 163; Palmer, 'Medicine', p. 60.
39. Nolte, 'Der kranke Fürst', p. 4.
40. Scheutz and Wührer, 'Dienst, Pflicht, Ordnung', pp. 17–19.
41. AT-OeStA, HHStA, HausA, Familienakten, 65.13, fol. 2^{v}.
42. Cf. Quaranta, 'Italian physicians', p. 566.
43. Fichtner, 'A Community of Illness', pp. 208–09; Mielke, 'Maximilian II', p. 864. A contribution on Maximilian's heartbeat by Tobias Heusinger will soon issue in the journal *Wiener medizinischen Wochenschrift*.
44. AT-OeStA, HHStA, HausA, Familienakten, 60.20, 12 October 1576, fol. 8^{r}. The *Consilium* used the expression 'continua cordis trepidatio'.

by kidney stones, intestinal ailments, hemorrhoids, gout, and phthisis, an inflammation of the lungs.[45]

Before Maximilian's death, on 12 October 1576, six learned physicians were involved in examining him, and discussing his health conditions and therapies. They included four imperial physicians—Crato von Craftheim, Andrea Camuzzi and Giulio Alessandrini, and the Flemish Nicolaus Biesius from Ghent (1516–73)—, and two physicians summoned on an *ad hoc* basis—Girolamo Mercuriale, and Benedetto Patini (1534–77), all of whom expressed different opinions. They were also joined by two lay female healers. This combination of professional and lay medical practitioners reflected the meeting of different types of knowledge and forms of medical practice that was common at the Viennese court.

In August 1573, Girolamo Mercuriale was called to Maximilian's bedside.[46] His consultation was published in his *Liber responsorum et Consultationum medicinalium*, issued in 1588. Mercuriale attributed Maximilian's heart palpitation to the ingestion of the poison contained in the mushrooms and small birds he had eaten. The poison had destroyed his natural temperament and injected 'a certain bad quality' in his heart, causing palpitation. Thereafter, the infected spirit reached all body parts—the brain, the lungs, the stomach, the liver, the kidneys, and the spleen—which also deteriorated. Mercuriale prescribed theriac and mithridatum, traditional compound medicines against poison.[47] In the same year, while Mercuriale was examining the emperor, a work on the latter's heart palpitation, entitled *Pro Divo Maximiliano Caesare semper Augusto. De cordis palpitatione consilium*, was published by Benedetto Patini, a learned physician from Brescia, author of a book on poisons published in 1572.[48] Patini also examined the Emperor in person: he scrupulously enumerated the patient's symptoms from a diachronic perspective, and listed in great detail all the remedies the imperial physicians had administered. According to Patini, Maximilian's palpitation did not depend on the vapors produced by the poison ingested, for, if it had been so, Maximilian would have been regularly affected by an accelerated heart rate until the power of the poison had run out. Patini assumed instead that the emperor's irregular heart rate had been sparked by watery humors which had filled up the membrane around his heart. Patini advised the emperor against the anti-venoms administered by Mercuriale and instead suggested warm thermal baths to eliminate the moist humors around the heart.[49]

Maximilian's disorders worsened during the imperial Diet of Regensburg (June to September 1576). Crato suggested taking four ounces of blood from the emperor, but Camuzzi deemed this blood excessive for a cardiopathic subject, since it would subtract vital spirit from the emperor's heart. Giulio Alessandrini agreed with Camuzzi on the prohibition of bloodletting. In contrast, Nicolaus Biesius was in favor of venesection, which would enlarge the veins to such an extent that medicinal decoctions, like those of guaiacum and sarsaparilla, could reach the internal body parts more quickly. Camuzzi did not approve of these decoctions since they would further damage the patient.[50]

This discussion was complicated by the contribution of two female medical experts, Duchess Anna of Saxony (1532–85), wife of Elector August of Saxony, and Agatha Streicher from Ulm (*c.* 1520–81), a middle-class healer. Both women were actively involved in the circulation of medical-pharmaceutical knowledge within German-speaking courts, and experienced considerable success as practitioners. Agatha, who enjoyed the trust of the upper class even though she was not part of it, is particularly interesting since scholars have tended to concentrate on the medical practice of aristocratic women. Alicia Rankin has studied the role of German noblewomen, renowned for providing home-based remedies to local communities as a form of charity and estate management.[51] Anna of Saxony developed considerable medical expertise, both engaging with pharmacy (*materia medica*) and searching for new cures. She had evinced a strong interest in medicine since the mid-1550s, producing distilled waters, medicinal oils, vinegars, and rose honey both in Dresden and in Annaburg, the site of an old princely hunting lodge in Lochau. Anna's remedies were sought-after within the

45. Lee, 'Medicine in Vienna', p. 167.
46. Emperor Maximilian II to Girolamo Mercuriale, 4 August 1573, in AT-OeStA, HHStA, Große Korrespondenz, 4 August 1573, 269^r.
47. Mercurialis, *Liber*, pp. 486–87. Mercuriale adopted the expression 'pravam quandam qualitatem'.
48. Patinius, *De venenis*.
49. Patinius, *Pro Divo Maximiliano*, pp. A4^v, B1^r and C2^r.
50. Camutius, *Excussio brevis*, pp. 36–37.
51. Rankin, 'Exotic materials'.

circle of her friends and acquaintances. By the late 1550s, she engaged in correspondence, mostly concerning pharmaceutical practices, with other women interested in the preparation of medicines.[52] Other noblewomen gained a reputation as skilled apothecaries, such as Philippine Wesler (1525/26–54), wife of Archduke Ferdinand II, and Eleonora from Toledo (1522–62), Spanish-born wife of Duke Cosimo I de' Medici.[53]

Despite her middle-class social background, Agatha had also successfully treated eminent German princes, both inside and outside her hometown of Ulm.[54] Count Günther of Schwarzburg recounted that Agatha had delivered him from gout; Franz Prinkenstein from Trento, the Habsburgs' envoy at the imperial Diet of Regensburg, extolled her healing methods, as did Georg Ilsung, provincial governor of Swabia.[55]

Her success was partially helped by the medical career of her brother, Johann Augustin Streicher, defined as 'doctor' in Ulm's municipal documents. He produced medicinal recipes, was an expert in uroscopy—as his manuscript treatise entitled *Iudicium urinarum* shows—and inclined towards Paracelsian doctrines. From 1561 to 1564, Augustin practiced medicine as a municipal physician mainly in Geislingen an der Steige (Baden-Württemberg), the native town of his wife, and in Ulm.[56] Agatha learnt medical practice from her brother and in this way, we may assume, also became acquainted with Paracelsian practices.

I will now focus on the involvement of Anna of Saxony and Agatha Streicher in the treatment of Emperor Maximilian II. In 1570, Maria of Austria, wife of Emperor Maximilian II, and Anna of Saxony met at a princely gathering in Vienna. On that occasion, Maria complained of the ailments from which her husband suffered, including gout. Upon her return to court in Dresden, Anna sent Maria a recipe to treat gout, which she had received from her mother, Dorothea of Saxony-Lauenburg.[57] In contrast to Anna's long-distance engagement in the emperor's health, Agatha intended to examine him in person. However, when she arrived at the Viennese court

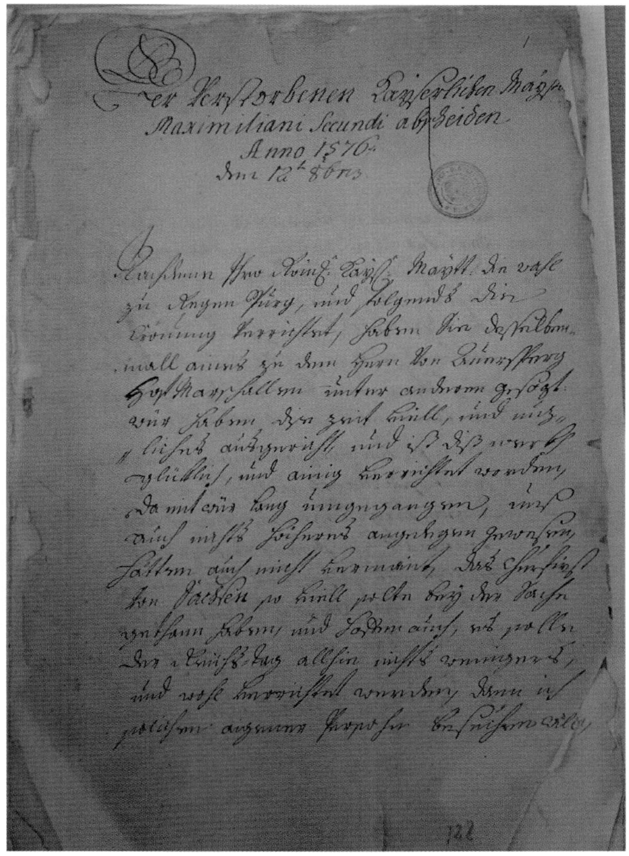
Der Verstorbenen Kayserlichen Mayst. Maximiliani Secundi abscheiden
Anno 1576.

3. First page of the Report on Emperor Maximilian II's death, 1576.

in September 1576, she was not allowed to see the patient, until a few days later, thanks to the intervention of the imperial physician Giulio Alessandrini.[58]

We can reconstruct Agatha's practice at the Viennese court from a report on the last days of Maximilian II's life. It was written on 12 October 1576, the date of his death.

Its author, whose identity is unknown, had accompanied the Emperor to the Diet of Regensburg. In its twenty-seven pages, this report provides detailed information about Maximilian's disorders and the autoptic examination of his body, and especially his lungs, heart, liver, spleen, kidneys, stomach, and intestines. Agatha is mentioned on the fifth page. She observed that 'dirty,

52. Rankin, *Panaceia's Daughters*, pp. 27, 31–32, 128–29; Rankin, 'Exotic materials', p. 536.
53. Seidl, 'Leibärzte', pp. 112–14; Strocchia, *Forgotten Healers*, pp. 16–17.
54. Vermeer, 'Ein „Iudicium Urinarum"', p. 2.
55. AT-OeStA, HHStA, HausA, Familienakten, 60.21, 26 September 1576, fol. 130r; cf. also Crato von Craftheim to Johannes Sambucus, 20 October 1576, in *Nützliche Sammlung*, p. 593.
56. Vermeer, 'Ein „Iudicium Urinarum"', pp. 2–4; Mielke, 'Maximilian II', p. 867; Sporhan-Krempel, 'Agatha Streicher um 1520-1581', pp. 20–21.
57. Rankin, *Panaceia's Daughters*, p. 128; Rankin, 'Exotic materials', p. 535.
58. 'Bericht über die Krankheit und Tod Maximilian's II', p. 102.

yellow and slimy water' had accumulated in the right side of the body, and she prepared a decoction to expel this noxious matter. She added that, if she had not administered this remedy to the emperor, the harmful water would have increased to such an extent that he would have been stricken by 'jaundice' and would have died within three days.[59] She thus recommended both a 'purging medicine' and 'the true balsam'. Alessandrini showed an open-minded attitude towards Agatha's medical skills: he carefully listened to her therapeutic proposal and convinced of the efficacy of her preparations, authorized her to administer them to the emperor.[60] Agatha's intervention thus convinced Alessandrini to prefer practice over theory, reflecting that he approved the remedies suggested by a female healer whose medical education was entirely empirical. Probably Alessandrini did not ignore Agatha's opinions, also because she had been summoned by the emperor in person.

In contrast, the imperial archiater Crato von Craftheim vigorously opposed her practice. He had been enjoying the emperors' favor for fifteen years and occupied the highest medical position at court. He thus felt entitled to criticize Agatha's prescriptions. He disagreed with her prohibition of wine-based drinks, believing that wine was the only thing capable of preserving the patient's strength. Furthermore, Crato's skeptical attitude reflected professional tensions between learned physicians and non-authorized practitioners. He even came to define Agatha as a 'very insolent and impudent woman,' full of 'noxious audacity.'[61]

Giulio Alessandrini also showed an interest in empirical therapies on another occasion. While he was writing his *De sanitate tuenda*, a work which explained what foods, drinks and climates were appropriate for people according to their natural temperaments, Alessandrini asked Tadeáš Hájek from Hájek (1525–1600), a Czech imperial physician, for information on the method to make white beer, i.e., a healthy beverage prepared in Bohemia based on wheat. Alessandrini intended to use this information to enrich the *regimina sanitatis* he was describing in his treatise. To meet Alessandrini's request, Hájek personally went to the 'Zythepsi,' i.e., 'brewers,' to gain simple ideas on how to prepare the beer.[62]

Interactions with medical empirics able to influence the relationship between theory and practice are also attested by Pietro Andrea Mattioli. The latter learned from midwives of Gorizia (the region inherited by the Habsburgs at the beginning of the sixteenth century) that the administration of quicksilver to women in labor did not have any negative consequences.[63] Furthermore, one of Mattioli's collaborators in Prague, the learned physician Georg Handsch (1529–78) from Leipa (not far from Prague), recorded hundreds of occasions when he obtained valuable information about female physiology and pathology from old women.[64]

Finally, it is necessary to understand whether Paracelsian doctrines, which were in vogue at the court of Prague during the reigns of Maximilian I, Ferdinand I, and especially Rudolf II, and involved many hands-on experiments, influenced the practice of Italian court physicians.[65] By patronizing Paracelsian physicians, alchemists, cabalists, magicians and prophetic mystics, Habsburg emperors aimed to consolidate their political authority and to demonstrate the universality of their sovereignty.[66] The Rudolfine court, in particular, was attended by the foremost international Paracelsians and alchemists: the physician Michael Maier from Rendsburg in Holstein, John Dee and Edward Kelley, Oswald Croll of Hesse, the Czech Matthias Borbonius, the Rulands, father and son, both named Martin, and the Polish Michael

59. AT-OeStA, HHStA, HausA, Familienakten, 60.21, 12 October 1576, fol. 130^{r-v}. The expressions used in the original source are respectively: 'unflätiges, gelbes, und schleimiges Wasser', and 'gelbesucht'.
60. Crato von Craftheim to Johannes Sambucus, 20 October 1576, in *Nützliche Sammlung*, pp. 594–95. Crato respectively used the expressions 'purgans medicamentum' and 'ver[um] balsam[um]'.
61. Ibid., pp. 593–94. Crato used the expressions 'impudentissima et confidentis mulieris' and 'nefariam audaciam'.
62. Hagecius, *De cervisia*, pp. 6–7. On white beer cf. Tomíček, 'Water', p. 444.
63. Matthiolus, *Epistolarum medicinalium*, p. 276.
64. Stolberg, 'Empiricism', pp. 513–14. In 1566, Handsch became personal physician to Archduke Ferdinand II at the court of Innsbruck. On Handsch, see Stolberg, *Gelehrte Medizin*, and Storchová, 'Handsch, Georg'.
65. Žemla, 'Adam Huber', pp. 537–39, and Purš, 'The Habsburgs', pp. 101–02.
66. Moran, 'Patronage', pp. 170, 175; Purš, 'The Habsburgs', p. 96; Trevor-Roper, *Renaissance Essays*, p. 18.

Sendivogius.[67] Tadeáš Hájek was also interested in Paracelsianism.[68]

The Paracelsian-alchemical doctrines widespread in the Bohemian territories elicited different reactions from Italian physicians, ranging from cautious curiosity to total rejection. Mattioli, for instance, was not a staunch Paracelsian, but had engaged with alchemical methods since 1528, when he began to collaborate with Giulio Alessandrini and Andrea Gallo in Trento to prepare chemical substances of mineral origin.[69] In both his *Discorsi* and *Opusculum de simplicium medicamentorum facultatibus*, written in Prague, Mattioli discussed distillation, melting, burning, calcinating, and the medical use of mercury and Georg Handsch left manuscripts with iatrochemical preparations obtained from Mattioli himself.[70] Antimony, a highly controversial drug widely associated with Paracelsus, was used generously by Mattioli and Gallo in Prague in the 1570s.[71] Likewise, on 28 April 1608, Gilberto Vosso twice administered a small quantity of *laudanum* to Maria Anna, Archduchess of Innerösterreich-Steiermark.[72] It was a sedative and analgesic remedy prepared by Paracelsus for the first time, by diluting opium in alcohol.

In contrast, Bartolomeo Guarinoni and Cristoforo Guarinoni-Fontana, both personal physicians to Rudolf II, condemned Paracelsian approaches and medicaments. Writing to Crato von Craftheim in 1585, Bartolomeo defined Paracelsian doctrines as 'obscure and contorted chemical reasoning'. He also complained that many physicians upheld Paracelsian thought as 'uncertain, inconsiderate, and evidently fanatical orientation.'[73] Cristoforo Guarinoni-Fontana stated that the health status of a Bohemian noblewoman, who suffered from fever and suppression of menstruation, was made worse by the medicaments a Paracelsian had previously administered to her. He agreed that Paracelsian medicaments were generally dangerous for living beings, but they became even more harmful if the body and its humors were not adequately prepared before they were administered.[74] The rigid hierarchical structure of court medical practitioners, and in particular the high socio-economic status enjoyed by Guarinoni and Guarinoni-Fontana, reflected in their salaries,[75] may also have contributed to their negative comments on Paracelsian remedies.

PATIENTS AND MEDICAL THEORY AND PRACTICE

The physicians' attitude towards theory and practice was influenced by the relationship with their patients. The significant social divide between court physicians—subjects and employees—and patients—rulers, patrons, and employers—could induce the former to reconsider the importance of classical medical sources to meet their patients' expectations. To remove bilious and pituitary humors from a count affected by a tertian fever, Giovanni Planerio followed the written medical tradition. In line with Hippocrates's *Aphorisms*, he administered a course of bloodletting, taking six ounces of blood, and diacatholicon, a purgative electuary with many ingredients. Then the count required him to repeat the bloodletting, since he believed that the previous evacuation had been too weak. Although Hippocrates did not recommend further bloodletting, Planerio drew three more ounces of blood.[76] Professional considerations prevailed over scientific ones; to maintain his patient's trust and his job, Planerio met his patient's request, even if it deviated from Hippocratic prescriptions.

On another occasion, the patient's opinion led the attending physician to question the medical tradition. In November 1559, Georg Handsch was treating an influential noblewoman, Herrin von Wartenberg (today

67. Cf. Evans, *Rudolf II*, pp. 205–07; Rampling, 'John Dee', p. 181; Purš and Smolka, 'Martin Ruland', pp. 581–606; Prinke and Zuber, 'Alchemical Patronage', pp. 325–26.
68. Purš, 'Tadeáš Hájek', pp. 423–57.
69. Ciancio, *'Per questa via'*, p. 164.
70. Žemla, 'Adam Huber', pp. 538–39.
71. Stolberg, 'Empiricism', p. 495.
72. AT-OeStA, HHStA, HausA, Familienakten, 65.13, 28 April 1608, fols 1^{v} and 2^{r}.
73. Bartolomeo Guarinoni to Crato von Craftheim, 19 August 1585, BUW, MS Akc. 1949/KN 611, no. 45, fol. 36^{v}. Guarinoni respectively used the expressions 'ambages chimicas' and 'dubiam, praecepitem ac plane fabulosam [viam]'.
74. Guarinonius, *Consilia medicinalia*, p. 702.
75. On Guarinoni's salary, see the account books in AT-OeStA, HHStA, HA, OHMA, SR, 183.52 (1575), 183.53 (1576); on Guarinoni-Fontana's salary, see Lee, 'Medicine in Vienna', p. 174. On the socio-economic status of both physicians, see Quaranta, 'Italian Physicians', pp. 556, 561, and 565.
76. Planerius, *Dubitationum*, fol. 48^{r-v}.

Stráž pod Ralskem, in the Czech Republic). To clean up the vicious humors from her womb, Handsch decided to apply a uterine enema-douche, an internal remedy considered by Galen as more effective than ingested remedies. In chapter eighty-nine of the *Ars medica*, Galen had stated that swallowed remedies lost their power in the stomach and intestines before reaching organs, such as the bladder and uterus. In contrast, the remedies that directly touched the affected body part worked far more rapidly, as Galen had asserted in the *De constitutione artis medicae*. Thus, an enema-douche, which stuck to the womb and worked through contact, would be efficacious.[77]

However, in December 1559, after a long discussion with Handsch, Herrin von Wartenberg, refused to take the remedy.[78] Since she exercised political power in Handsch's native region, he feared that her negative reaction would damage his family both professionally and personally.[79] On 24 November 1559, Handsch had expressed this concern in a letter to Mattioli, asking for his opinion on the suitability of an enema-douche. He added that he would patiently wait for and accept his opinion without questioning it, even if it was negative.[80] This reflects his respect for Mattioli's judgment but also suggests that his self-confidence in the efficacy of the remedy may have been undermined by his female patron.

Handsch affirmed that he 'did not want to be like a goose which clamors for something among swans',[81] suggesting fear of being criticized and of appearing an unconventional physician compared to his colleague Mattioli who, up to then, had not treated the condition with an enema-douche.[82] In his eyes, this risk was concrete since even Hippocrates, the father of medicine, had not been able to avoid being attacked. He also noted that Hippocrates complained that 'in medicine, there [was] more blame than honor, because of a population's unfair and malignant prejudices'.[83] Thus, two social factors impinged on Handsch's view of the relationship between theory and practice, and made him reconsider his scientific beliefs based on classical medical sources: the fear that a possible error in treatment would make him lose the favor of his female patron and that his scientific reputation would be affected negatively.

The impact that the patient's opinion had on Handsch is in line with other studies, which emphasize the subservient attitude of learned physicians towards their patients. Mary Lindemann, for instance, has pointed out that, although physicians gathered information about bodily signs and symptoms, they acted more according to patients' wishes.[84]

Sometimes, however, physicians ignored patients' objections and did not yield to their pressure. Cristoforo-Guarinoni Fontana was summoned to the bedside of Wilhelm Ursinus von Rosenberg, High Burgrave of the Kingdom of Bohemia. Wilhelm experienced serious symptoms, including dropsy and goiter, which, following Galen, he blamed on the watery humors which had accumulated in the veins of the liver and spleen. Furthermore, the patient could no longer walk or even be transported by cart, so that he had to be carried on a stretcher. He was also hit by a temporary loss of consciousness, which, according to the Galenic texts, could occur immediately before death, so that Guarinoni-Fontana predicted the patient would soon die. The physician stayed true to his opinion, although Wilhelm and his family persistently asserted that his health was improving. Wilhelm's relatives attributed this improvement to the treatment of a proto-chemist, probably the renowned theosopher and alchemist Heinrich Khunrath.[85]

Guarinoni-Fontana defied these opinions and continued to maintain that Wilhelm was seriously ill. This also occurred when, in February 1563, Ferdinand II, Archduke of Austria and King of Bohemia, suffered from a putrid and malignant fever. His attending physician, Pietro

77. Georg Handsch to Pietro Andrea Mattioli and Johann Willebroch, 24 November 1559, in ÖNB, HAN, MS 9650, fol. 53^{r-v}.
78. Georg Handsch to Johann Willebroch, 24 December 1559, in ÖNB, HAN, MS 9650, fol. 56^{r}.
79. Georg Handsch to Pietro Andrea Mattioli and Johann Willebroch, 24 November 1559, in ÖNB, HAN, MS 9650, fol. 53^{r}: 'Domina in patrem et patriam meam habet imperium, eius iussa mihi capessere fas est'.
80. Ibid.
81. Ibid.: 'Ego [...] nolim tanquam anser inter olores quicquam obstrepere'.
82. Ibid., fol. 53^{v}.
83. Georg Handsch to Johann Willebroch, 24 December 1559, in ÖNB, HAN, MS 9650, fol. 56^{v}. Handsch wrote: 'in medicina plus subesse reprehensionis, quam honoris propter iniqua et maligna vulgi praeiudicia'.
84. Lindemann, *Medicine and Society*, pp. 238 and 273–75.
85. Cristoforo Guarinoni-Fontana to Agostino Lucido, 5 December 1591 and 27 October 1592, in Guarinonius, *Consilia medicinalia*, respectively p. 697 and 716.

Andrea Mattioli, recommended a decoction of rhubarb and manna which, according to the classical medical authors, could expel putrid humors through the intestine.[86] The Archduke, however, refused this medicine since he believed that it would weaken and even damage him. Mattioli did not give up his therapeutic approach, for, with 'persuasive skills and flatteries,' he convinced the Archduke to ingest the purgative remedy, and insisted upon its effectiveness, relying on ancient medical writers.[87]

Mattioli's stubbornness shows that he expected the purgative decoction to work. At the patient's bedside, he began listing all the improvements he had observed in the Archduke's health condition. On 13 February 1563, he wrote: 'While vapors disappear, pains, sufferings and hallucinations are also relieved'.[88] On 17 February, the physician confirmed the same positive impression: 'His Royal Highness is healthier than before; that melancholic peak has not reappeared [...], he sleeps sufficiently and eats, and he is now stronger'.[89] Finally, on 20 February, Mattioli observed that the purgative remedies had successfully expelled melancholic humors, and both the color of face and pulse appeared natural.[90]

Mattioli's devotion to both his therapeutic prescriptions and the written medical tradition they represented may be explained by the necessity to be consistent in his treatment, as a change of mind could, in the Archduke's eyes, undermine his position as imperial physician.

CONCLUSIONS

Italian physicians who served the Habsburg family in the sixteenth century regularly reached the limits of both medical literature and practice. On the one hand, many passages of the Hippocratic-Galenic corpus turned out to be incomplete and/or susceptible to different interpretations. On the other, the data physicians gleaned from the observation of the bodily symptoms and signs guaranteed neither correct diagnoses nor efficacious therapies. With such uncertainty, circumstantial factors were decisive in the relationship between theoretical and practical knowledge.

While in published and handwritten correspondence novel ideas were often discussed, physicians also tended to express opinions closer to classical medical sources to avoid acrimonious disputes which could undermine their professional reputation. In contrast, when physicians looked for solutions to increase the chances of patients' recovery, they were more inclined to abandon the remedies handed down by classical medical sources and turn to remedies proposed by proto-chemists and women medical practitioners.

Irrespective of the fact that the physicians' opinions complied with either the ancient medical tradition or empirical practice, they made sure to provide solid arguments for their diagnoses and therapeutic choices. To this end, they relied on logical thinking, medical literature, practical observations, or a combination of these alternatives. On a case-by-case basis, they chose a plausible way to meet the broad variety of their socio-professional needs, i.e., keeping their role at court, dismantling real or potential criticism by other physicians, making learned medicine more acceptable to patients, and improving their health status.

The physicians' relationship with theoretical and practical knowledge was also influenced by their interactions with Habsburg political power. The necessity of physicians to respect the choices of the imperial family concerning treatment could clash with the physicians' need to ascertain its outcomes. Prescriptions were mainly based on classical sources, which physicians tried to impose on their patients, even when they refused them, arguing for the importance of theoretical knowledge. Even so, Italian physicians (as well as their therapeutic approach and its consistency) were constantly monitored by the imperial family, its close entourage, and court officers. This scrutiny influenced their decisions, often forcing them to navigate between theoretical and practical knowledge. Thus, the production, transformation, and dissemination of medical knowledge at the Habsburg courts were intimately connected to the court environment and the multiple interests it represented.

86. AT-OeStA, HHStA, HausA, Familienakten, 60.15, 8 February 1563, fol. 4^r; 17 February 1563, fol. 9^r.
87. Ibid., 13 February 1563, fol. 7^r. Mattioli used the terms 'persuasionibus, et blanditiis'.
88. Ibid.: 'Atqui remittentibus vaporibus illis, remittuntur quoque moerores, tristitiae, et falsae imaginations'.
89. Ibid., 17 February 1563, fol. 9^r: 'Paroxismus ille Melancholicus hactenus non rediit amplius, satis bene dormit, ac etiam comedit, et vires quoque meliuscule habent'.
90. Ibid., 20 February 1563, fol. 11^r.

WORKS CITED

Printed Primary Sources

'Bericht über die Krankheit und Tod Maximilian's II., erstattet Philipp II. den 13. October 1576 vom Marquis d'Almazan, seinem Gesandten am Wiener Hofe', in *Quellen zur Geschichte des Kaisers Maximilian in Archiven gesammelt und erläutert*, ed. by Matthias Koch, 2 vols (Leipzig: Voigt und Günther, 1857–61), II (1861), pp. 101–07.

Camutius, Andreas, *Excussio brevis praecipui morbi, nempe cordis palpitationis Maximiliani secundi* (Florence: typis Georgii Marescoti, 1580).

Acta graduum academicorum ab anno 1538 ad annum 1550, Fonti per la storia dell'Università di Padova 3, ed. by Elda Martellozzo Forin (Padua: Antenore, 1971).

Guarinonius, Christophorus, *Consilia medicinalia* (Venice: Thomam Baglionum, 1610).

Hagecius, Thaddaeus, *De cervisia, eiusque conficiendi ratione, opusculum* (Frankfurt am Main: Andreas Wechel, 1585).

Leonicenus, Nicolaus ed., *Claudii Galeni De arte curativa ad Glauconem* (Lyon: Apud Gulielmum Rouillium, 1549).

Matthiolus, Petrus Andreas, *Epistolarum medicinalium libri quinque* (Prague: In Officina Georgii Melantrichii, 1561).

Mercurialis, Hieronymus, *Liber responsorum et consultationum medicinalium* (Basel: Per Conradum Valdkirch, 1588).

Nützliche Sammlung Verschiedener Meistens ungedruckter Schrifften, Berichte, Urkunden, Briefe, Berichte, ed. by Christian Gottlieb Buder (Franckfurt–Leipzig: Christian Heinrich Cuno, 1735).

Patinius, Benedictus, *De venenis, quae in humanis fiunt corporibus* (Brescia: apud Vincentium Sabium, 1572).

Patinius, Benedictus, *Pro Divo Maximiliano Caesare semper Augusto De cordis Palpitatione Consilium* (Brescia: apud Vincentium Sabium, 1573).

Planerius, Ioannes, *Dubitationum et solutionum in III Galeni de diebus criticis liber unus. Eiusdem. Collegia nonnulla ad varios morbos Viennae habita* (Venice: Apud Iacobum Vitalem, 1574).

Weinrich, Martinus, *Fama posthuma Martini Weinrichii, philosophi et medici clarissimi, physices et eloquentiae professoris in illustri Gymnasio Vratisl[aviensi] ad D[ivam] Elisabeth[am] in annum XXXV. primarii et celeberrimi*, [Wroklau, 1612].

Secondary Sources

Amsler, Nadine, 'The Work of Many Bodies: Wet Nurses and Dynastic Reproduction at German Courts, c. 1650–1750', *European History Quarterly* 53/3 (2023), pp. 391–406.

Andretta, Elisa, 'Les multiples visages d'un archiatre pontifical du XVIe siècle. Activités et fonctions de Michele Mercati au Palais Apostolique', in *Être médecin à la cour (Italie, France, Espagne, XIIIe–XVIIIe siècle)*, ed. By Elisa Andretta and Marylin Nicoud (Florence : Edizioni del Galluzzo, 2013), pp. 161–82.

Bachmann, Hans, 'Dr. Johann Peter Merenda. Aus dem Leben eines Innsbrucker Hofarztes, 1542 bis 1567', *Tiroler Heimatblätter* 28 (1953), pp. 5–10.

Bonnard, Jean-Baptiste, 'Male and Female Bodies according to Ancient Greek Physicians', *Clio. Women, Gender, History*, 37 (2013), pp. 1–18.

Brumana, Angelo, '*Si serviendum est, principibus serviendum*. Medici bresciani alla corte degli Asburgo nel XVI secolo', *Misinta*, 43 (2015), pp. 41–48.

Bylebyl, Jerome J., 'The Manifest and the Hidden in the Renaissance Clinic', in *Medicine and the Five Senses*, ed. by William Frederick Bynum and Roy Porter (Cambridge: Cambridge University Press, 1993), 40–60.

Cavallo, Sandra, *Artisans of the Body in Early Modern Italy* (Manchester–New York: Manchester University Press, 2007).

Ciancio, Luca, '*Per questa via s'ascende a magior seggio.* Pietro Andrea Mattioli e le scienze mediche e naturali alla corte di Bernardo Cles', *Studi Trentini. Storia*, 94 (2015), pp. 159–84.

Dannenfeldt, Karl H., 'The Introduction of a New Sixteenth-Century Drug: *Terra Silesiaca*', *Medical History*, 28 (1984), 174–88.

De Renzi, Silvia, 'Medical Competence, Anatomy and the Polity Seventeenth-century Rome', in *Spaces, Objects and Identities in Early Modern Italian Medicine*, ed. by Sandra Cavallo and David Gentilcore (Malden, MA: Blackwell, 2008), pp. 79–95.

Divišová, Bohdana, 'Ärzte mit dem Nachnamen Guarinoni—oder: All die kaiserlichen Guarinoni', *STUDIA RUDOLPHINA. Bulletin Centra pro výzkum umění a kultury doby Rudolfa II.*, 11 (2011), pp. 89–101.

Être médecin à la cour (Italie, France, Espagne, XIIIe–XVIIIe siècle), ed. by Elisa Andretta and Marylin Nicoud (Florence: Edizioni del Galluzzo, 2013).

Evans, Robert J., *Rudolf II and His World. A Study in Intellectual History (1576-1612)* (London: Thames & Hudson, 1997; 5th ed.).

Fichtner, Paula S., 'A Community of Illness: Ferdinand I and His Family,' in *Kaiser Ferdinand. Aspekte einer Herrscherlebens*, ed. by Martina Fuchs and Alfred Kohler (Münster: Aschendorf, 2003), pp. 203–16.

Findlen, Paula, 'The Formation of a Scientific Community: Natural History in Sixteenth-century Italy,' in *Natural Particulars. Nature and the Disciplines in Renaissance Europe*, ed. by Anthony Grafton and Nancy G. Siraisi (Cambridge, MA: MIT Press, 1999), pp. 369–400.

Garbellotti, Marina, 'Al servizio della comunità. Medici, chirurghi e speziali nel Principato vescovile di Trento nell'età moderna', in *Medicina e sanità in Trentino nel Cinque-Seicento tra saperi, società e scambi culturali*, ed. by Giovanni Ciappelli and Alessandra Quaranta (Trento: Università degli Studi di Trento. Dipartimento di Lettere e Filosofia, 2019), 127–51.

Garbellotti, Marina, 'Confini giurisdizionali in tempo di epidemia. L'ufficio di sanità di Trento tra potere cittadino e potere principesco nel Seicento', in *Questioni di confine e terre di frontiera in area veneta. Secoli XVI–XVIII*, ed. by Walter Panciera (Milano, Hoelphi: 2009), pp. 269–86.

Garbellotti, Marina, *Le risorse dei poveri. Carità e tutela della salute nel principato vescovile di Trento in età moderna* (Bologna: Il Mulino, 2006).

Girolamo Mercuriale, Johann Crato von Krafftheim. Une correspondance entre deux médecins humanistes, ed. by Jean-Michel Agasse and Concetta Pennuto (Geneva : Librairie Droz, 2016).

Herrmann, Sabine, *Tomaso Rangone. Arzt, Astrologe und Mäzen im Italien der Renaissance* (Göttingen: Vandenhoeck & Ruprecht, 2017).

Herrmann, Sabine, 'Ärzte am Hof von Mantua. Karrierewege, Anforderungen und Aufgaben', in *Höfe und Experten. Relationen von Macht und Wissen in Mittelalter und Früher Neuzeit*, ed. by Marian Füssel, Antje Kuhle, and Michael Stolz (Göttingen: Vandenhoeck & Ruprecht, 2018), pp. 121–34.

Lee, Crystal M., 'Medicine in Vienna in the Sixteenth and Seventeenth Centuries' (unpublished doctoral thesis, University of Virginia, 1994).

Lindemann, Mary, *Medicine and Society in Early Modern Europe. New Approaches to European History* (Cambridge: Cambridge University Press, 1999).

Medicine at the Courts of Europe 1500–1837, ed. by Vivian Nutton (London–New York: Routledge, 1990).

Heinz-Peter Mielke, 'Maximilian II. Und das Schwenkfeldertum', in *Forschungen zur Reichs, Papst- und Landegeschichte. Peter Herde zum 65. Geburtstag von Freunden, Schülern und Kollegen dargebracht*, II, ed. by Karl Borchardt and Enno Bünz (Stuttgart: Hiersemann, 1998), 863–69.

Heusinger, Tobias, 'Das zitternde Herz des Kaisers', in *Wiener medizinischen Wochenschrift*, forthcoming.

Moran, Bruce T., 'Patronage and Institutions: Courts, Universities, and Academies in Germany; an Overview: 1500-1750', in *Patronage and Institutions: Science, Technology and Medicine at the European Courts, 1500–1750*, ed. by Bruce T. Moran (Rochester: Boydell Press, 1991), pp. 169–83.

Nicoud, Marilyn, *Le prince et les médecins: pensée et pratiques médicales à Milan (1402–1476)* (Rome: Collection de École française de Rome, 2014).

Nolte, Cordula, '*der leib der hochst schatz*—Zu fürsterlicher Körperlichkeit, Gesunderhaltung und Lebenssicherung (1450–1550)', in *Fürstin und Fürst. Familienbeziehungen und Handlungsmöglichkeiten von hochadeligen Frauen im Mittelalter*, ed. by Jörg Rogge (Ostfildern, Thorbecke Verlag, 2004), 45–92.

Nolte, Cordula, 'Der kranke Fürst. Vergleichende Beobachtungen zu Dynastie- und Herrschaftskrisen um 1500, ausgehend von den Landgrafen von Hessen', *Zeitschrift für Historische Forschung*, 27 (2000), pp. 1–36.

Palmer, Richard, 'Medicine at the Papal Court in the Sixteenth Century', *Medicine at the Courts of Europe 1500–1837*, ed. by Vivian Nutton (London–New York: Routledge, 1990), pp. 49–78.

Patronage and Institutions: Science, Technology and Medicine at the European Courts, 1500–1750, ed. by Bruce T. Moran (Rochester: Boydell Press, 1991).

Pomata, Gianna, '*Praxis historialis*: The Uses of *Historia* in Early Modern Medicine', in Historia. *Empiricism and Erudition in Early Modern Europe*, ed. by Gianna Pomata and Nancy G. Siraisi (Cambridge, MA: MIT Press, 2005), pp. 105–46.

Prinke, Rafał T., and Zuber, Mike A., 'Alchemical Patronage and the Making of an Adept: Letters of Michael Sendivogius to Emperor Rudolf II and His Chamberlain Hans Popp', *Ambix*, 65.4 (2018), pp. 324–55.

Purš, Ivo, 'The Habsburgs on the Bohemian Throne and Their Interest in Alchemy and the Occult Sciences', in *Alchemy and Rudolf II. Exploring the Secrets of Nature in Central Europe in the 16th and 17th Centuries*, ed. by Ivo Purš and Vladimír Karpenko (Prague: Artefactum, 2016), pp. 93–128.

Purš, Ivo, 'Tadeáš Hájek of Hájek and His Alchemical Circle', in *Alchemy and Rudolf II. Exploring the Secrets of Nature in Central Europe in the 16th and 17th Centuries*, ed. by Ivo Purš and Vladimír Karpenko (Prague: Artefactum, 2016), pp. 423–57.

Purš, Ivo, and Smolka, Josef, 'Martin Ruland the Elder, Martin Ruland the Younger, and the Milieu of Emperor's Personal Doctors', in *Alchemy and Rudolf II. Exploring the Secrets of Nature in Central Europe in the 16th and 17th Centuries*, ed. by Ivo Purš and Vladimír Karpenko (Prague: Artefactum, 2016), pp. 581–606.

Quaranta, Alessandra, 'Italian Physicians at the Habsburg Courts (1550–1620). Hiring Processes, Professional Networks and Integration into the Court Space', *European History Quarterly*, 53.4 (2023), pp. 549–578.

Rampling, Jennifer M., 'John Dee and the Alchemists: Practising and Promoting English Alchemy in the Holy Roman Empire', *History and Philosophy of Science*, 43 (2012), pp. 498–508.

Rankin, Alisha, *Panaceia's Daughters: Women as Healers in Early Modern Germany* (Chicago: University Chicago Press, 2013).

Rankin, Alisha, 'Exotic Materials and Treasured Knowledge: The Valuable Legacy of Noblewomen's Remedies in Early Modern Germany', *Renaissance Studies*, 28.4 (2014), pp. 533–55.

Rankin, Alisha, *The Poison Trials: Wonder Drugs, Experiment, and the Battle of Authority in Renaissance Science* (Chicago: University of Chicago Press, 2021).

Scheutz, Martin, and Wührer, Jakob, 'Dienst, Pflicht, Ordnung und Gute Policey. *Instruktionsbücher am Wiener Hof im 17. und 18. Jahrhundert*', in *Der Wiener Hof im Spiegel der Zeremonialprotokolle (1652–1800)*, ed. by Irmgard Pangerl,

Martin Scheutz, and Thomas Winkelbauer (Innsbruck–Viena–Munich–Bozen: Studienverlag, 2007), pp. 15–228.

Seidl, Katharina, 'Leibärzte und medizinische Praxis am Hof Erzherzog Ferdinands II. im Spiegel der Ambraser Sammlungen', in *In fürstlicher Nähe. Ärzte bei Hof (1450-1800)* (Innsbruck: Innsbruck University Press, 2021), ed. by Elena Taddei and Marina Hilber, pp. 111–26.

Siraisi, Nancy G., 'Giovanni Argenterio and Sixteenth-Century Medical Innovation. Between Princely Patronage and Academic Controversy', *Osiris*, 2nd ser., 6 (1990), pp. 161–80.

Sporhan-Krempel, Lore, 'Agatha Streicher um 1520-1581', in *Baden-Württembergische Portraits. Frauengestalten aus fünf Jahrhunderten*, ed. by Elisabeth Noelle-Neumann (Stuttgart: Deutsche Verlags-Anstalt, 1999), pp. 16–22.

Stolberg, Michael, *Gelehrte Medizin und ärztlicher Alltag in der Renaissance* (Berlin–Boston: De Gruyter, 2021).

Stolberg, Michael, 'Empiricism in Sixteenth-Century Medical Practice: The Notebooks of Georg Handsch', *Early Science and Medicine* 18 (2013), pp. 487–516.

Storchová, Lucie, 'Handsch, Georg', in *Companion to Central and Eastern European Humanism*, ed. by Lucie Storchová, Vol. 2: *Czech Lands*, Part 1 (Berlin: De Gruyter, 2020), pp. 512–22.

Strocchia, Sharon T., *Forgotten Healers. Women and the Pursuit of Health in Late Renaissance Italy*, (Cambridge, MA: Harvard University Press, 2019).

Tomíček, David, 'Water, Environment, and Dietetic rules in Bohemian Sources of the Early Modern Times', in *Bodily and Spiritual Hygiene in Medieval and Early Modern Literature. Explorations of Textual Presentations of Filth and Water*, ed. by Albrecht Classen (Berlin—Boston: De Gruyter, 2017), pp. 441–457.

Trevor-Roper, Hugh, *Renaissance Essays* (London: Secker and Warburg, 1985).

Vermeer, Hans J., 'Ein Iudicium Urinarum" des Dr. Augustin Streicher aus dem Cod. Wellc. 589', *Sudhoff Archiv*, 54.1 (1970), pp. 1-19.

Vlachová, Jana, 'Known and Unknown Creators of the Illustrations for the Prague editions of Mattioli's Herbal (1562, 1563)', *Huntia*, 18.4 (2021), pp. 157–70.

Wernisch, Martin, 'Der Adiaphoristische Streit in Böhmen. Ein Beitrag zum Verständnis des spezifischen Verlaufs der böhmischen Reformation', in *Reformation als Kommunikationsprozess. Die böhmischen Kronländer und Sachsen* (Norm und Struktur. Studien zum sozialen Wandel in Mittelalter und Früher Neuzeit 51), ed. by Petr Hrachovec, Gerd Schwerhoff and Winfried Müller (Vienna–Cologne–Weimar: Böhlau, 2021), pp. 401–48.

Žemla, Martin, 'Adam Huber of Riesenpach (1545-1613) and his Translation of the Book on Regimen within the Context of the Prague Medical Milieu', *Early Science and Medicine*, 21 (2016), pp. 531–56.

3

The Role of Medicinal Remedies in Seventeenth-Century Medical Treatment: The Case of Rome*

Sandra Cavallo

Early modern medical history has recently witnessed a flurry of research on *materia medica*. These studies have highlighted the growing availability of new and old medical ingredients in European markets, the increased employment of minerals, metals and chemicals in medicine, the expansion of techniques for making medicinal remedies and the participation of women and men, empirics and qualified practitioners, in the production and commercialization of medicinal preparations.[1] Much work has been done, in other words, on the expanded offer of *materia medica*, its supply and transformation, and on the agents of such changes.

Much less attention has been paid to the uses of these drugs, i.e., to their place in early modern therapeutic practice. Yet, the success enjoyed in this same period by printed recipe collections that propose medicinal preparations for various afflictions has led to assume that pharmaceutical remedies acquired a decisive role in cures, replacing the Galenic-inspired dietetic and evacuative measures that had informed responses to disease for centuries.

In his groundbreaking *Science and the Secrets of nature,* for example, William Eamon, argues that 'the predominance of medical recipes in books of secrets... is an indication of important changes in the medical economy and medical practice', 'the demand for drugs to treat specific ailments as opposed to complex regimens for living accelerated in this period'.[2] According to this narrative, the growing availability of medicinal preparations not only undermined dietetic treatments (i.e. the role of diet, sleep, exercise, environment and emotional state in the recovery of health) but changed more broadly therapeutic practice, leading to a more direct form of treatment (similar in conception to our own), in which the remedy was intended to target the disease head on. This change, it is said, went hand in hand with the demise of humoral pathology: diseases were increasingly understood as distinct, recognizable entities, defined by specific symptoms, whose effects could be directly countered by specific drugs.[3] Between the mid-sixteenth and mid-seventeenth centuries, it is argued, new anatomical knowledge, the discovery of the circulatory system, the systematic use of microscopes and the triumph of empiricism, which led to massive experimentation with drugs, seriously undermined the Galenic view of the human body. Classical humoral physiology was challenged by the emergence of alternative physiological theories that construed the body as dominated by chemical, hydraulic and mechanical processes.[4] Even those, like Michael Stolberg, who document the persistent use of evacuative treatments in all sorts of illnesses, argue that drugs acquired a new role in treatment, as specific remedies were increasingly employed to cure specific diseases.[5]

But was this really the case? To what extent did the increased availability of medicinal remedies and the

* I am grateful to Elisa Andretta, John Henderson and Sharon Strocchia for their insightful comments on a first version of this essay.

1. Among the studies focusing on Italy, Bellorini, *The World of Plants*; Gentilcore, 'The Impact'; Pugliano, 'Natural History'; Minuzzi, *Sul filo dei segreti.*
2. Eamon, *Science*, p. 138.
3. Cook, 'Markets and Cultures'; Stolberg, *Experiencing Illness*, esp. pp. 24–27.
4. Valuable syntheses of this view are Nutton, 'Renaissance Galenism' and Donato, 'Galen in the Age of Change'.
5. Stolberg, *Learned Physicians*, esp. pp. 181, 223.

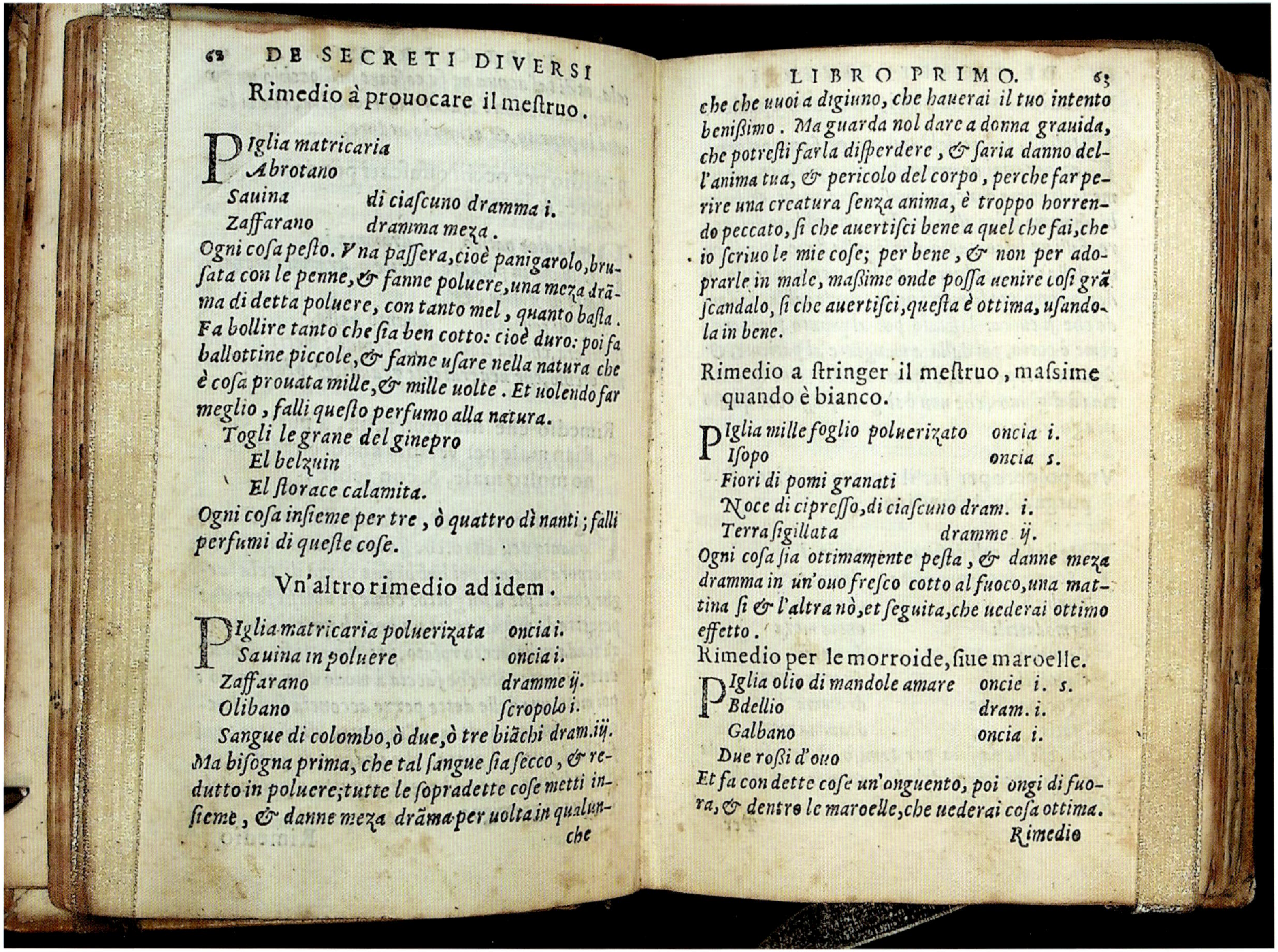
62 DE SECRETI DIVERSI
Rimedio à prouocare il meſtruo.

Piglia matricaria
Abrotano
Sauina di ciaſcuno dramma i.
Zaffarano dramma meza.

Ogni coſa peſto. Vna paſſera, cioè panigarolo, bruſata con le penne, & fanne poluere, una meza drãma di detta poluere, con tanto mel, quanto baſta. Fa bollire tanto che ſia ben cotto: cioè duro: poi fa ballottine piccole, & fanne uſare nella natura che è coſa prouata mille, & mille uolte. Et uolendo far meglio, falli queſto perfumo alla natura.

Togli le grane del ginepro
El belzuin
El ſtorace calamita.

Ogni coſa inſieme per tre, ò quattro dì nanti; falli perfumi di queſte coſe.

Vn'altro rimedio ad idem.

Piglia matricaria poluerizata oncia i.
Sauina in poluere oncia i.
Zaffarano dramme ij.
Olibano ſcropolo i.
Sangue di colombo, ò due, ò tre biãchi dram. iij.

Ma biſogna prima, che tal ſangue ſia ſecco, & reduttoin poluere; tutte le ſopradette coſe metti inſieme, & danne meza drãma per uolta in qualunche

LIBRO PRIMO. 63
che che uuoi a digiuno, che hauerai il tuo intento beniſsimo. Ma guarda nol dare a donna grauida, che potreſti farla diſperdere, & ſaria danno dell'anima tua, & pericolo del corpo, perche far perire una creatura ſenza anima, è troppo horrendo peccato, ſi che auertiſci bene a quel che fai, che io ſcriuo le mie coſe; per bene, & non per adoprarle in male, maſsime onde poſſa uenire coſi grã ſcandalo, ſi che auertiſci, queſta è ottima, uſandola in bene.

Rimedio a ſtringer il meſtruo, maſsime quando è bianco.

Piglia mille foglio poluerizato oncia i.
Iſopo oncia s.
Fiori di pomi granati
Noce di cipreſſo, di ciaſcuno dram. i.
Terra ſigillata dramme ij.

Ogni coſa ſia ottimamente peſta, & danne meza dramma in un'ouo freſco cotto al fuoco, una mattina ſi & l'altra nò, et ſeguita, che uederai ottimo effetto.

Rimedio per le morroide, ſiue maroelle.

Piglia olio di mandole amare oncie i. s.
Bdellio dram. i.
Galbano oncia i.
Due roſsi d'ouo

Et fa con dette coſe un'onguento, poi ongi di fuora, & dentro le maroelle, che uederai coſa ottima.
Rimedio

4. Page from an extremely popular recipe book (*Secreti diversi et miracolosi*, first ed.1563, followed by seventeen further editions), which, as was common in this textual genre, mechanically associates remedies and health conditions.

emergence of new theories of physiology and pathology in the medical literature have the claimed effects and dramatically change therapeutic approaches? The argument I have outlined above is logical but largely speculative. Many have noted in passing that even the most prominent representatives of the new medical philosophies, from William Harvey to Giovanni Battista Morgagni, continued to use 'traditional' cures in their practice (although the rationale for these cures was perhaps explained in ways that now drew more on the language of salts and alkali than that of humors).[6] In any case, research on this issue has been episodic and limited to the therapeutic practice of only a few prominent figures. We still know very little about the everyday cures prescribed by ordinary doctors.[7] As William Eamon has recently noted, 'the history of therapeutics is still the least understood part of the history of medicine'.[8]

In what follows, I hope to contribute to our awareness of medical treatment in this period of great intellectual change by examining the cures adopted by a newly ennobled Italian family, the Spadas, over the course of the seventeenth century. Originally from Romagna, they settled in Rome in the 1630s and, through marriage, obtained a marquisate in 1636.[9] The rich epistolary exchange between different family members is filled with references to the health problems that arose in the household and how they were treated.[10] Since they cover the entire seventeenth century, these letters, together with the detailed reports (dated 1663 and 1686) on the final illnesses of two family members, enable us to verify whether the ways in which disease was understood and handled in practice underwent significant changes during this period. Did medicinal remedies prevail over 'traditional' Galenic treatments, which quickly became obsolete?

I will also consider the theory of disease and related therapeutic recommendations that emerge from two widely read medical tracts: Benedetto Vittori's *Prattica d'esperienza* and Paolo Zacchia's *De mali hipocondriaci*. The comparison between these texts, written 80 years apart, should reveal any significant progression from one therapeutic model to another. Combining sources that illustrate practice and theory respectively, I will address some key (but generally overlooked) questions concerning how the function of medicinal preparations was understood. Were they perceived as curative and a preferred alternative to dietetic and evacuative therapies, as often assumed? Did the increased use of chemical remedies mean that a new, non-humoral view of the body and of disease had become prevalent? If not, should we assume that cures inspired by the humoral paradigm remained unchanged over the centuries? Or should we look for less radical changes that nonetheless had a significant impact on the patient's experience?

The present exploration will offer valuable insights into the precise nature of Galenic therapies in seventeenth-century Rome. I do not propose to generalize from the therapeutic experiences of the Spadas, but to offer material useful for future comparison. Surely, the cures they received were representative of the therapeutic approach adopted in Rome by families of similar rank. Indeed, they relied on the services of well-established professionals, who enjoyed the trust of an ample, distinguished clientele. In the second half of the seventeenth century, once the family had settled in Rome, the practitioners in charge of their health were members of a medical elite that combined academic posts with service in the major hospitals of the city and the Papal court. For decades, the physician consulted when a member of the family was ill (even if just to get a second opinion on independently adopted cures) was Gabriele Fonseca (*c.*1586-1668), personal physician and secret chamber assistant of Pope Innocenzo X and a reader of practical medicine at the University of Rome.[11] His scientific contributions were not significant (he published only one treatise, *Medici Oeconomia,* in 1623), but he is notable for his openness to the use of new drugs, having experimented early on with Peruvian bark (*cinchona*) in his

6. e.g., Bresadola, 'Pazienti e Curatori'; Nutton, 'Renaissance Galen', p. 478; 'Donato, 'Galen', pp. 496–98; Bertoloni Meli, 'Mechanistic Pathology'; ibid., *Mechanism, Experiment, Disease*, esp. p. 343.
7. Notable exceptions are, with regard to Italy, Bartolini, 'Consulti medici', Calabritto, 'Medicina practica' and, on the Holy Roman Empire, Stolberg, *Learned Physicians*, pp. 181–212.
8. Eamon, 'How to Read', p. 42. Similar remarks are made by Philip Rieder and François Zanetti in their Introduction to *Materia Medica*, p. 8.
9. For further information on the Spadas, see Cavallo and Storey, *Healthy Living,* chapter 2.
10. On the value of family correspondence for the study of medical practice, see my 'Family Letters'.
11. Further biographical details can be found in Fiorentini and Nelson Novoa, 'Gabriel de Fonseca'.

treatment of the Pope's nephew.[12] Even if not a protagonist of novel currents in medical thought, Fonseca showed an interest in new trends. His library, whose inventory has recently been published, contains the work of prominent figures from the previous two generations who had given significant impetus to the study of medical botany, the medicinal properties of minerals and metals, and the renewal of pharmacopeia.[13] Contemporary advocates of iatrochemical medicine, such as Pierre Jean Fabre (1588-1658) and Pietro Castelli (1570-1661), are also represented. As well as being a renowned botanist and a supporter of chemical remedies, the latter championed an alternative view of digestion as a fermentation process.[14] How far did these readings affect Fonseca's medical practice?

Fonseca was sometimes replaced in his duties to the Spadas by the younger Giovanni Tiracorda. A doctor at the Santo Spirito hospital, Tiracorda served as personal physician of as many as five consecutive popes and is reputed to have been a mentor of Giovanni Maria Lancisi. When Fonseca died, his post in the service of the Spadas was filled by the distinguished Girolamo Brasavola (1628-1705), another long-time physician of the papal household and a reader of theoretical medicine at La Sapienza.[15] Clearly these were all learned and well-informed practitioners, and they would have been keenly aware of changes in the intellectual trends of the day. Brasavola was himself an advocate of new medical theories and championed views of the body inspired by atomism and chemistry.[16] How far were these innovative ideas translated into practice and to what extent did they affect the treatments prescribed by these practitioners?

Even the Spada family—whom, as I have shown elsewhere, often resorted to self-treatment, thanks, in particular, to the medical expertise of Maria Spada—read about medicine.[17] Their library, inventoried in 1661 at the death of Cardinal Bernardino, contains twenty-five medical, pharmaceutical and alchemical volumes, as well as eleven books of secrets. Compared with their doctor's library, the Spadas' was more oriented towards the sixteenth century and less up to date, but it also contained books published at the turn of the century (Gerard Dorn, Pietro Bono, Andrea Libavio, Milius, and Baldo Baldi) that promoted chemical and alchemical medicines.[18]

The Spadas therefore seem to have been aware of and intrigued by these new trends in medical thought. The epistolary description of their everyday medical practice will clarify the extent to which these titles had an impact on the treatments adopted by the family.[19]

THE CONTINUOUS ROLE OF DIETETICS

To what extent were regimens supplanted by medicinal remedies in the early modern period? The evidence from the Spada letters suggests that dietetic measures, often called *regola del vivere* (rules of life) by contemporaries, remained a permanent element of cures throughout the seventeenth century. At certain times of the year, medical treatment could even be entirely based on life regimens, since the environmental conditions were not deemed favorable to the success of what was considered the most crucial form of healing: evacuation through purging, bloodletting or other means.

We must bear in mind that 'dietetics' here refers to the management of all six non-naturals, not just diet: sleep, exercise, evacuations, the air one breathed, and the passions one experienced were also supposed to have a significant impact on health and disease. A clear example of the importance attributed to these factors is offered by the cures prescribed to Signora Daria Albicini, Paolo Spada's wife, who was suffering from a breast tumor in

12. *Gabrielis a Fonseca lusitani*. Maehle, 'Peruvian Bark'.
13. Examples include Antonio Musa Brasavola (1500-?), Andrea Cesalpino (1524/25-1603), Michele Mercati (1541-1593). Their professional biographies can be found in *Dizionario Biografico degli Italiani*. The inventory of doctor Fonseca's library has been published in Nelson Novoa, 'Libros y saberes'.
14. See Clericuzio, 'Chemical Medicine'.
15. For information about posts at the Papal court, see Marini, *Degli archiatri pontifici*.
16. Favino, 'Sostanza e materia'.
17. Cavallo, 'The Domestic Culture of Health'.
18. 'Inventario dei beni del cardinale Bernardino Spada', in ASRo, Notai del Tribunale dell'Auditore Camerale, Testamenti e Donazioni, vol. 5933. 23.11.1661, pp. 760–775.
19. Clearly, the presence of certain titles in a library is not, by itself, evidence of an influence on practice: we cannot assume that their owners subscribed to their contents, or that these books were even read. They may have been donated or purchased for curiosity and then forgotten, acquired to display intellectual status, or bought out of obligation to authors who were friends or acquaintances.

Brisighella, where the family resided at the time.[20] In the winter of 1612, both the local doctor and the more distinguished physician consulted by Paolo in Rome (where he was serving as tax collector for the Papal States), limited themselves to recommend that she 'eats healthy food but with parsimony and does not drink more than 3 pounds in weight of light white wine per day, or half the portion of clear and good red wine', but also that she 'shields herself from the cold and the air while it is so chilly' and stays 'in a cheerful and peaceful state of mind'.[21] Similar recommendations were made when the tumor swelled: she was told to rest in bed, follow a very strict diet, and have enemas.[22]

Nearly all the non-naturals are evoked in these prescriptions: food and drink, air temperature, rest, evacuations, and the control of passions. Exercise is the only aspect of healthy living not represented. Probably Daria was too feeble to be expected to take walks (the preferred form of physical activity). The inclusion of exercise in the prescribed cure features commonly in the letters of other members of the family, especially in the second half of the seventeenth century. In October 1680, for example, Maria Spada, sixty-five and long tormented by a 'flux' in her knees, legs and thighs that made it difficult for her to move, was forcing herself to go out every day, on the doctor's recommendation, to take some air and 'do a bit of exercise' so as to 'dissipate and divert the swelling that affects her legs every evening'.[23] Taking walks, largely employed in the early modern period as a means to prevent disease, was therefore also perceived as a form of treatment capable of healing ('dissipate and divert') certain illnesses.[24]

Like Maria, Daria wholeheartedly believed in the medical benefits of dietetic treatments. She therefore carefully complied with the doctors' prescriptions, also regarding her diet, even if this entailed considerable sacrifice: 'my meal is on my own by the fire so that I am not tempted by the things that are on the table. In the morning [it consists of] a light broth or a soup of bread, in the evening a thrush or some offal, or a little bit of capon, [and] a cooked quince'.[25] In addition, she drank only a light white wine that her husband had chosen for Lent, and she drank it in moderation.[26]

The treatment of Daria's tumor was initially limited to the management of the non-naturals because it was deemed impossible to adopt more radical cures in winter. Concerns about the adverse effects of extreme air temperatures were a key consideration and determined the therapeutic calendar. An attempt to treat her with a light purge in November had failed, and in mid-January the local doctor's proposal to let blood from Daria's feet had met with her hostility and her husband's scepticism, as he 'did not believe in the effect of cures administered in this season'.[27] The tumor could not be 'solve[d]' because 'the cold is so opposed to this type of matter', but 'it will certainly resolve with the coming of the mild weather' when it would be possible to apply what was deemed the most efficacious treatment: a vigorous purge.[28] It was therefore decided that in the spring, Daria would undergo more radical evacuative cures, which would induce the expulsion of the vicious and excessive humors responsible for her problem.[29] Before then, stated the doctors, medical treatment had to remain 'conservative' because 'this season' was 'not good for healing this kind of infirmity'.[30]

20. The information is contained in fifty-two letters exchanged between Paolo and Daria between November 1611 and March 1612.
21. 'cibarsi di roba buona ma con parsimonia e quindi di non bere più di libre 3 di peso il giorno di vin bianco piccolo, o metà di rugo quando sia chiaro e buono'; 'di defendersi dal freddo e dall'aere mentre sta in questo rigore'; 'e di stare allegramente e consolatamente'. ASRo, Fondo Spada Veralli (henceforth FSV), FSV, B.589, 21.1 and 11.2.1612.
22. Ibid., 4.1.1612.
23. 'da lunedì in qua sono uscita ogni giorno a pigliare un poco d'aria e fare un poco di esercitio', 'con tutto che le mie ginocchia e gambe non siano spicciate e libere dal dolore', 'e questo lo faccio per consiglio del medico per vedere di dissipare e divertire il gonfiore che ogni sera ho nelle gambe'. Ibid., B.410, 30.10.1680.
24. On the preventive functions of exercise, see Cavallo and Storey, *Healthy Living*, chapter 5.
25. 'il mio mangiare è sola davanti al fuoco per che non abbia a venirmi voglia di cose che sono in tavola, la mattina un brodeto o panacela, la sera un tordo o coratelle o un poco di capone, una mela cotogna cotta'. ASRo, FSV, B.589, 28.1.1612.
26. Ibid.
27. Ibid., 30.11.1611; 'io credo poco alli medicamenti che si fanno in questa stagione che è tanto horrida che mai più fu in Roma maggior freddo', ibid., 14.1.1612; 'E' vero che il sig, Gnocco scrisse che mi cavassi sangue ma non l'ho fatto e non voglio fare niente con questi freddi', ibid., 21.1.1612.
28. '[la risipola] sebbene adesso vi pare che andasse adagio a risolversi perché i freddi son così nemici a simil materia, si risolverà al certo ai tempi dolci'. Ibid., January 1612. See also ibid., 8.2.1612.
29. Ibid., 11 and 15.2.1612.
30. 'né per questo inverno pensino ad altro che a conservarvi per potervi poi guarire indubitatamente a primavera', ibid., 21.1.1612; 'non sendo questa stagione bona da guarire simili infermità', ibid., 1.2.1612. See also ibid., 11.2.1612.

Belief in the seasonality of cures, therefore, seems to have been commonplace among both laypeople and professionals. It was also reiterated in highly popular vernacular medical advice tracts.[31] Air temperature and quality were thought to play a key role not only in triggering disease but in preventing (or facilitating) recovery. The severe cold was even held responsible for the worsening of a morbid condition. Daria's husband was, for example, sad to hear that she was in greater pain due to the cold weather, but considering the extremely low temperatures that winter, he was also unsurprised that her tumor was giving her more discomfort than usual.[32]

There is no sign in these testimonies of a decline in the importance attributed to environmental and behavioral factors and their impact on the body. If anything, the care that early modern people took to manage air quality and temperature, as well as the other non-naturals increased and became more sophisticated in this period.[33] The enduring reverence in which Hippocrates was held in Europe from the mid-sixteenth century (when Greek and Latin editions of the Hippocratic corpus started to multiply) was partly responsible for this growing attention to the effects of life habits, climate, and the seasons on health that we encounter both in medical advice books and in lay testimonies.[34] And even if the adoption of an Hippocratic outlook, with its emphasis on environmental conditions that similarly affected the health of everyone living in the same region, certainly inflicted a blow to concerns about unique individual complexions, this did not undermine the value attributed to dietetic measures, as often assumed. These simply became less individualized.[35] Regimens were clearly still regarded as forms of therapy and their place was not ceded to pharmaceutical remedies. Indeed, there is almost a complete absence of references to medicines in the cures prescribed to Daria during the five months in which she was fighting her disease. The possible adoption of a pharmaceutical treatment crops up only once during this period, when Daria travelled to Rimini in mid-December to consult another practitioner. His prescription consisted of both topical and oral remedies. Yet, it seems unlikely that Daria ever pursued this cure, given that, on her return, the prescription met with the disapproval of the local doctor and the scorn of her husband.[36] As we observed above, they saw medicines as ineffective in cold weather. Subsequently, there is no further mention of these cures.

Dietetic measures were not, however, presented as exclusive of other cures in Daria's overall treatment, but as components of a therapeutic process in which purging and pharmaceutical remedies would also participate, but at a later stage: medicaments would certainly be used in spring, to trigger the planned, resolutive purge. As Daria's condition worsened, however, it was decided not to wait any longer and proceed with the salvific evacuative treatment. Laxative potions and venesections were thus ordered in late February.[37] However, we lack a specific account of the outcome of these cures, since Daria rarely wrote to Paolo at this point. Sadly, the story then ended abruptly with Daria's death around 17 March 1612, the date of Paolo's last letter to her.

THE THERAPEUTIC PRIMACY OF PURGING IN THE TESTIMONIES OF THE SPADAS

Humoral principles were still dominant, in the second half of the seventeenth century, in the Spada household: recovery from illness was only understood to occur once the cause of the pathology—an excessive accumulation of piteous, bilious, phlegmatic, and more generally degenerated humors—was let out of the body via intestinal evacuation, bloodletting, sweating, vomiting, or a combination of these means. Although it is sometimes presented in scholarship as a distinct form of therapy, bloodletting was also seen to fulfill an evacuative function. Thus, the words 'evacuation' and 'purging' were used interchangeably by the Spadas and referred to all ways of

31. e.g., Fioravanti, *Capricci medicinali*, p. 55^{v}.
32. ASRo, FSV, B.589, 4 and 11.1.1612.
33. See the numerous examples in Cavallo and Storey, *Healthy Living*. Stolberg argues that the role of dietetics in therapies was much less significant North of the Alps. See his *Learned Physicians*, pp. 204–214.
34. On the popularity enjoyed by Hippocrates in the early modern period, see Nutton, 'Hippocrates in the Renaissance'; Maclean, 'The Reception of Hippocrates'.
35. I discuss these issues in my 'Habitat, Habit and Changing Ideas of Complexion'.
36. ASRo, FSV, B.589, 10 and 17.12.1611.
37. Ibid., 22 and 29.2.1612.

expelling the morbid matter and fluids that had concentrated in certain parts of the body.[38]

In this broad sense, purging was indeed the most common cure adopted in the household. Superficial ailments such as swellings, scrapes, and sores were sometimes treated simply with topical remedies prescribed by the surgeon. Virginia Spada, suffering from an inflammation of the eyes believed to have been caused more by the heat than anything else, was treated with locally applied lentiscus water.[39] Even in the case of minor ailments, however, the use of purging was frequent. Hence, when Maria Spada suffered from an inflammation of the eyes thought to originate from an internal disorder (an overheated liver), she was advised to induce a purge with quinine and then undergo a light evacuation of blood using leeches.[40] Children, too, were purged. The young daughter of Virginia Spada, aged seven, was given 'the medicine' to provoke intestinal evacuation just because she had some neck pain and a slight fever. This was done even though the ailment was deemed 'of no consequence' by those attending to her.[41]

Bloodletting, too, was applied almost universally. Only very young children were exempted. The brothers Ciriaco and Guido Spada (aged ten and nine), in bed with what was suspected to be rubella, were first given clysters and then bled (albeit in a much milder forms than for adults).[42] By contrast, the two-year-old Andrea, in bed with fever and a lack of appetite thought to be caused by teething and eating undercooked food, was spared bloodletting. He was instead cured by enemas accompanied by *fomenti* (hot cloths or cloths soaked in hot water) and ointments, both applied topically to his stomach.[43] Meanwhile, the sores in his mouth were treated locally with an extract of vitriol (*spirito di vetriolo*) and he was made to drink 'porcupine water'.[44] The same caution used towards children extended to the elderly. When the aged Bernardino fell ill with the disease that eventually led to his death, doctor Fonseca consulted with other three doctors to decide whether it was too risky to bleed him, 'the patient being sixty-eight years old'.[45] Age and gender also determined what kind of bloodletting was applied. From the age of fifty-five, Maria Spada was only bled mildly, with leeches.[46] She was not even treated with venesection during her last illness.[47]

The evacuative therapies adopted in the Spada household generally followed a relatively rigid order, whatever the disease. Bowel evacuation was normally the initial step and was first stimulated by an enema and then by the ingestion of laxative substances: from the mildest ones such as angelica water, manna, peach flower syrup, serum, or sweet almond oil, to the stronger rhubarb and thermal waters like those of Nocera or Tettuccio (which, when taken in large quantities, had a purgative effect). Venesection, which was done on the side of the body opposite to the affected one, often followed bowel evacuation. When the ailment was thought to be caused by noxious food, emetics were also administered to make the patient vomit. Cardinal Bernardino Spada, in bed with belly pain after a meal of snails, was prescribed broths with theriac water and oxymel (a mix of sugar and vinegar) to make him sick.[48] Spontaneous evacuations were also encouraged: having observed that Bernardino was sweating profusely, doctors ordered a sudorific remedy that would boost the natural discharge of the morbid matter.[49] To complete the evacuative process, vesicants were often used: these were poultices made of caustic substances that were meant to attract the vicious humors to the surface and trigger the formation of blisters that, once broken, enabled the expulsion of those vicious humors.[50] Vesicants were applied, for example, to Eugenia Spada's husband, who suffered from

38. For a similar equivalence in Galen's work, see Kuriyama, 'Interpreting the History of Bloodletting', p. 31.
39. ASRo, FSV, B.607, 4 and 5.8.1661.
40. Ibid., 4 and 7.5.1669.
41. 'non era cosa di considerazione'. Ibid., B.1115, 16.10.1669.
42. Ibid., B.607, 6 and 7.5.1661.
43. Ibid., B.1115, 2 and 25.6.1667, 12 and 16.7.1662.
44. This was possibly a concoction in which the precious porcupine stone (a variety of bezoar, renowned for its medicinal powers) had been boiled or macerated. On porcupine stones, see Crimi, 'Guarire a corte' and Peter Borschberg, 'The Euro-Asian Trade'.
45. 'trattandosi di soggetto di età di 68 anni'. 'Della infermità e morte', in ASRo, FSV, B. 463, 1661. Cap. XXXII.
46. Ibid., B.607, 7.5.1669; 24.5.1670; B.1115, 20.11.1671.
47. Ibid., B.483, pp. 169–170.
48. 'Della infermità e morte', in Ibid., B.463, 1661. Cap. XXXII, paragraph 6.
49. 'Diario dell'infermità della quale morsi il Cardinal Spada fatto d'ordine del monsignor Commendatore da Lorenzo Fontana Aiutante di Camera di Sua Ecc. e rivisto dal sig. Medico Piacenti', in Ibid., 26 October 1661.
50. On *vescicatori*, see Salvi, *Il chirurgo*, pp. 46–49.

a persistent high fever that brought about his death in only twelve days. This additional form of evacuation was attempted once he had been purged and bled and had taken comforting remedies like the *boccon di giacinto* (hyacinth bites).

Different forms of evacuation thus combined to bring the expulsive process to completion. What then was the role of pharmaceutical remedies? Medicinal preparations were key to these treatments but rather than being used as alternative to evacuative therapy, they were seen as an instrument of its success. On the one hand, as we have seen, they were used, to induce bowel movements, or other forms of discharge. But in the case of the severely ill, internal and external medicines were also often administered to fulfill another function: as 'restorative' remedies, meant to reinforce the cardinal organs that had been weakened by the long, purgative cures. Indeed, it was acknowledged that when prolonged, evacuative treatments put considerable strain on the sick body. The seriously ill Bernardino was thus advised to take *bocconi di giacinto*, a solid medicine thought to be particularly efficacious because it contained gem powder. This remedy was considered comforting to the stomach and heart and restorative of their natural heat, which had been consumed by the illness and the strong cures adopted to fight it.[51] Likewise, to reinforce its depleted natural heat, warm compresses called *pittime* were sometimes applied to the heart.[52]

On the other hand, medicinal preparations were also used to render evacuations more efficacious. The process by which morbid matter was expelled from the body was not always successful; it was thus carefully monitored. Doctors closely scrutinized the patient's feces, urine, blood, and vomit. If these evacuations did not look as expected the intestinal purge and bloodletting were repeated but the patient was also given remedies that would ease the process. For example, if the blood extracted from the patient appeared too watery or thick, medicaments were administered that would thicken or soften the blood, enabling it to do its job of draining the unhealthy material. Likewise, if the faeces appeared full of undigested matter, remedies were deployed that favored the internal processing of this matter and ultimately eased its natural expulsion. Indeed, thanks to their specific humoral qualities (refreshing, warming, drying, moisturizing, thickening, softening, and so on), certain medicaments were supposed to make the morbid matter that caused the pathology removable. Correspondents therefore wrote of taking, together with purgatives, remedies that would 'cool down the blood that was a bit scorched', 'refresh and dry up the blood', 'refresh the liver', or 'sweeten the blood so as to reach the expected result'.[53]

The medicinal preparations used by the Spadas, therefore, played important functions within the framework of humoral medicine. Their extensive use did not preclude a humoral understanding of disease since they were not believed to carry the power to heal by themselves but were expected to support the primarily expulsive healing process in different ways. As we have seen, many medicaments were meant to stimulate the evacuation of the bilious, phlegmatic, or melancholic matter that caused various pathologies by inducing intestinal purging, vomiting, sweating, or attracting the morbid humors to the surface. In other cases, medicinal remedies were meant to strengthen the natural heat of the body (especially the heart) that had been weakened by both the disease and the repeated purges. A third function of pharmaceutical preparations was, as we have just observed, that of supporting the evacuative process indirectly, by altering the humoral qualities of the blood, liver, or other body parts so that the vicious matters could dissolve or be expelled spontaneously through various channels.

It should also be noted that remedies of different types (for internal or external use, made from plant, mineral and animal substances, and with metallic or chemical ingredients) were used indifferently and often simultaneously. To treat her breast rhagades, for example, Eugenia Spada made use of plant extracts like mastic oil, minerals such as lead ointment, and metal derived infusions of litharge (pulverized lead oxide). Moreover, the remedies used by the Spadas were mostly distillates, extracts, and essences, hence created through chemical processes.

In the cures adopted by the Spadas, we therefore encounter the same integration of natural and chemical remedies found in other geographical areas in the same

51. ASRo, FSV, 'Diario dell'infermità', 22 September, 1661. On hyacinth compounds, see Castelli, *Antidotario,* p. 96.
52. ASRo, FSV, B.1115, 12 and 13.8.1662.
53. Ibid., B.618, 30.4.1678; 15.3.1679; 12.4.1679; 22.4.1679; 'dargli qualche cosa da rinfrescare per essere il sangue un poco brugiato'; 'dargli qualche cosa da rinfrescare, e essiccare il sangue'; 'pigliare qualche altra cosa da rinfrescare il fegato e il sangue'; 'piglierà alcune cose per addolcire il sangue a effetto di conseguire quel che si vorrebbe'.

period.[54] As other scholars have observed, however, the significant adoption of what were then defined as chemical medicines does not entail the emergence of a iatrochemical understanding of the body and its diseases.[55] The vocabulary utilized by the Spadas to describe the action of such medicaments and the logic underpinning it were entirely humoral. These remedies, in other words, were not believed to operate according to chemical processes but were appreciated for their humoral qualities. By carrying qualities contrary to those characterizing the disease, they eased the evacuative process.

Dietetic measures also normally complemented the cures prescribed to the Spadas or adopted independently by them. From the start of the infirmity, the patient was kept on a very lean diet of broths with eggs or sweet almond soups. This regime often lasted for long stretches of time. Eugenia, for example, complained of hunger pangs after twelve days on a restricted diet, during which she ate only soup and boiled meat for lunch, and nothing but soup for dinner.[56]

Rest was considered just as fundamental to the cure's success. Orazio Spada, frequently troubled by stomach-aches, was advised to purge with the aid of mild laxatives like angelic water and manna, to drink broths and Tettuccio water, but also 'to refrain from attending to any sort of activity, and even ban the use of the pen'.[57] When the ailment persisted, a change of air was also contemplated, as this might facilitate the purge. This same solution was suggested to the young Virginia Spada, who was 'continuing the purge but [did] not see the expected benefits,' as 'moving to somewhere nearby [Rome] may do the trick.'[58]

The composite treatment adopted to cure various members of the Spada family thus reveals a distinctive trait of therapy in this period: various types of evacuation, medicinal remedies, and dietetic prescriptions were not alternative types of treatment but part of the same therapeutic cycle and complementary to each other. We do not find that the extensive use of medicinal remedies replaced these other forms of therapy and led to their decline. It was only if evacuation was successful that the sick person would fully recover and be healed. Even though evacuative operations were preceded, accompanied, and followed by the ministration of internal, external, natural, and chemical medicines, as well as by baths in thermal, medicated, or sea water, these remedies are never described as straightforwardly curative; theirs was an ancillary function. The evidence from the Spada household suggests that in seventeenth-century Rome, the modern idea of responding to disease by taking a remedy that could resolve the affliction by itself was still alien to the dominant way of thinking.

THERAPIES IN THE MEDICAL LITERATURE

How far do the cures adopted in the Spada household match the therapeutic advice found in medical treatises? In many ways, they closely resemble the instructions in Benedetto Vittori's highly popular *Prattica d'esperienza*, a text directed at a broad audience that discusses the nature of various diseases, as well as their cures and their rationale.[59] This text interests us because it was published for the first time in 1550 and thus would not have been affected by newer trends in medical treatment that allegedly assigned a greater role to curative drugs at the expense of dietetic and evacuative measures. Additionally, this was one of some twenty-five medical books in the Spada library and was therefore potentially known to members of the family. I will also consider another, equally popular text, also present in the library: *De mali hipocondriaci*, which was published in vernacular in 1639 by the distinguished Roman physician, Paolo Zacchia. Written nearly a century after Vittori's, this text should ostensibly offer a more "modern" perspective on disease causation and the appropriate therapies.[60] In fact, as we shall see, Zacchia's therapeutic advice contains some

54. Floury-Buchalin, 'Les querelles'; Stolberg, *Learned Physicians*, pp. 363–77.
55. Ibid. For Italy, see Palmer, 'Pharmacy'; Clericuzio, 'Chemical Medicine'.
56. 'son già 12 giorni che sto a regola e sto tanto a regola che non posso starci di più, e non mangio altro che minestra e lesso e la sera minestra sola, e patisco perchè ho appetito'. ASRo, FSV, B.1115, 9.8.1662.
57. 'con riguardo dill'otio, e di non applicarsi quei giorni a cosa veruna e con dar di bando anco alla penna'. Ibid., B.618, 5.10.1678.
58. Ibid., 7.4.1679.
59. Vittori (1481-1562) was a distinguished university lecturer in Padua and Bologna. His *Medicatio empirica singolorum morborum* had seven editions in Latin between 1550 and 1598 and two in Italian, under the title *Prattica d'esperienza* (1570 and 1624).
60. Paolo Zacchia (1584-1659), known especially for his contribution to legal medicine, was also proto-physician of the Papal States several times over. Although Zacchia's text, unlike Vittori's, is devoted to a single health condition, hypochondria is described as an illness with so many variations

interesting novelties compared to Vittori's: the two texts diverge in the importance attributed to the non-naturals in healing practices, in the range and vigor of the recommended evacuative therapies, and in the value of metal and chemical remedies. However, these are not the radical shifts in the role attributed to remedies postulated by some scholars but variations within an essentially humoral paradigm. The therapies recommended in these texts repropose the coexistence of the dietetic, expulsive, and pharmaceutical measures commonly adopted in the Spada household.

Recommendations about the management of the non-naturals are far more abundant in Zacchia than in Vittori: the former devotes a chapter to each of them, and advice about the time and length of sleep, suitable exercise, the desirable quality of the air and the passions that patients should avoid (or favor) is also interspersed throughout the book. Zacchia's increased awareness of the role of the non-naturals in treating illness is likely a reflection of the greater significance that this theme had acquired in medical writing from the late sixteenth century onwards.[61] For Vittori, diet is an important element of treatment for only some diseases, namely those that generate fever: hence, when discussing putrid fever, the author includes eight pages of detailed instructions on the different foods to be administered to the sick day by day for fourteen days, depending on the evolution of the symptoms and the constitution of the infirm.[62] In Zacchia, by contrast, the therapeutic use of foods is mentioned far more regularly. Here, diet is an integral component of any treatment: the text devotes four full chapters to the foods and a page to the drinks recommended for the various types of hypochondriacs.[63] Advice about diet and related cooking recipes is also scattered throughout the work. Zacchia even theorizes the therapeutic superiority of diet over medicaments, since by altering the humors with foods instead of remedies the prudent physician will obtain an important result: 'his patients will treat themselves according to the commandments of their doctors with less annoyance and will not notice that they are being treated'.[64] For him, the use of diet is therefore preferable to that of medicines.[65]

The increased medicinal value attributed to food seems justified when one considers that Zacchia, writing nearly a century after Vittori, was able to capitalize on the increased knowledge of the medicinal properties of plants (and foods more generally) that had been accumulated in the late sixteenth and early seventeenth. centuries.[66] At the same time, a significant continuity characterizes the way in which the virtues of foods are understood in the two texts: for both Vittori's and Zacchia's these lie in the humoral qualities of edible substances, which should be opposed to those of health complaints. As Zacchia states, 'diseases must be cured with those things that are contrary to the disease and its cause'.[67] For example, in the case of rubella and smallpox (conditions characterized by over-heated blood), Vittori recommends avoiding victuals that 'augment the blood' (i.e., wine and foods with a hot complexion such as meats, eggs and spices), and opt instead for a diet based on 'foods that refresh and hydrate' (spinach, pumpkin, endive, cucumber, watermelon, and barley water).[68]

Faith in the therapeutic value of diet, however, did not preclude the use of medicines. On the contrary, these two forms of treatment went hand in hand. As in the Spada household, resort to medicinal remedies—both internal and external and administered in a variety of ways (as drinks, pills, powders, poultices, hot compresses,

that the comparison between the two works is acceptable if one wants to use it to highlight the differences between the two authors' ideas about the body, disease and its treatment.

61. On this literature and its chronology, see Cavallo and Storey, *Healthy Living*, chapter 1.
62. Vittori, *Prattica*, pp. 170ʳ–173ᵛ. For another example, see the description of the eight foods allegedly ideal for a sufferer from ethic fever, ibid., pp. 232ʳ–233ᵛ.
63. Zacchia, *De' mali*, chapters IX-XII and chapter XIII on drinks.
64. 'I suoi pazienti con minor tedio si medicheranno stando ubbidienti ai comandamenti dei loro medici, e non si accorgeranno di essere curati'. Ibid., p. 136.
65. 'quando sia possibile far sì che gli stessi cibi abbian forza di medicamenti, dobbiamo piutosto di quei cibi che dei medicamenti servirci'. Ibid. pp. 134–35.
66. See the development of a specific and extremely popular literature on the virtues of different foods, especially Pisanelli, *Trattato della natura de' cibi* (at least 28 editions between 1583 and 1676); Durante, *Il Tesoro della sanità*, containing a large section on foods (37 editions between 1586 and 1679). See also Boldo, *Libro della natura;* Romoli, *La singolare dottrina*; Bertaldi, *Regole.* Another developing textual genre, herbals, often contained information about the medicinal properties of edible plants and herbs.
67. 'il curare dei mali si ha da fare con le cose al male e alla causa di essi contrarie'. Zacchia, *De' mali*, p.133.
68. Vittori, *Prattica*, p. 255ᵛ.

ointments, baths)—is extremely frequent in both Vittori and Zacchia's prescriptions. The great majority of these medicinal preparations, however, are not described as curative, but are seen to indirectly contribute to the healing process by promoting evacuative procedures in different ways.

The range of functions attributed to remedies in the Spada household is confirmed by Zacchia, who however classifies remedies in four, rather than three categories. He explains that the role of medicines, like that of diet, is twofold: *evacuante* and *alterante*. While the preparations in the former category directly provoke evacuations, those in the latter make them possible. That is, they enable the expulsion of noxious humors by modifying the so-called first qualities (hot, cold, humid, and dry) and second qualities (thick, thin, open, and closed) of organs and fluids.[69] In Vittori's, too, many of the recommended remedies are purgative while others favor the digestion of the morbid matter (*materia del male*), thus easing its expulsion and 'resolution'.[70] In the case of pleurisis or *postema delle coste* (a cluster of pus at the ribs), for example, different remedies are employed at different stages of the affliction to prepare the body for an evacuative outcome. From day four, they aim to 'thin the matter already flowing and descended' and 'soothe and soften the chest' to facilitate spitting, given that 'the treatment of *postema* resides in the easiness of spitting.'[71]

A third category of remedies is constituted by lenitive preparations meant to mitigate pain and comfort the affected organs. For example, those ill with rubella or smallpox—conditions that offend the nose, eyes, throat, and chest—are advised 'to wet the eyes with rose water, to relieve the nose by inhaling barley water, to touch the nose and eyes with gold, and to soothe the throat by keeping candy sugar in the mouth'.[72] These medicaments therefore target symptoms by alleviating the pain and discomfort felt in various parts of the body. Like all other types of drugs, they do not aim to cure the cause. Indeed, by being illnesses 'that proceed from abundance,' smallpox and rubella 'can only be cured by evacuation.'[73]

Alongside soothing individual organs, comforting remedies are also recommended to strengthen bodies weakened by repeated purgative cures. These can be seen as a fourth category of drugs, which we have found to be used also by the Spadas for this purpose.

In short, in advice texts, as in actual practice, medicinal preparations fulfilled different functions but they were not meant to target specific diseases directly. Evacuation remains the main aim of the cure, and healing can only occur when a complete removal of the overabundant or undigested humors has taken place.[74] Compared with the practices in the Spada household, however, the range of possible evacuations is broader in the texts, especially in Vittori. Here, the pores of the head, mouth, and nose are also evacuative conducts. Alongside diuretics, emetics, and sudorifics, patients are therefore given pills that favor the purging of phlegmatic material 'from the head' through insensible perspiration, or a 'powder to be scattered on the head' and then brushed off in the morning that was meant to absorb the matter that would otherwise descend to the chest and cause asthma.[75] So-called *masticatori* (substances that the patient should chew and then spit out) are also prescribed to help expel the dangerous matter through saliva; and remedies that stimulate sneezing are suggested to enable the same process through the nose.[76]

Regarding bloodletting, this form of purging features more frequently in Vittori than in Zacchia, who wrote eighty years later. Zacchia is particularly skeptical of venesection from the arms or feet and instead favors less invasive locations (for example, haemorrhoidal veins or the space between the little finger and the ring finger) and less strenuous methods (leeches or cups rather than the lancet). He also praises the removal of the morbid matter through lesions deliberately created by *rottori* (cauters) or vesicants.[77] Overall, he is an advocate of soft medication. Hence, he insists that the laxatives employed to purge the

69. Zacchia, *De' mali*, p. 133.
70. See, for example, the massages, pills, syrups, and *rottorio* prescribed to this end in the case of paralysis in Vittori, *Prattica*, pp. 11^r–12^r.
71. 'nella qual facilità di sputo veramente consiste tutta la cura della postema'. Ibid., p.41.
72. 'ci si bagni gli occhi con acqua di rosa, si rimedi al naso col tirar acqua d'orzo, e si tocchi naso e occhi con oro, e si rimedi la gola con tener in bocca zucchero candito'. Ibid., p. 257^r.
73. 'percioché son malattie per abbondanza: onde l'evacuatione farà la cura loro'. Ibid., pp. 254^v–255^r.
74. A tripartite distinction between evacuative, comforting, and altering remedies is also made by André Du Laurens. See Suciu, 'La pharmacie du mélancholic', pp. 110–111.
75. Vittori, *Prattica*, p. 37^v.
76. Ibid., pp. 4^v, 5^v.
77. Zacchia, *De' mali*, pp. 125, 128–130.

body should be mild. He declares himself an 'enemy' of evacuative oral remedies (even those normally considered *piacevolissimi* like manna, rhubarb, and sena), especially those (also used by the Spadas) administered as solids, since they operate in a more violent way than fluids. Pills or *boccone* should therefore only be given to patients with a very strong constitution. In his view, the same effect can be obtained using enemas, emetics, or natural diuretics, or by making the patient sweat with the aid of substances imported from the Indies that only drain excessive heat and do not detrimentally impact the natural heat of the organs.[78]

Zacchia's cautions against the use of purgative medicines and venesection, combined with the great stress he lays on the curative power of food, seem to signal a shift towards gentler forms of therapy—albeit within a humoral understanding of disease and cure—that does require further attention. Critics of excessive venesection are documented in both Italy and other European countries in the late sixteenth and early seventeenth centuries.[79] However, these critical voices have frequently been associated with a more general abandonment of the humoral paradigm and a break with its arsenal of dietetic and evacuative therapies, a development which I have not encountered in my sources. Indeed, Zacchia was simply proposing to replace certain forms of evacuation with less vigorous ones, and to reinforce (rather than diminish) the reliance on regimens in medical treatment.

This author also recommends metal and chemical remedies much more commonly than Vittori. Indeed, in Zacchia's therapeutic advice we encounter frequent mentions of sulphureous and ferrous waters, antimony, and especially *acciaro* (pulverized steel), a remedy also used by the Spadas. Resorting to these substances seems to have become more common in the seventeenth century, both in actual practice and learned medical advice. However, this did not alter Zacchia's explanation of disease causation. Compared to what has been observed in other European contexts in this period, his text does not contain references to an iatrochemical model of the body and its pathologies. Physiological processes are not explained as chemical reactions (triggered by processes of distillation, separation, fermentation, or calcination) but in humoral terms. The spagyric vocabulary is alien to the lexicon of this author.[80]

CONCLUSION

This comparison between the therapies recommended by widely read medical texts authored by distinguished physicians and the vivid testimonies of how the sick members of a noble Roman family were actually cured during the seventeenth century has suggested that, both in theory and in practice, the significant increase in the number and range of drugs administered to patients did not correspond to a decline in the therapeutic use of regimens, bloodletting, and purging, as is often assumed. If anything, reliance on the six non-naturals in preventing and fighting disease increased in this period, and some aspects of healthy living received even greater attention. Even if used more extensively, pharmaceutical remedies did not acquire a dominant and directly curative role in therapies but continued to accompany and complement healing practices that are normally generically defined as 'galenic' or 'traditional' because they subscribed to a humoral understanding of physiology and pathology. Indeed, by exploring their function, we have seen that medicines were primarily employed to trigger and assist various forms of evacuation.

These findings challenge the idea that a shift occurred during this period in which drugs acquired the power to heal by themselves and diseases were increasingly conceptualized as well-defined entities that attacked the body from the outside, rather than as endogenous mutations that interfered with the normal functioning of organs. Indeed, the attribution of a curative function to drugs is supposed to go hand in hand with a new view of disease, which was no longer expected to be cured by the expulsion of corrupted matter derived from over-abundant or undigested humors.

78. Ibid., pp. 137–38.
79. Among these, Marco Cornacchini (active at the turn of the sixteenth century) and Pietro Castelli (d.1661) were both strongly influenced by Hippocratic and Paracelsian thinking. See Clericuzio, 'Chemical Medicine'. On these authors, see their entries in *Dizionario Biografico degli Italiani*.
80. A language that conflates Galenic and chemical terminology can instead be observed in seventeenth-century England. Wear 'Medical Practice', pp. 294–320. A far more complex mix of lexical fields (humoral, mechanistic, chemical, and nervous) has been seen to develop in eighteenth-century France. See Rieder, *La figure du patient*; Pilloud, *Les mots du corps*, pp. 175–186.

The fact that diseases have specific names has been seen as evidence for the emergence of this ontological view of illnesses.[81] However, this more specific terminology was not a sign of departure from the humoral paradigm. An analysis of medical treatises of great appeal, such as those of Vittori and Zacchia, reveals that disease names were in fact umbrella terms covering a range of conditions that were distinguished by their humoral characteristics. Hypochondria, for example, required different treatments depending on whether one of its symptoms, flatulence (*ventosità*), was caused by cold and moist matter, thick, cold and moist matter, hot and moist matter, or cold and dry matter. In other words, humoral variants of a disease were grouped together under the same label. Likewise, scabies could be caused by an excess of sanguine, choleric, melancholic, or phlegmatic humors, and each of these 'types' of scabies required a different treatment.[82] An ontological interpretation of disease was alien to the theoretical framework that informed both these treatises.

In the Spada correspondence, too, there are no signs that a view of disease that 'grabs', 'assails' or 'invades' the body was becoming dominant.[83] Even if the pathogenic process could initially be triggered by external factors (like exposure to cold or hot weather, or exhaustion caused by a long journey) the illness was not perceived as a foreign agent. The condition could originally derive from an external cause (corrupted air, for example) but it was the subsequent unnatural concentration of certain humors, or humoral qualities, in parts of the body that was believed to produce the morbid symptoms.

This does not mean, however, that therapies inspired by the humoral paradigm remained static over the centuries. Change did occur, but it was subtle and did not reflect a shift from a humoral to a chemical or mechanistic view of the body, and even less from a physiological to an ontological understanding of disease. The comparison between two popularizing medical texts published eighty years apart has highlighted significant variations in the therapeutic practice recommended by learned doctors that are also evident in the Spada letters. On the one hand, we have noted the easy penetration of chemical and metal-based remedies into early modern healing practices; yet these new drugs were appreciated as expressions of the now better-known virtues of nature rather than as products of an alternative, Paracelsian philosophy. On the other hand, we have observed how regimens—the impact of air on health, in particular—were given a greater role in healing practices over the course of the seventeenth century. Another novelty is represented by Zacchia's polemical support of milder types of evacuation and bloodletting than those more commonly used. He recommends limiting the use of venesection and strong laxatives and suggests specific dietary programs as a preferable alternative. Humoral treatment, often represented as unchanging over the centuries was therefore subject to significant variations. Regrettably, only a few scholars have showed interest in the specific forms taken by 'Galenic' cures in different periods or regions.[84]

These trends are evident in the cures prescribed in the 1680s to Maria Spada (nearly seventy-year-old), who was first affected by 'apoplectic accidents' (strokes) and paralysis, then by dropsy. The case is of particular interest since the Spada doctor at the time was Girolamo Brasavola, a man regarded as an innovator in medical theory.[85] Maria's medical treatment was certainly less invasive than the one administered to another member of the family, Bernardino, twenty-five years earlier, when he was more or less her age. In the report on her final infirmity, there is no mention of bloodletting (a treatment that had been repeatedly applied to Bernardino). Instead, the cure consisted of an intestinal purge, the ingestion of thermal waters, and a preparation based on *acciaro*. Later, diuretics were also administered.

Maria's treatment was therefore significantly mild, even though its aim was still freeing the body from the plethora that impeded the regular working of the organs: it was maintained that an abundance of serum in the blood had put pressure on the lungs, risking suffocation. In keeping with tradition was also the idea that the spasms in Maria's chest and belly were 'caused by the womb' (hence the label 'uterine'). Undoubtedly, the language used to describe her condition and symptoms was quite precise and clearly reflected an advanced anatomical knowledge. Yet, this did

81. Stolberg, *Experiencing Illness*, esp. p. 25.
82. Vittori, *Prattica*, pp. 157v–158r.
83. These terms are taken from Stolberg, *Experiencing Illness*, p. 24. See also, Stolberg, *Learned Physicians*, pp. 221–25.
84. Bartolini, 'Consulti medici'; Weston, *Medical Consulting,* esp. ch.7; Rieder, *La figure du patient*, pp. 445–475.
85. Brasavola was the author of a lost medical treatise containing a recently recovered chapter on fermentation informed by atomistic theory and corpuscular philosophy. Favino, 'Sostanza e materia'.

not alter the overall Galenic representation of disease and treatment.

The persistent, or even enhanced importance of the non-naturals is also confirmed: the cause of Maria's afflictions was attributed entirely to her altered emotional state: 'It was acknowledged that more than anything else, the marchioness was affected by the passions of the soul', as she had recently lost both her daughter Virginia and her daughter-in-law Vittoria.[86] These events were believed to have caused an 'agitation of the mind' (*agitazione di mente*) that made her symptoms reappear and worsen, and also led to an unusual retention of urine. The importance that emotions have acquired in the etiology of Maria's illnesses contrasts with the passing mention of the need to stay cheerful that had characterized the medical advice given to Daria several decades earlier. The impression that the emotional state had acquired a greater role in the understanding of disease is also suggested by some of the Spada letters of the late seventeenth century: here, melancholy and hypochondria are repeatedly invoked as deriving from dangerous states of mind that need to be avoided or dispelled.[87] It has not been possible to explore this shift in greater depth in the limited space of this essay. If confirmed, however, the growing attention paid to feelings and passions as causes of pathologies could be yet another sign of the dynamic character of humoralism in the period examined.

The medical treatment administered to Maria Spada in the 1680s suggests that the therapies prescribed by doctors like Brasavola, who adhered in their academic writings to advanced currents of medical thought, were not as innovative as one might expect. Indeed, the medical views found in the Latinate texts that these doctors directed to the scientific community diverge considerably from those that characterize their everyday medical activities. Clearly, these texts cannot be taken as an indication of actual practice. As we have seen, a much more reliable depiction of what was going on at the patient's bedside is offered by popularizing, vernacular medical texts like Vittori's and Zacchia's.

The question remains, however, as to how we should explain this gap between vernacular and academic theory, and between the latter and actual practice. It can be argued that doctors depended on patients' narratives for their diagnoses and were expected to discuss their assessment of the case and its cures with medically informed laypeople who relied on a model of the body and disease deeply informed by humoral thinking. These exchanges necessarily relied on a lexicon and set of concepts comprehensible to non-professionals. The richness of patients' medical culture could therefore be an obstacle to translating new ideas into actual practice.[88] It is precisely because they were to be intelligible to patients and lay carers, that texts directed to the medical consumer (like Vittori's and Zachia's), provide a more reliable window on both the cures that were prescribed and how they were explained to patients. Only the demise of the medically knowledgeable patient would make it possible for doctors to apply the theories they were perfecting in their academic writings. However, it is also possible that the development of views of physiology and pathology alternative to the humoral ones was not accompanied by a parallel development of alternative therapies. Indeed, concepts like obstruction, immoderate amounts, healing through expulsion, and curing via opposite seem to have remained key to therapeutic thinking, even if applied to a body now being described in new ways. More work is needed to provide more robust answers to the questions raised in these pages.

WORKS CITED

Printed Primary Sources

Bertaldi, Lodovico, *Regole della sanità et natura dei cibi di Ugo Benzi senese*... (Turin: Domenico Tarino, 1620).

Boldo, Bartolomeo, *Libro della natura et virtù delle cose, che nutriscono, e delle cose non naturali* (Venice: Domenico and Giovan Battista Guerra, 1576).

Castelli, Pietro, *Antidotario romano latino e volgare* (Rome: Giuseppe Corvo, 1675).

Durante, Castore, *Il tesoro della sanità* (Rome: Zanetti, 1586).

Fioravanti, Leonardo, *Capricci medicinali* (Venice: Spineda, 1629) (first ed. 1561).

86. 'La marchesa più che altro si riconosceva offesa dalle passioni d'animo'. ASRo, FSV, B.483, 1686, p.169v. Maria's ailments were described as 'passions' and of a 'uterine' nature also by her daughter Eugenia; the best cure for them was *svario*, i.e. diverting the woman's mind from sad thoughts. Ibid., B.624, 29.11.1683, 4.9.1685.

87. Ibid., B.618, 5.10.1678; B.1115, 27.9.1679, 14.10.1679. 16.10.1680.

88. For similar considerations see Rieder, *La figure du patient*, esp. p. 503.

[Fonseca, Gabriele], *Gabrielis a Fonseca lusitani olim in pisana academia publici professoris nunc Romae medicinam exercentis Medici Oeconomia In qua omnia que ad prefecti medicimunus attinent brevibus explanantur* (Rome: Andream Phaeum, 1623).

Pisanelli, Baldassarre, *Trattato della natura de' cibi et del bere* (Rome: Bartholomeo Bonfadino, 1583).

Romoli, Domenico, *La singolare dottrina* (Venice: Giovan Battista Bonfadino, 1593).

Salvi, Tarduccio, *Il chirurgo. Trattato breve* (Rome: G.B. Robletti, 1642).

Vittori, Benedetto, *Prattica d'esperienza* (Vicenza: Antonio Megietti 1624) (first Italian ed. 1570).

Zacchia, Paolo, *De' mali hipocondriaci* (Rome: Vitale Mascardi 1644).

Secondary sources

Bartolini, Donatella, 'Consulti medici seicenteschi "secondo porterà il bisogno di lubricar il corpo"', *Medicina & Storia*, 15 (2008), 11–28.

Bellorini, Cristina. *The World of Plants in Renaissance Tuscany: Medicine and Botany* (Aldershot: Ashgate, 2016).

Bertoloni Meli, Domenico, 'Mechanistic Pathology and Therapy in the Medical Assayer of Marcello Malpighi', *Medical History*, 51:2 (2007), 165–80.

Bertoloni Meli, Domenico, *Mechanism, Experiment, Disease. Marcello Malpighi and Seventeenth-Century Anatomy* (Baltimore: Johns Hopkins University Press, 2011).

Borschberg, Peter, 'The Euro-Asian Trade in Bezoar Stones (approx. 1500 to 1700)', in *Artistic and Cultural Exchanges between Europe and Asia, 1400-1900*, ed. by Michael North (London: Routledge, 2010), pp.29–43.

'Brasavola, Antonio, detto Antonio Musa', *Dizionario Biografico degli Italiani* (online), vol. 14, 1972, by Giuliano Gliozzi, https://www.treccani.it/enciclopedia/brasavola-antonio-detto-antonio-musa_(Dizionario Biografico)

Bresadola, Marco, 'Pazienti e Curatori nella Pratica di Marcello Malpighi', in *Storia, Scienza e Società*, ed. by Paola Govoni (Bologna: CIS, 2006), pp. 17–45.

Calabritto, Monica, '*Medicina practica, consilia*, and the illnesses of the head in Girolamo Mercuriale e Giulio Cesare Claudini. Similarities and differences of the sexes', *Medicina e storia*, 11 (2006), 63–83.

'Castelli, Pietro', *Dizionario Biografico degli Italiani Treccani*, vol. 21, 1978, by Augusto De Ferrari. https://www.treccani.it/enciclopedia/pietro-castelli_(Dizionario-Biografico)/

Cavallo, Sandra and Tessa Storey, *Healthy Living in Late Renaissance Italy* (Oxford: Oxford University Press, 2013).

Cavallo, Sandra, 'The Domestic Culture of Health', in *The Routledge History of the Domestic Sphere in Europe 16th to 19th Centuries*, ed. by Joachim Eibach and Margareth Lanzinger (London, New York: Routledge, 2020), pp. 455–74.

Cavallo, Sandra, 'Habitat, Habit and Changing Ideas of Complexion in Early Modern Italy,' in *Charity, Medicine, and Religion in Late Medieval and Early Modern Italy: Essays in Memory of Philip R. Gavitt*, ed. by Beth Petitjean and George Dameron (Toronto: University of Toronto Press, 2024), pp. 209–32.

Cavallo, Sandra, 'Family letters', in *Early Modern Medicine: A Source-Centered Introduction*, ed. by Olivia Weisser (London: Routledge, 2024), pp. 226–41.

'Cesalpino, Andrea', *Dizionario Biografico degli Italiani* (online), vol. 24, 1980, by Augusto De Ferrari. https://www.treccani.it/enciclopedia/andrea-cesalpino/

Clericuzio, Antonio, 'Chemical Medicine and Paracelsianism in Italy 1550-1650', in *The Practice of Reform in Health, Medicine and Science 1500-2000*, ed. by Margaret Pelling and Scott Maldelbrote (Ashford: Ashgate 2005), pp. 59–79.

Cook, Harold J., 'Markets and cultures: medical specifics and the reconfiguration of the body in early modern Europe,' *Transactions of the RHS*, 21 (2011), 123–45.

'Cornacchini, Marco', *Dizionario Biografico degli Italiani* (online), vol. 29, 1983, by Ivo Comparato. https://www.treccani.it/enciclopedia/marco-cornacchini_(Dizionario-Biografico)/

Crimi, Giuseppe, 'Guarire a Corte: Appunti sulla Farmacopea nella Corrispondenza dei Gonzaga', in *Cultura alimentare a Mantova fra Cinquecento e Seicento: Storie di cibi e banchetti nei carteggi gonzagheschi.—(I Gonzaga digitali 3)*, ed. by Andrea Canova and Daniela Sogliani (Torrossa com., 2018), pp.109–126.

Donato, Maria Pia, 'Galen in the Age of Change (1650-1820)', in *Brill's Companion to the reception of Galen*, ed. by in Petros Bouras-Vallianatos and Barbara Zipser (Leiden/Boston: Brill, 2019), pp. 487–507.

Eamon, William, *Science and the Secrets of Nature: Books of Secrets in Medieval and Early Modern Culture* (Princeton: Harvard University Press, 1994).

Eamon, William, 'How to Read a Book of Secrets', in *Secrets and knowledge in medicine and science 1500–1800*, ed. by Elaine Leong and Alisha Rankin (Ashgate: Farnham, 2011), pp. 23–46.

Favino, Francesca, 'Sostanza e materia in uno scritto inedito di Girolamo Brasavola', *Medicina nei Secoli*, 15/2 (2013), pp. 247–67.

Fiorentini, Roberto and James Nelson Novoa, 'Gabriel da Fonseca. Un medico portoghese nella Roma del Seicento', in *Archivio della Società romana di storia patria*, 143 (2020), 277–311.

Floury-Buchalin, Cécile, 'Les querelles autour des remèdes chimiques et exotiques dans la littérature du xvii siècle', in Rieder and Zanetti (eds), *Materia medica*, pp. 131–46.

Gentilcore, David, 'The Impact of New World Plants, 1500-1800: the Americas in Italy', in *The New World in Early Modern Italy,*

1492-1750, ed. by Elizabeth Hodorowich and Lia Markey (Cambridge: Cambridge University Press, 2017), pp. 190–205.

Kuriyama, Shigehisa, 'Interpreting the History of Bloodletting', *Journal of the History of Medicine and Allied Sciences*, 50/1 (1995), 11–46.

Maclean, Ian, 'The Reception of Hippocrates by Physicians at the End of the Seventeenth Century. A Comparative Study', in *The Worlds of Knowledge and the Classical Tradition in the Early Modern Age*, ed. by Dmitri Levitin and Ian Maclean (Leiden/Boston: Brill, 2021), pp. 217–74.

Maehle, Andreas-Holger, 'Peruvian Bark: From Specific Febrifuge to Universal Remedy', in Andreas-Holger Maehle, *Drugs on Trial, Experimental Pharmacology and Therapeutic Innovation in the Eighteenth-Century*, Clio Medica Online, Volume 53 (1999), pp. 223–309.

Marini, Gaetano Luigi, *Degli Archiatri Pontifici* (Rome: Pagliarini, 1784).

'Mercati, Michele', *Dizionario Biografico degli Italiani* (online), vol. 73, 2009, by Elisa Andretta. https://www.treccani.it/enciclopedia/michele-mercati_(Dizionario-Biografico)/?search=MERCATI%2C%20Michele

Minuzzi, Sabrina. *Sul Filo dei Segreti. Farmacopeia, Libri e Pratiche Terapeutiche a Venezia in Età Moderna* (Milan: Edizioni Unicopli, 2016).

Nelson Novoa, James W., 'Libros y saberes en la biblioteca de un médico cristiano nuevo portugués en la Roma del Barroco', in *Bibliotecas en la Monarquía Hispánica durante la Primera Globalización (siglos XVI-XVIII)*, ed. by Natalia Maillard Álvarez and Manuel Fernandez Chaves (Zaragoza: Prensas de la Universidad de Zaragoza, 2021), pp. 63–91.

Nutton, Vivian, 'Hippocrates in the Renaissance,' *Sudhoff s Arch Z Wissenschaftsgesch Beih.*, 27 (1989), 420–39.

Nutton, Vivian, 'Renaissance Galenism 1540-1640: Flexibility or an Increasing Irrelevance?', in *Brill's Companion to the reception of Galen*, ed. by Petros Bouras-Vallianatos and Barbara Zipser (Leiden/Boston: Brill, 2019), pp. 472–86.

Palmer, Richard, 'Pharmacy in the Republic of Venice in the Sixteenth Century,' in *The Medical Renaissance of the Sixteenth Century*, ed. by Andrew Wear, Roger K. French and Ian M. Lonie (Cambridge: Cambridge University Press 1985), pp. 100–117.

Pilloud, Séverine, *Les mots du corps. Expérience de la maladie dans les lettres de patients à un médecin du 18 siècle: Samuel Auguste Tissot* (Ganève: Editions BHMS, 2013).

Pugliano, Valentina, 'Natural History in the Apothecary's Shop', in *Worlds of Natural History*, ed. by Helen Ann Curry, Nicholas Jardine, James A. Secord, and Emma C. Spary (Cambridge: Cambridge University Press, 2018), pp. 44–60.

Rieder, Philip, *La figure du patient au XVIII siècle* (Geneva, Drosz, 2010).

Rieder Philip and Zanetti François (eds), *Materia medica: Savoirs et usages des médicaments aux époques médiévales et modernes* (Geneva: Librairie Droz, 2018).

Stolberg, Michael, *Experiencing Illness and the Sick Body in Early Modern Europe* (Basingstoke: Palgrave Macmillan, 2011).

Stolberg, Michael, *Learner Physician and Everyday Medical Practice in the Renaissance* (Berlin/Boston: De Gruyter, 2023).

Suciu, Radu, 'La pharmacie du mélancholic: à propos de quelques médicaments mélanagogues en usage à la fin de la Renaissance', in Rieder and Zanetti eds, *Materia medica,* pp. 105–118.

Wear, Andrew, 'Medical Practice in late Seventeenth-and Early Eighteenth-Century England: Continuity and Union', in *The Medical Revolution of the Seventeenth Century*, ed. by Roger French and Andrew Wear (Cambridge: Cambridge University Press, 1989), pp. 294–320.

Weston, Robert, *Medical Consulting by Letter in France 1665-1789* (Farham, Ashgate 2013).

4

Between Land and Sea: Medicine and Galley Slavery in Early Modern Livorno*

Lucia Dacome

In November 1564, Francesco Orsi, a physician from Pisa, was asked to examine 145 ailing captives who had just arrived on the Tuscan galleys in Portoferraio to ensure that they had no transmissible disease. Since Orsi found nothing of concern, the captives were disembarked. Upon medicating them, the physician noticed that they were primarily affected by three ailments: fever, wet cough, and dysentery. However, he realized that they could not be healed because a major pre-condition for their recovery was missing: the circumstances in which they were kept did not allow for any proper handling of the six non-naturals.[1] The non-naturals were those environmental factors whose management was considered crucial in maintaining and restoring health.[2] In their traditional formulation, they usually included air, food and drink, rest and exercise, sleep and waking, excretion and retention, and the passions of the soul. In keeping with their principles, Orsi stressed the need to improve the captives' conditions, lest they die, but received from the *comito* (galley officer) a horrifying reply. The officer said that he did not care if they died. In fact, he did not care if 10,000 died. He saw enslaved individuals die every day. He also noted, cynically, while laughing, that a greater number of deaths amounted to a reduced expense for 'the Duke' and shockingly invited Orsi to kill several of them in order to carry out autopsies on their bodies: the physician was welcome to 'shoot two or three of them to see what they have inside'.[3] Orsi replied 'gladly', but remarked that that was not necessary because he already knew what to expect, namely, water-soaked lungs and a rotten liver due to drinking 'gross and salty water', as he had seen in the cadavers of captives in the expedition 'of the Pignone'.[4] Orsi's reply to the galley officer's atrocious proposal is also shocking in that it does not communicate any sense of outrage. It further reveals that Orsi had already dissected captives with like symptoms in similar circumstances and knew what to expect.

This essay begins with this unsettling exchange to explore the relationship between medical practice and medical theory in the context of galley slavery. It focuses

* I am very grateful to the editors of this volume, Sandra Cavallo and John Henderson, as well as to Joseph Berkovitz and Lavinia Maddaluno, for helpful comments on earlier versions of the essay. I also wish to thank Andrea Addobbati, Franco Angiolini the late Clara Errico, Lucia Frattarelli Fischer, Michele Montanelli, Cesare Santus, and Stefano Villani, for fruitful conversations, valuable insights, and archival suggestions. I am indebted to Esther Atkinson for impeccable research assistance and editorial suggestions and insights, and to Myriam Iuorio for adroit archival assistance. Special thanks go to Daniela Tazzi who has enthusiastically supported this project from its very beginning and has generously offered invaluable help and archival guidance. Earlier versions of this essay were presented at Villa I Tatti (2019), the Annual Congress of the Mediterranean Studies Association (2019), and King's College London (2023). I wish to thank audiences at these events for their helpful feedback. Research for this essay was supported by a Victoria College Research Grant (2017); the Jackman Humanities Institute (2018); Villa I Tatti–The Harvard Center for Italian Renaissance Studies (2019); a SSHRC Institutional Grant (2018); and a SSHRC Insight Development Grant Fund # 505096 (2018–2024).

1. ASFi, MdP, 510b, 1383^r, Letter of Francesco Orsi, 22 December 1564; also cited in Corsini, 'Il servizio', II, pp. 815–16.
2. On the non-naturals in the early modern period, see Emch–Dériaz, 'The Non-Naturals'; Cavallo and Storey, *Healthy Living*; *Conserving Health*, ed. by Cavallo and Storey. On the longer history of the non-naturals, see also Niebyl, 'The Non-Naturals'; García-Ballester, 'On the Origin', pp. 105–15; *Lifestyle and Medicine*, ed. by Kennaway and Knoeff.
3. ASFi, MdP, 510b, 1383^r, Letter of Francesco Orsi, 22 December 1564. Unless otherwise stated, translations are my own.
4. Ibid.

on Livorno, where galley slavery developed as the result of Medicean Tuscany's investment in the corsair war.[5] Cosimo I de' Medici's efforts towards creating a Tuscan fleet dated back to the mid-1540s. In 1561, the Order of the Knights of Saint Stephen was then established on the model of Malta's Knights of Saint John with the approval of Pope Pius IV. The knighthood was aimed at defending the Tuscan coast (as well as the Catholic faith) and engaged in military operations and corsair activities against Barbary corsairs and the Ottoman Empire.[6] Stationed in Livorno, its fleet set off to confront 'enemy' vessels, mainly from the Muslim Mediterranean world, and raid the coasts of North Africa and the Eastern Mediterranean, enslaving the individuals captured along the way.[7] Since slavery was purportedly predicated on religious difference, it targeted the religious other, who was regarded, at least in principle, as 'enslaveable'. Consequently, enslaved individuals belonged to different religious groups, including Jews, Eastern Christians, and Protestants, but were primarily Muslims, arriving in the city from across the Ottoman Empire and beyond. While women and children were usually sold in the slave market, and often entered the world of domestic slavery, most men became property of the prince and were coerced to row on the galleys of the Tuscan fleet alongside forced laborers (*forzati*, namely convicts condemned to forced labor) and *buonavoglie* (or *bonavoglie*, paid oarsmen who often served on the galleys to pay off their debts), who were usually Catholic.[8] At the turn of the seventeenth century, the 'Bagno' was created in Livorno as a purpose-built edifice to house and control unfree rowers and prevent their escape (fig. 5).[9] Including health-related spaces, like a hospital and an apothecary shop, it became the primary location for medical practitioners to attend its many unfree residents who were subjected to extreme conditions that made them prone to illness, injury, disability, and death. The Bagno brought together the management of captives' health with their subjection to the perils of enslaved life. This essay explores the unfolding of medical practice in an environment like galley slavery characterized by the convergence of violence and health management.

The story of Orsi and the galley officer allows us to peer into the relationship between medical practice and medical theory in this setting. The galley officer's heinous comments shed light on the role of health management in the Tuscan slave economy. The harsh conditions of bondage, systematic exposure to violence, and involvement in galley warfare exposed captives to the constant risk of sickness and impairment. Yet, as implied by the galley officer's words, enslaved individuals who could not row due to ill health and disability were considered a financial burden. Accordingly, galley regulations highlighted the need to preserve and recover captives' health. The shocking exchange between the physician and the galley officer further draws attention to Orsi's concern for the lethal consequences of improperly managing the non-naturals as well as his familiarity with autopsy as a way of exploring the causes of death. This essay considers these aspects of medical practice in the context of Livorno's galley slavery. It argues that the concentration of enslaved individuals subjected to extreme conditions called for special medical intervention.

We do not know how representative the exchange between Orsi and the galley officer might have been. But it sheds light on the tension between the extraordinary violence of enslavement and the economic pressure to attend to captives' fitness and health. While the role of medicine and the involvement of medical practitioners in the world of slavery have been examined in the Atlantic context, their place in the history of Mediterranean slavery and, in particular, in the Italian lands, remains

5. On slavery in Livorno see, for instance, Salvadorini, 'Traffici'; Toaff, 'Schiavitù'; Angiolini, 'Slaves'; Frattarelli Fischer, 'Il bagno'; Calafat and Santus, 'Les avatars'; Nadalo, 'Negotiating'; Rosen, 'Pietro Tacca's *Quattro Mori*'; Ostrow, 'Pietro Tacca'; Frattarelli Fischer, *L'Arcano*, pp. 45, 55, 63–69, 105–07, 132–35 et passim; Tommasino, 'Bulghaith'; Bonazza, *Abolitionism*, esp. Chapter 3; Errico and Montanelli, *Il bagno*; Santus, *Il 'Turco'*; Herzig, 'Slavery'; Bartels, 'Prisoners'; Bonazza, 'Collective'; Herzig, 'Enslavement'. See also Brege, *Tuscany*, esp. pp. 94–96 and 224–25; Terpstra, 'Found'; Wilbourne, *Voice*.
6. On the Order of the Knights of Saint Stephen and the Tuscan fleet see, for instance, Guarnieri, *I Cavalieri*; Angiolini, *I cavalieri*; Lo Basso, *Uomini*, pp. 337–68; Poole-Jones, 'The Medici'; Silva, '"To the Victor"'; Brege, *Tuscany*, Chapter 6.
7. It is worth noting that part of the enslaved population was also traded in Livorno's slave market.
8. *Buonavoglie*'s debts were often contracted in gambling sites opened by the Grand Duke in the port.
9. The term *bagno* echoed the Turkish *banyol*, the site where captives were kept in Istanbul. In 1598, the architect Giorgio Vasari the Younger included a section on the 'Bagno, or Serraglio' in his work *La città ideale* dedicated to Ferdinando I de' Medici, where he referred to the presence of a *bagno* in Malta, Algiers, and other places; see Vasari, *La città*, p. 182. On the (uncertain) origins of the term 'Bagno', see Frattarelli Fischer, 'Il bagno', p. 79; Calafat and Santus, 'Les avatars', pp. 478–79; Nadalo, 'Negotiating', p. 278; Rosen, 'Pietro Tacca's Quattro Mori', p. 39; Santus, *Il 'Turco'*, pp. 34–35.

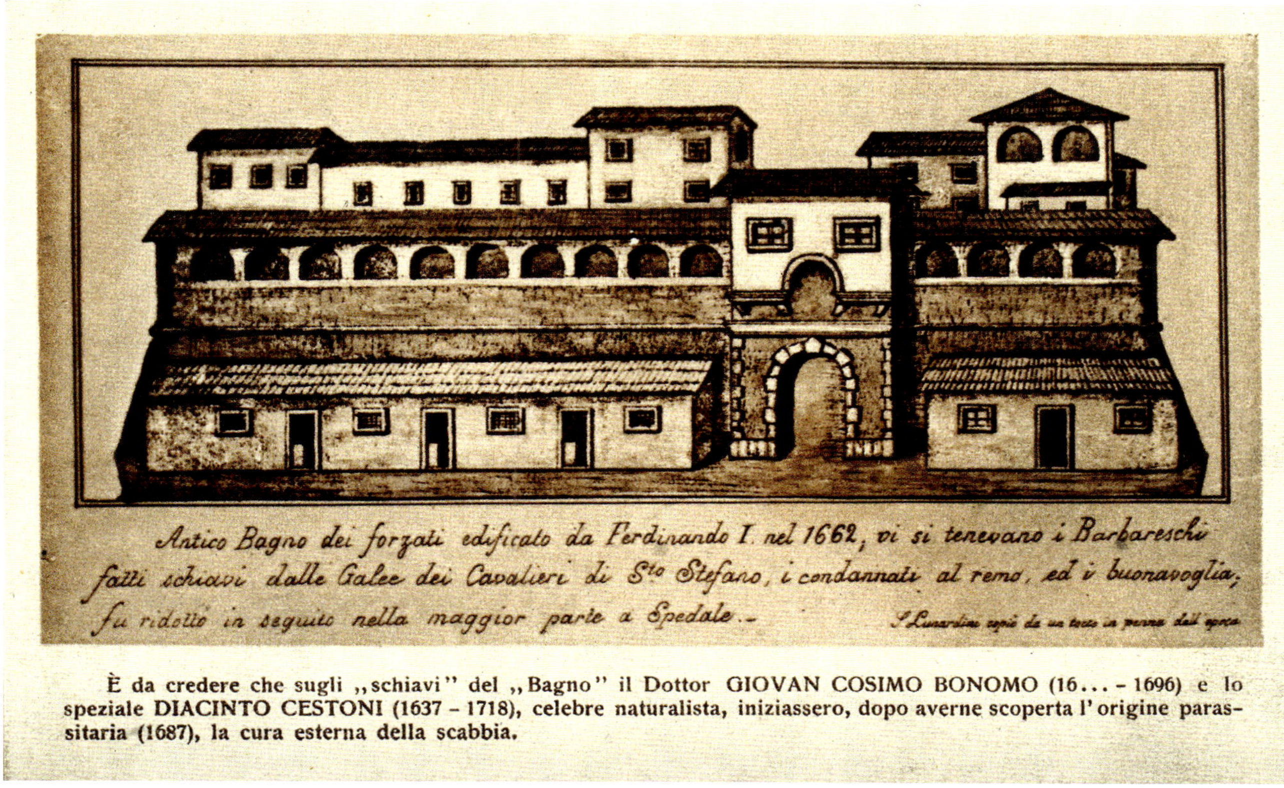

5. Early drawing of the Bagno reproduced in a postcard with a note mentioning that, purportedly, the new treatment of scabies proposed by Doctor Giovanni Cosimo Bonomo and apothecary Diacinto Cestoni was first administered to the 'slaves' of the 'Bagno'.

under-studied.[10] Works on Mediterranean slavery have highlighted the role of ransom and the logic of reciprocity as key differentiating factors from the dynamics of Atlantic slavery.[11] The infrastructure of ransom and reciprocity that governed Mediterranean slavery also affected its medical world. For one thing, health-related considerations played a significant part in decisions about ransom. For another, the fear that accusations of medical neglect of enslaved individuals could have repercussions for Christian captives in Muslim Mediterranean lands led to showcasing special investment in health care as characteristic of galley slavery's provisions.

Drawing attention to health-related considerations and the medical management of enslaved individuals does not mean, of course, downplaying the level of brutality to which they were regularly subjected, which is well represented by the vignette of the encounter between Orsi and the galley officer seen above. Rather, it invites us to consider the different uses of medical practice and its entanglements with medical theory in a setting characterized by the presence of numerous individuals coerced to live and labor in extreme conditions. This essay argues that galley slavery came to define a special site of both health-damaging and health-managing, an arena where health was simultaneously pursued and

10. For the Atlantic context, see, for instance, Savitt, *Medicine*; Fett, *Working Cures*; Mustakeem, *Slavery*; Cooper Owens, *Medical Bondage*; Paugh, *The Politics*; Roberts, 'To Heal'; Schiebinger, *Secret Cures*; Turner, *Contested Bodies*; Murphy, 'Re-writing'. On slavery and medicine in the Mediterranean world, see, Shefer Mossensohn, 'Medical Treatment'; Blumenthal, *Enemies*, pp. 66–70 et passim; Ferragud, 'The Role'; Blumenthal, 'Domestic Medicine'; Barker, *That Most Precious Merchandise*, esp. Chapter 4. On medicine and slavery in the Italians lands, see Corsini, 'Il servizio'; Bono, *Schiavi musulmani*, pp. 200–11.

11. See, for instance, Bono, *Schiavi musulmani*, esp. Chapter 5; Fiume, *Schiavitù mediterranee*; Bono, *Schiavi*; Hershenzon, *The Captive Sea*. In this context, at least part of the enslaved population could hope to be ransomed, and some could maintain a level of, however mediated, contact with their communities. See also Matar, *Mediterranean*.

undermined, and accordingly brought about a special type of medical attention. In the Bagno and its hospital, medical practitioners engaged in observing, inspecting, assessing, curing, controlling, and collecting information about enslaved individuals. Following their activities brings into focus the fashioning of Livorno's galley slavery as a site of health-related environmental concerns and systematic observation of bodies and diseases. Investigating this medical world further allows us to catch a glimpse of the dynamics of medical practice in a setting in which captives were in turn the bearers of medical knowledge, and their habits and skills—as well as their bodies—became the object of medical attention. The last part of the essay turns to enslaved individuals' health-related practices and habits that drew the interest of local medical practitioners. In particular, it considers a famous case of observation, translation, and experimental re-elaboration of a healing practice that was common among captives, resulting in a new account of an ailment like scabies and new treatment.

Finally, exploring the context of the encounter between enslaved individuals and medical practitioners sheds light on the maritime or, more precisely, the 'coastal' dimension of medicine in early modern Italy. In recent years, historians have highlighted how Italy's maritime history has often been overlooked by the historiography.[12] Such a historiographic lacuna has also characterized the history of medicine, which has largely concentrated on urban and inland environments. A focus on the medical world of galley slavery underscores the peculiarities of medicine as it was practised between land and sea, and in the context of the convergence of conflict and exchange that characterized coastal encounters in the Mediterranean world.[13] While doing so, it presents a particularly interesting point of entry into the shifting dynamics of medical practice and theory in early modern Italy.

GALLEYS AS SITES OF MORBIDITY

From afar, galleys presented an imposing spectacle. Decorated by artists, they stood out as remarkable maritime creatures (fig. 6).[14] In numerous depictions, they are featured elegantly navigating in the open sea or anchored in ports with their silhouette and decorations drawn against the horizon (fig. 7). Between 1664 and 1688, Ignazio Fabroni, a Pistoiese nobleman and knight of the Order of Saint Stephen, depicted many such scenes, as well as life during galley expeditions, in striking drawings where the violence of enslavement and the harsh conditions endured by unfree rowers are singularly toned down (figs. 6 and 8).[15]

In fact, galleys were crowded, dirty, and dangerous places where hundreds of individuals were forced to row while being chained to benches, confined to a minimal space, and exposed to the elements. The dimensions of the galleys could vary but were often between forty and fifty-five meters long and four to six meters wide.[16] Much of the central space was occupied by twenty-five to thirty rows of benches where five, six, or even seven rowers were busy pulling the oar or resting (fig. 8).[17] The number of rowers on each galley was high and could reach 300 or more. On 26 July 1620, for instance, the six grandučal galleys included a total of 1683 rowers (1075 captives, 489 forced laborers, and 119 *buonavoglie*).[18] After part of the fleet was sold in 1647, the number of rowers continued to be high. On 16 November 1678, for instance, the remaining four galleys counted 1050 'healthy' rowers (534 captives, 343 forced laborers, and 173 *buonavoglie*).[19]

Rowers could sometimes count on a drape for protection from the rain, cold, wind, and sun (fig. 6).[20] However, they were subjected to extreme conditions that jeopardized their fitness and health. In a rare first-hand account, William Davies, a British surgeon who was enslaved by the Tuscan fleet at the end of the sixteenth

12. See, for instance, Fogu, *The Fishing Net*.
13. For an early study of the Tuscan fleet's medical world, see Corsini, 'Il servizio'. Chizzolini's 'Medicare' was published when this article was in production and regrettably could not be considered here. On the need to engage with 'healthscaping' processes in premodern global contexts beyond urban and European-centred histories of early public health, see Geltner and Coomans, 'The Healthscaping Approach'.
14. Pampalone, 'Pier Leone Ghezzi'; Agostini, *Istantanee*, pp. 63–64; Martin and Weiss, *The Sun*.
15. See BNCF, Rossi Cassigoli, MS 199. On Fabroni and his drawings, see, for instance, Agostini, *Istantanee*; Pomini, 'Image Making'.
16. Bono, *Schiavi musulmani*, p. 155; Agostini, *Istantanee*, p. 64.
17. See Corsini, 'Il servizio', I, pp. 287–88; Bono, *Schiavi musulmani*, pp. 155–56; Lo Basso, *Uomini*, esp. pp. 13ff; Santus, *Il 'Turco'*, 162n44.
18. ASFi, Carte Strozziane, 148, fol. 340^{r}.
19. ASFi, MP, 2439, fol. 371^{r}.
20. Ibid., fols 474^{v} and 671^{v}; Pantera, *L'armata*, p. 223. See also Corsini, 'Il servizio', I, 287; Agostini, *Istantanee*, p. 71.

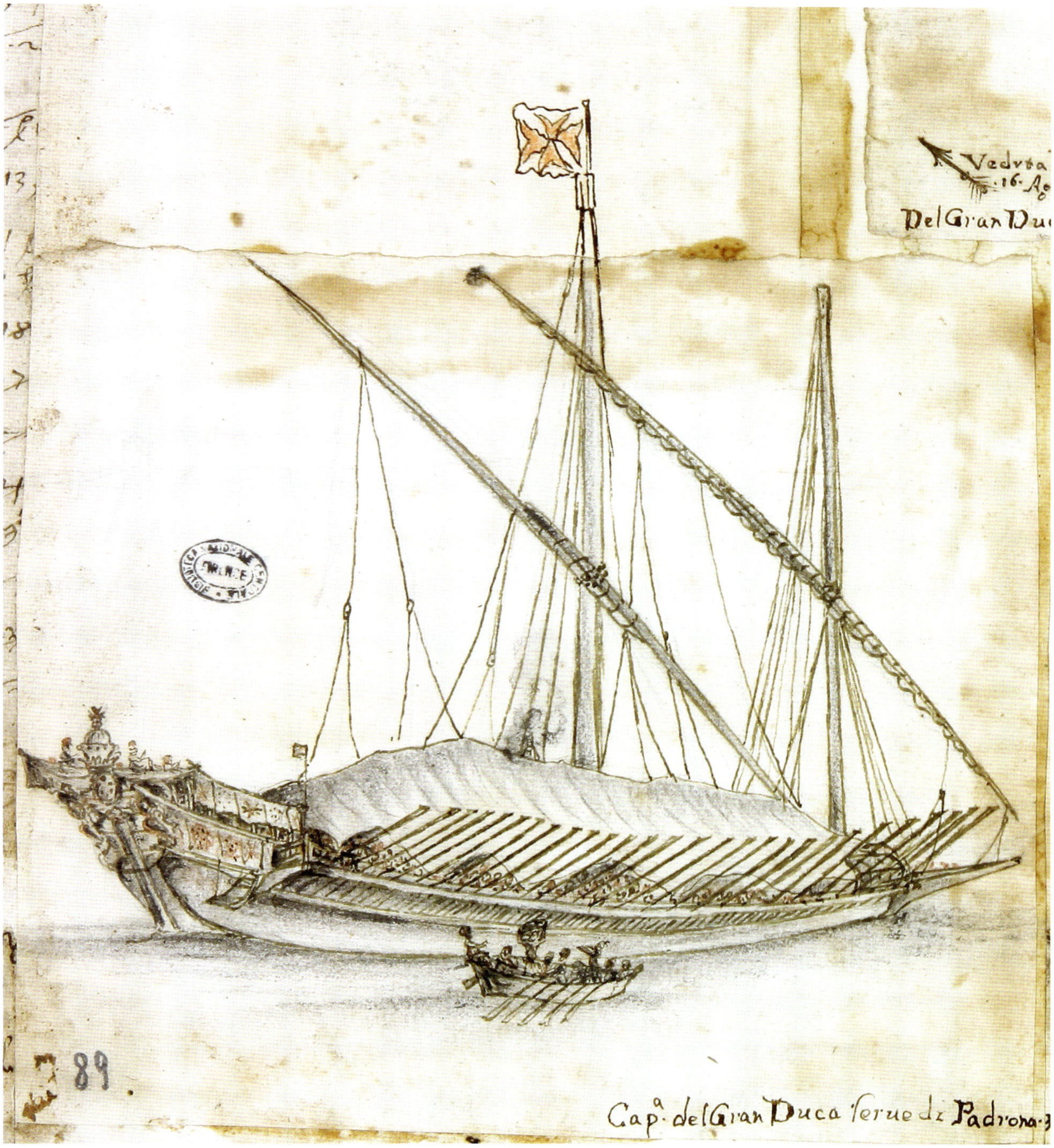

6. 'The Grand Duke's *Capitana* galley serving as *Padrona* galley', from Ignazio Fabroni, 'Album di ricordi di viaggi e di navigazioni sopra le galere toscane dall'anno 1664 all'anno 1687'.

century, reported the miseries he had to endure as a captive of the Grand Duke:

> [...] I was made a Gally slaue to row at an Oare, where our former diet lessened, but blowes increased, to the losse of many of our liues. We were shauen Head and Beard euery eight or tenth day, being alwaies naked, but onely a payre of linnen bréeches and chaines continually [...] The miserie of the Gallies doth surpasse any mans iudgement or imagination, neyther would any man thinke that such torture, or torment were vsed in the world, but onely they that

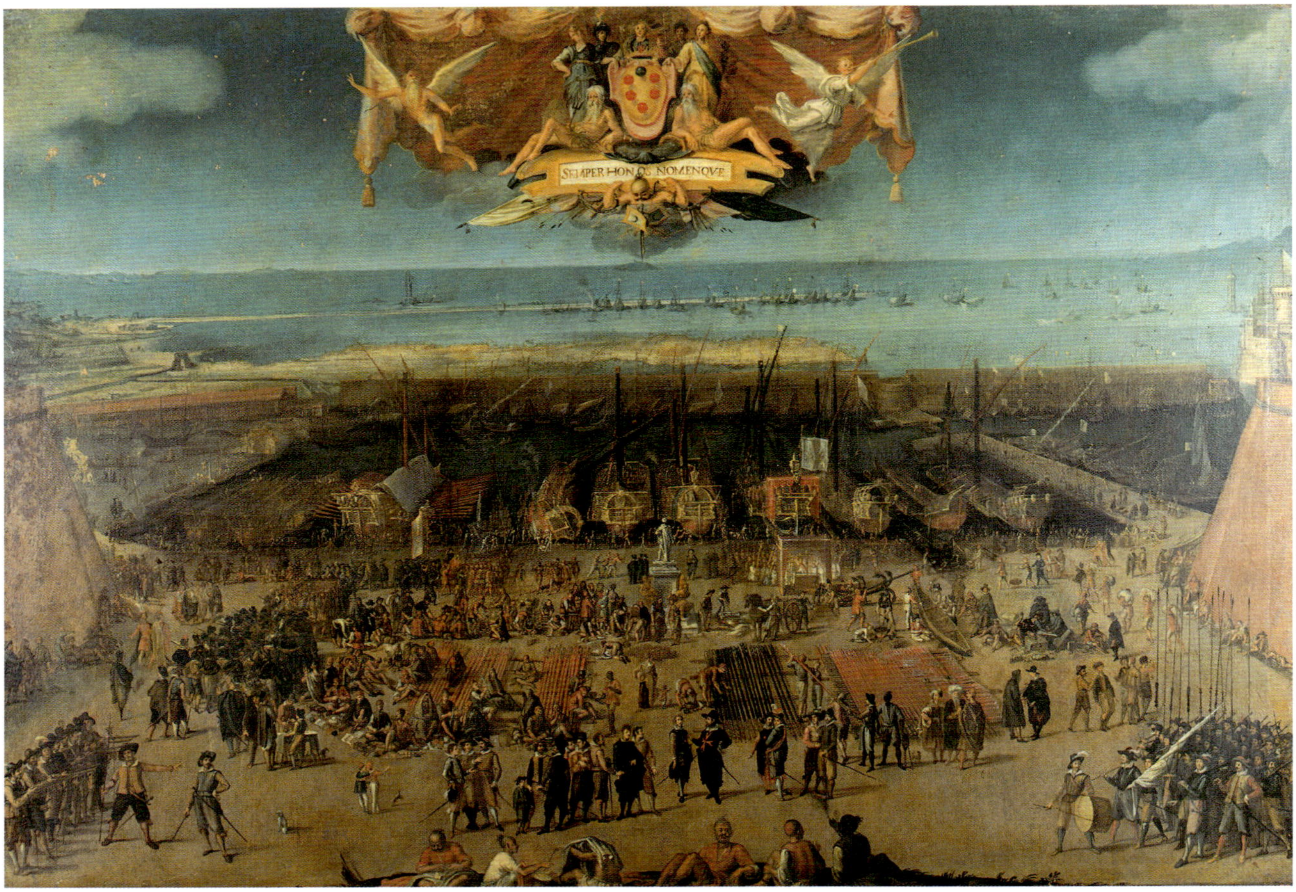

7. View of the Port of Livorno and the Galleys of the Order of Saint Stephen.

> féele it, the extreamitie of miserie causeth many a slaue to kill themselues, or else séeke to kill their Officers.[21]

Davies was Protestant and noticed that the Grand Duke did 'offend the Turks' more than 'all Christendom'.[22] A century later, the Capuchin father Filippo Bernardi still characterized the lives of Livorno's unfree rowers in terms of coercion to strenuous labor, a meagre diet, exposure to violence, and adverse weather conditions.[23] Not surprisingly, galley expeditions were hotbeds of disease and demanded regular medical care. Galley morbidity affected not only unfree rowers but everybody on board. In the autumn of 1716, for instance, the Livorno apothecary Diacinto Cestoni (1637–1718) noticed that the granducal galleys had returned full of sick people, and many had died not in battle but of disease. In fact, almost everybody on board was sick, regardless of whether they were officers, soldiers, forced laborers, or enslaved individuals.[24] Even more, the conditions under which unfree rowers labored made them especially liable to being injured and falling ill. Since the health and fitness of captives were crucial to the Tuscan slave economy, their importance was emphasized in statutes and regulations, and a complex medical apparatus was deployed both on the galleys and on the mainland to attend to the unfree workforce.

The statutes of the Order of the Knights of Saint Stephen postulated the need to have sufficient

21. Davies, *A True Relation*, section 4, n.p. On Davies, see, for instance, Neri, *Uno schiavo*; Brege, *Tuscany*, pp. 94–95.
22. Davies, *A True Relation*, section 4, n.p. The term 'Turk' was broadly used to refer to enslaved individuals from the Islamic world.
23. APCFi, MS 282, Bernardi, 'Relazione', p. 3.
24. Biblioteca Marucelliana, MS Redi 75, Letters nos 538 and 539.

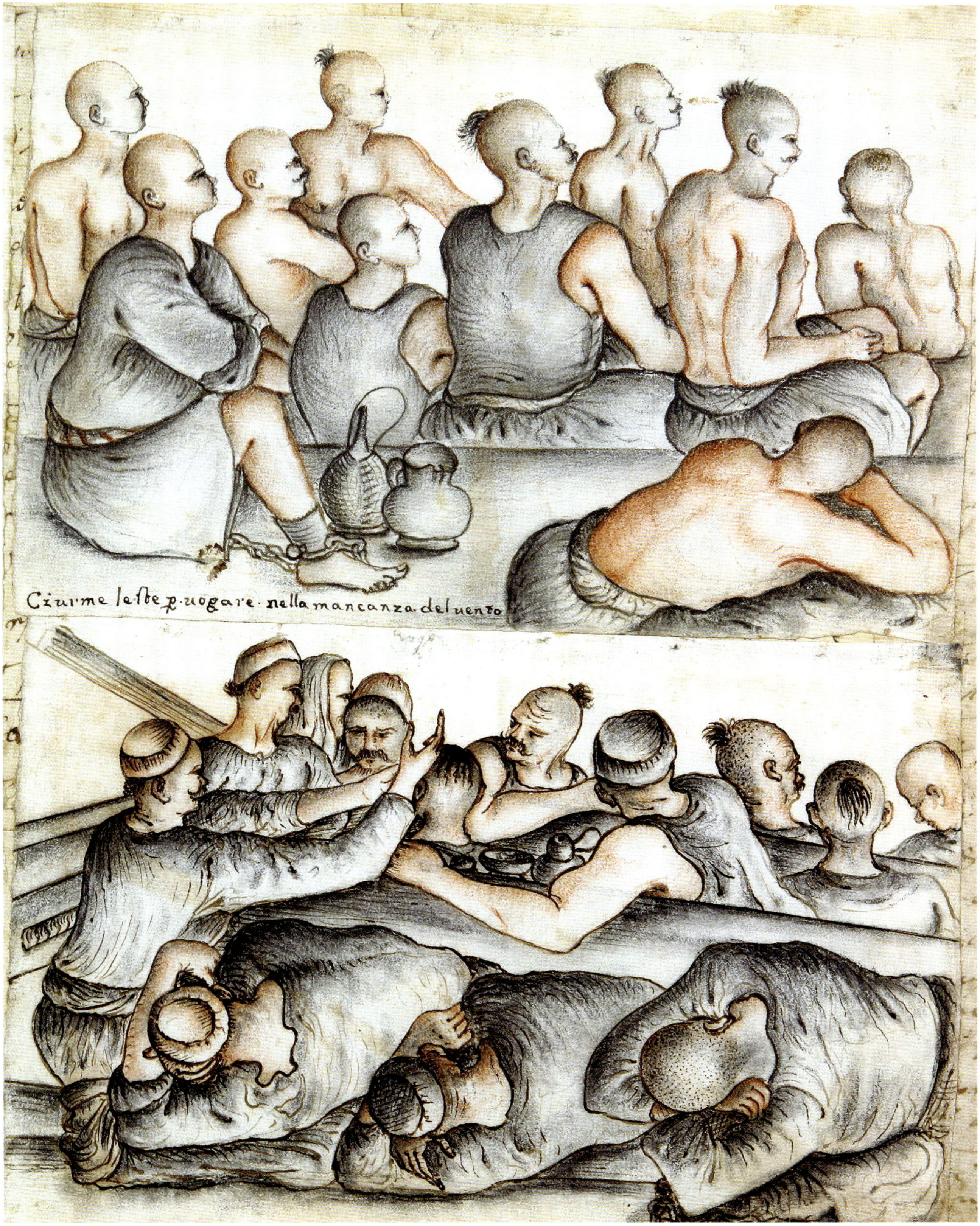

8. 'Oarsmen ready to row in the absence of wind' (above) and 'Oarsmen's other positions' (below), from Ignazio Fabroni, 'Album di ricordi di viaggi e di navigazioni sopra le galere toscane dall'anno 1664 all'anno 1687'.

medicaments and food on board the galleys as a condition for being allowed to leave the port.[25] Likewise, from the outset the regulations that governed galley life established that sick rowers had to receive regular medical assistance, fresh and good food, and remedies.[26] While 'healthy' rowers survived on a meagre diet, sick rowers could rely on richer provisions that included wine, meat, and bread.[27] In keeping with humoral principles, galley medical practice entailed the prescription of a proper diet and the administration of fresh medicaments as well as bloodletting. Since rowers were at constant risk of wounds and injuries, medical practice also required extensive engagement in various other surgical tasks. Reflecting traditional medical hierarchies, the galley medical apparatus included physicians, apothecaries, barbers (later replaced by surgeons), and carers like assistants to the barbers called *barbierotti* (or *barberotti*) and apothecary assistants called *spezialotti*, both chosen for the most part from among the enslaved population. Even before the establishment of the Order of the Knights of Saint Stephen, the presence of barbers and physicians was recorded on the Tuscan galleys in the 1550s.[28] From at least 1570, apothecaries also joined the medical practitioners on board the vessels.[29] Operating in different capacities and positions, these practitioners participated in the galley health care system in a variety of ways. While, in principle, only one physician and one apothecary were employed for the whole fleet, each galley crew included one barber who engaged in a wide variety of duties.[30] Unlike physicians and apothecaries, barbers were not employed on a permanent basis but were hired year after year at the time of navigation.[31] Still, they played a vital role in the galleys' medical world.

In 1614, Pantero Pantera's influential *L'armata navale* (1614), purportedly the first comprehensive work in Italian on naval warfare, noticed that barbers employed on the galleys were 'very necessary to cure the sick and wounded'.[32] They had to be skilled in surgery so as to be able not only to dress wounds but also treat fractures, bone dislocations, tumors, catarrhs, abscesses, and 'other accidents of life'. They then had to follow the orders received from the physician, carry out bloodletting through venesection or cupping, supervise the administration of food to the sick, ensure its quality, and take care of those who had no appetite. Moreover, they had to oversee the administration of medicines, syrups, poultices, ointments, and other remedies.[33] In short, barbers were very busy carers, practising in close contact with the sick and engaging in all kinds of tasks. They were assisted by *barbierotti* whose duties included traveling back and forth to the shore to collect what was needed for ailing rowers as well as preparing food, feeding the sick, and administering medicines.[34] Over time, barbers were replaced by surgeons, who could rely on more permanent employment and remained central to the medical management of galley navigation.[35] Like barbers before them, surgeons had to supervise the fulfillment of physicians' prescriptions and the administration of food to the sick, in addition to attending to wounds and injuries and engage in other surgical tasks.[36] Although surgeons were subordinated to physicians, the sheer need for surgical expertise on board allowed them to acquire more prominence within the galleys' system of care. It also afforded them some privileges initially granted only to physicians, such as finding accommodation within the Bagno. In fact, the need for surgical skills on galleys was such that even physicians were supposed to be versed in surgery and able to treat the wounded.[37] As physicians often looked for dispensation from navigating, they argued that in the case of short expeditions involving only

25. *Statuti, e costituzioni*, p. 94.
26. See ASFi, MP, 2132, Part I, Folder 6, 'Considerazioni sopra il ristretto delle spese delle Galere', no. 20; ASFi, MP, 2077, fol. 579^{v}.
27. See, for instance, ASFi, MP, 2077, fol. 705^{r}.
28. Ibid., fols 71^{v}–72^{r} and 150^{v}. See also Corsini, 'Il servizio', I, pp. 285–86.
29. Corsini, 'Il servizio', I, p. 455.
30. On galley physicians, apothecaries, and barbers in the Tuscan fleet, see Corsini, 'Il servizio', I, pp. 297–308 and 438–57.
31. Ibid., I, p. 306.
32. Pantera, *L'armata*, p. 126. Although Pantera was a naval commander based in Civitavecchia at the service of the papal fleet, his text offered a template for other Italian fleets.
33. Ibid.
34. Ibid., p. 136.
35. See, for instance, ASFi, MP, 2086, fol. 502^{v}. On surgeons in the Tuscan fleet, see Corsini, 'Il servizio', I, pp. 308–21.
36. Ibid., I, p. 296.
37. Pantera, *L'armata*, p. 111.

one galley, a 'skilled and experienced' surgeon could appropriately replace them.[38]

During galley expeditions only one physician was supposed to serve the whole fleet. Positioned on one of the chief galleys, either the *Capitana* or the *Padrona*, the physician had to travel on smaller boats to the other galleys to attend to the sick.[39] In practice, this principle was not always considered feasible and fell under scrutiny. When a galley physician became critically ill in 1636, the city's governor and admiral Giulio Montauto highlighted the need to have a physician, as well as a surgeon, stationed on each galley.[40] Moreover, after the fleet experienced conspicuous losses, in August 1686 two galley physicians, Romano Romanelli and Clemente Cosci, boarded the galleys. And when Romanelli fell ill, Cosci replaced him.[41] Regardless, the matter of physicians' privileges during navigation remained contentious. Throughout Tuscany's engagement in the corsair war, physicians remained reluctant to navigate, often asking for dispensation.[42] Over time surgeons too grew increasingly disinclined to serve in galley expeditions and sought to be exonerated.[43] In 1729, a shortage of surgeons led the Bagno administration to employ a young surgeon without much experience, being aware that there was 'the risk of causing more damage than help'.[44]

Galley physicians operated in different capacities.[45] During galley navigation, they had to treat the sick and wounded, prescribe medicaments, ensure that they were fresh and not corrupted, and, if needed, check the quality of food. In a rare portrait of a galley physician, Ignazio Fabroni depicted Clemente Cosci in the act of holding a flowered plant while reading a booklet, perhaps related to the plant's medicinal properties (fig. 9).[46] On shore, physicians also served in the galley hospital and prescribed preventive measures to keep the enslaved population fit and healthy. Together with surgeons, they were systematically involved in the observation of captives' bodies. They were called to examine enslaved individuals at the time of their arrival or purchase, as well as during their stay, and carried out autopsies after their death. They checked their state of fitness and health and searched for the signs of transmittable diseases, such as the plague (*mal contagioso*) or the great pox (*mal franzese*), which was widespread among the rowers. Physicians and surgeons also served as expert witnesses in the case of criminal offences, reported unfree rowers wounded in fights, and regularly inspected enslaved individuals' bodies to assess their ability or, rather, inability to row as part of the process that informed deliberations about purchase and ransom. In all these capacities, they fully participated in the dynamics of galley slavery. They engaged in a system of scrutiny and control where medical observation and inspection played an important part in the management of the enslaved population.

Thus, galleys operated as complex and extensive sites of medical practice, places where medical practitioners worked in close contact with individuals subjected to extreme conditions that made them prone to disease and disability. Yet, even with the deployment of this composite medical apparatus, galleys remained sites of morbidity characterized by sickness and death. Measures were taken to try to mitigate this situation. For instance, galley regulations prescribed that rowers had to be properly dressed. Moreover, they specified that galleys should not navigate in the winter.[47] This recommendation was reflected in the fact that galley navigation was usually limited to the warmer periods of the year (usually between April/May and late September/early November). Still, early on enslaved individuals were forced to live and sleep on the galleys throughout the year. They were constantly exposed to adverse weather conditions and an insalubrious environment that led to the proliferation of disease. Once

38. ASFi, MP, 2106, Letter of Luigi Montorsi, 10 December 1706. See also Corsini, 'Il servizio', I, p. 452.
39. ASFi, Carte Strozziane, 148, fol. 161ʳ; Corsini, 'Il servizio', I, p. 296. The apothecary who joined galley expeditions was also usually positioned on the *Capitana*.
40. ASFi, MP, 2084, Letter of Giulio Montauto, 25 February 1636 [i.e., 1637, in keeping with the Florentine calendar or 'Florentine style', according to which the year started on 25 March, and which will similarly be noted hereafter]. See also Corsini, 'Il servizio', I, p. 444.
41. ASFi, MP, 2100, Letter of Lorenzo Gonieri, 22 August 1686.
42. See, for instance, ASFi, MP, 2439, fols 334ʳ, 337ᵛ, 705ʳ, 718ʳ; ASFi, MP, 2101, Letter of Romano Romanelli, 22 August 1691; ASFi, MP, 2284, Letter of Romano Romanelli, 15 August 1695; ASFi, MP, 2105, Letter of Vitolino Vitolini, 25 May 1702.
43. See, for instance, ASFi, MP, 2113, Letters of Giuseppe Prini, 26 June 1724 (and attached note) and 14 August 1724.
44. ASFi, MP, 2115, Letter of Vincenzio Benci, 18 April 1729.
45. Corsini, 'Il servizio', II, pp. 652–59.
46. Agostini, *Istantanee*, p. 78.
47. ASFi, MP, 2132, Part I, Folder 6, 'Considerazioni sopra il ristretto delle spese delle Galere' [no folio number].

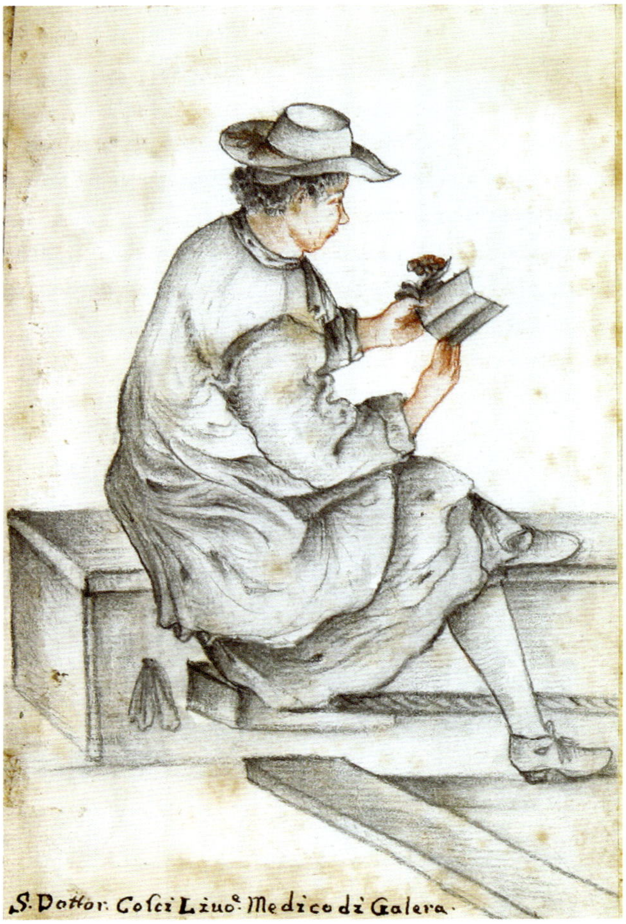

9. Ignazio Fabroni's drawing of 'Dr. Cosci from Livorno, galley physician'.

they fell sick, they had a slim chance of survival. In 1564, a similar situation led Orsi to highlight that lack of proper management of the non-naturals would cause his enslaved patients to die. As we have seen, Orsi's request for better conditions for the captives he attended was met with an atrocious proposal. A few decades later, the establishment of the Bagno promised to offer a roof and purportedly improved living conditions to Livorno's unfree rowers when the galleys did not navigate during the winter months. It also introduced a new reality in the medical world that revolved around galley slavery in the Italian lands.

THE BAGNO AS A SITE OF HEALTH MANAGEMENT

At the turn of the seventeenth century, the Bagno was built to house the increasing numbers of enslaved individuals arriving in the city as the result of the corsair war.[48] Between 1558 and 1610, the galleys of the Order of the Knights of Saint Stephen reportedly enslaved 9628 individuals.[49] In 1607, the raid of Bona alone resulted in the enslavement of some 2000 individuals.[50] Created to keep this large and diverse unfree labor force in check, the Bagno accommodated captives from across the Ottoman Empire and beyond, including regions like Morocco and sub-Saharan Africa, along with forced laborers and *buonavoglie*.[51] Although the Bagno was erected as an isolated edifice 'surrounded by high walls like a fortress', it was located right at the core of the city center and occupied a large area.[52] Placed in between the port and the main square that hosted the Duomo, the building developed around a central yard that had at its center a large cistern with drinkable water and, on one side, a well with salty water that was used to wash clothes.[53]

Over time, the Bagno became an ever more complex institution. In addition to the dormitories, which were assigned according to each galley, it comprised several mosques and churches, administrative offices, apartments for galley physicians and officers, and residences for clergymen, such as cells for the Capuchin friars who were entrusted with the Bagno's moral surveillance and spiritual guidance.[54] It also included health-related spaces: a hospital that constituted the core of the Bagno's health care provision and an apothecary shop that was supposed to provide a regular supply of fresh medicaments and served both the Bagno's residents and the local free population. Moreover, adjoining the building were the

48. APCFi, MS 282, Bernardi, 'Relazione', p. 6.
49. ASFi, Carte Strozziane, 145, fol. 46^{v}.
50. Ibid., fol. 3^{r}.
51. On the Bagno and its structure, see APCFi, MS 282, Bernardi, 'Relazione', pp. 5–14. See also Bono, *Schiavi musulmani*, pp. 164–66; Frattarelli Fischer, 'Il bagno'; Calafat and Santus, 'Les avatars', esp. pp. 475–79; Nadalo, 'Negotiating'; Rosen, 'Pietro Tacca's *Quattro Mori*', pp. 39–42; Errico and Montanelli, 'Il bagno'; Frattarelli Fischer, *L'Arcano*, pp. 63–65 et passim; Santus, *Il 'Turco'*, esp, pp. 33–40.
52. APCFi, MS 282, Bernardi, 'Relazione', p. 6.
53. Ibid.
54. Ibid., pp. 6–9.

stufe (hot rooms), which were visited by new unfree residents before being admitted and were then used by them on a regular basis for the purpose of health and cleanliness.[55] The Biscotteria, which employed enslaved individuals, also bordered the Bagno.[56] And both inside and along its external walls a number of shops and taverns provided sites where enslaved individuals engaged in commercial activities— such as barbershops, coffee shops, and shops selling, for instance, iron or garments and woollens made by them.[57]

From the outset, the Bagno operated as a site of both contact and conflict: a place of widespread brutality and coerced labor and, at the same time, an arena of encounter and exchange. It also became a venue governed by health-related concerns and considerations. In fact, surprising as it may sound, in the self-celebratory narratives of some of its advocates, the Bagno was presented as a 'unique privilege' enjoyed by Tuscany's enslaved population (as opposed to other sites of galley slavery where in principle captives could not move from the galleys).[58] This was because in the colder season it provided a shelter for unfree rowers, who would have otherwise been forced to live and sleep on the galleys, a situation that, as we have seen, led to the proliferation of diseases and high mortality rates. Conversely, the Bagno purportedly promised to offer improved health-related and environmental conditions to Livorno's unfree population. Such characterization clearly omitted the Bagno's reality as a site of systematic exposure to violence. But it also echoed the fact that, since captives needed to be healthy and fit to row, the Tuscan court became invested in their health.

Health-related considerations also marked the management of both the galleys' and the Bagno's physical spaces. Although early modern medical views of disease were neither static nor homogeneous, they largely associated the spreading of disease with exposure to poisonous air and contact with infected bodies and materials.[59] Likewise, bad smell was associated with 'corrupt' air and, by implication, disease and its transmission.[60] Not surprisingly, calls for cleanliness were part of the routines of both the galleys' and the Bagno's maintenance and administration. When moored in the port, galleys had to be cleaned every month.[61] Regulations related to the Bagno further prescribed that both the courtyard and the rooms be kept clean, and that waste causing bad smell be regularly disposed of 'for the sake of health'.[62] In a context marked by widespread morbidity and constant fear of epidemics, the salubriousness of the Bagno's environment became an object of primary concern. After a period during which many residents had fallen ill with tertian fever, the walls of the Bagno were newly painted and residents' mattresses were remade to prevent infection.[63] And when the presence of numerous animals, including dogs, rams, and 'filthy animals', created a 'bad smell and dirt', the administration asked the Grand Duke permission to remove all of them from the Bagno.[64]

As we have seen, when Orsi asked for a better management of the non-naturals to allow for the recovery of his enslaved patients, he received a heinous reply. Over the course of the seventeenth century, however, increased attention to the non-naturals, such as air, became part of the health management of the Bagno's unfree population.[65] The concern for air quality also informed the considerations that marked the seasonal relocation of rowers from the Bagno to the galleys and back at the beginning and end of the period of galley navigation. In the late spring or early summer, when the weather turned hot and the air became insalubrious, rowers were moved to the galleys. Conversely, the cooling of the air in the late summer or early autumn marked their return to the

55. See, for instance, ASFi, MP, 2132, Part I, 7, 'Costitutioni, et ordinationi dell'offitio del Capitano del Bagno', Chapter 31; ASFi, MP, 2086, fol. 1259^r.
56. The Biscotteria was a bakery that produced the 'round bread' sold to the local populations as well as *biscotto*, a type of bread that constituted a fundamental part of the diet of unfree rowers; see APCFi, MS 282, Bernardi, 'Relazione', p. 14. See also Errico and Montanelli, *La biscotteria*; Santus, *Il 'Turco'*, p. 38.
57. See, for instance, APCFi, MS 282, Bernardi, 'Relazione', pp. 6–7.
58. Ibid., p. 8.
59. See, for instance, Carmichael, 'Contagion Theory'; *Imagining Contagion*, ed. by Carlin; Cohn, *Cultures of Plague*; Cavallo and Storey, *Healthy Living*; Henderson, *Florence Under Siege*; Inì, 'Materiality'.
60. On smell and its health-related implications in the pre-modern period see, for instance, Palmer, 'In Bad Odour'; McVaugh, 'Smells'; Rawcliffe, '"Delectable Sightes"'; Dugan, *The Ephemeral History*, Chapter 4; Cavallo and Storey, *Healthy Living*, Chapter 3; Cavallo, 'Health'; Rombough, 'Air'.
61. ASFi, MP, 2104, Letter of Vitolino Vitolini, 23 August 1700.
62. ASFi, MP, 2132, Part I, folder 7, 'Costitutioni, et ordinationi dell'offitio del Capitano del Bagno', no. 9.
63. ASFi, MP, 2086, fols 749^r–750^r (Letter to Matteo Prini, 10 November 1684). See also Corsini, 'Il servizio', II, p. 667.
64. ASFi, MP, 2101, Letter of Lepido Petrocci, 18 October 1690.
65. On air management in the early modern period, see Cavallo and Storey, *Healthy Living*, esp. Chapter 3; Cavallo, 'Health'; Rombough, 'Air'.

Bagno.[66] In keeping with humoral views that hot air was a harbinger of disease, heat generated particular concern and was associated with the development of bad smells.[67] On 27 May 1699, for instance, the increasing heat prompted the decision to relocate the rowers to the galleys after it was noticed that a bad odor came out of the Bagno's dormitories when the doors were opened in the morning.[68] In the following decades, environmental considerations continued to inform the relocation of rowers. On 5 July 1713, the concern that heat may affect rowers' sleep led the superintendent Giuseppe Prini to consider relocating them from the Bagno to the galleys.[69] And on 18 July 1724, Prini again observed that it was high time to move the rowers to the galleys 'due not only to the heat but also the discomfort and the various small animals'.[70] Even these few examples show how environmental considerations informed the health management of large numbers of enslaved individuals.[71] Notably, while relocating unfree rowers from the Bagno to the galleys marked for them the beginning of a time of intense coerced labor, it was presented as a response to health-related environmental concerns. Even more, the galley hospital became a special site where such concerns were played out.

PROPERLY COVERED IN BED: THE GALLEY HOSPITAL

The hospital formed the high point of the Bagno's health care provisions. Reflecting the medical infrastructure deployed on the galleys, it involved physicians, surgeons, apothecaries, and *barbierotti*. Here unfree sick rowers purportedly found better treatment as well as regular medical assistance, with physicians and surgeons regularly calling in to check them, *barbierotti* attending to them as carers, and apothecaries providing fresh medicaments.[72] The establishment of 'galley hospitals' accompanied much of the history of galley slavery. To start with, old or disused galleys, customarily called *pulmonare*, usually served as infirmaries in the centers of galley slavery.[73] In Livorno, however, a galley hospital was reportedly erected by Cosimo I as early as 1547.[74] From the outset, it became the core of particular care and attention, and provisions were made for 'everything that needs to be done in the hospital of the galleys'.[75] Initially located outside the Bagno, the hospital underwent different phases and was later integrated into the building. In 1646, the Grand Duke Ferdinand II expressed the intention to move it to one of the Bagno's best rooms.[76] His successor Cosimo III ordered the construction of a new hospital inside the Bagno whose works started in 1673 and were reportedly completed the following year.[77] On 23 October 1677, the commissioner Lorenzo Gonieri received the order to transfer patients from the 'old' hospital to the new one.[78] And in January 1690 Cosimo III's son Ferdinando and his wife Violante Beatrice of Bavaria visited the hospital's new *fabrica*.[79]

In his 'Relazione', the Capuchin father Filippo Bernardi noticed that, like the 'old' hospital, the new hospital initially gathered 'both Christians and Turks', but was subsequently divided into two sections with the creation

66. See, for instance, ASLi, Confraternite, 226, Note of 22 October 1681; ASFi, MP, 2439, fols 328^r, 340^r, 884^r, 886^r; ASFi, MP, 2104, Letter of Vitolino Vitolini, 9 October 1699; ASFi, MP, 2108, Letter of Giuseppe Prini, 22 September 1713.
67. See, for instance, ASFi, MP, 2100, Letter of Lorenzo Gonieri, 9 May 1689.
68. ASFi, MP, 2104, Letter of Vitolino Vitolini, 27 May 1699.
69. ASFi, MP, 2108, Letter of Giuseppe Prini, 5 July 1713.
70. ASFi, MP, 2113, Letter of Giuseppe Prini, 18 July 1724.
71. On growing attention to the importance of environmental factors in the pursuit of health and its relation to the revival of Hippocratic views in the early modern period see, for instance, Cavallo and Storey, *Healthy Living*, esp. 78–80; *Conserving Health*, ed. by Cavallo and Storey; De Renzi, 'Seats and Series'.
72. See, for instance, ASFi, Carte Strozziane, 148, fol. 155^v; ASFi, MP, 2113, Letter of Giuseppe Prini, 14 February 1723 [i.e. 1724].
73. Pantera, *L'armata*, p. 111.
74. Biblioteca Labronica, MS 85, IV, pp. 198–99. This hospital was reportedly demolished in 1605 (p. 198).
75. ASFi, Carte Strozziane, 148, fols 155^r–156^v.
76. ASFi, MP, 2132, Part I, Folder 4, Note of 8 March 1646.
77. Biblioteca Labronica, MS 85, V, pp. 64 and 66.
78. ASLi, Confraternite, 224, Letter of Ferdinando Bardi, 23 October 1677. In early 1679, the transferral of patients from the more capacious 'old' hospital located outside the Bagno to the new one inside the building was discussed again in the correspondence between the Bagno administration and the court; see, for instance, ASFi, MP, 2439, fols 419^{r-v}.
79. ASFi, MP, 2101, Letter of Lepido Petrocci, 21 and 22 January 1689 [i.e., 1690]. See also Corsini, 'Il servizio', II, p. 660.

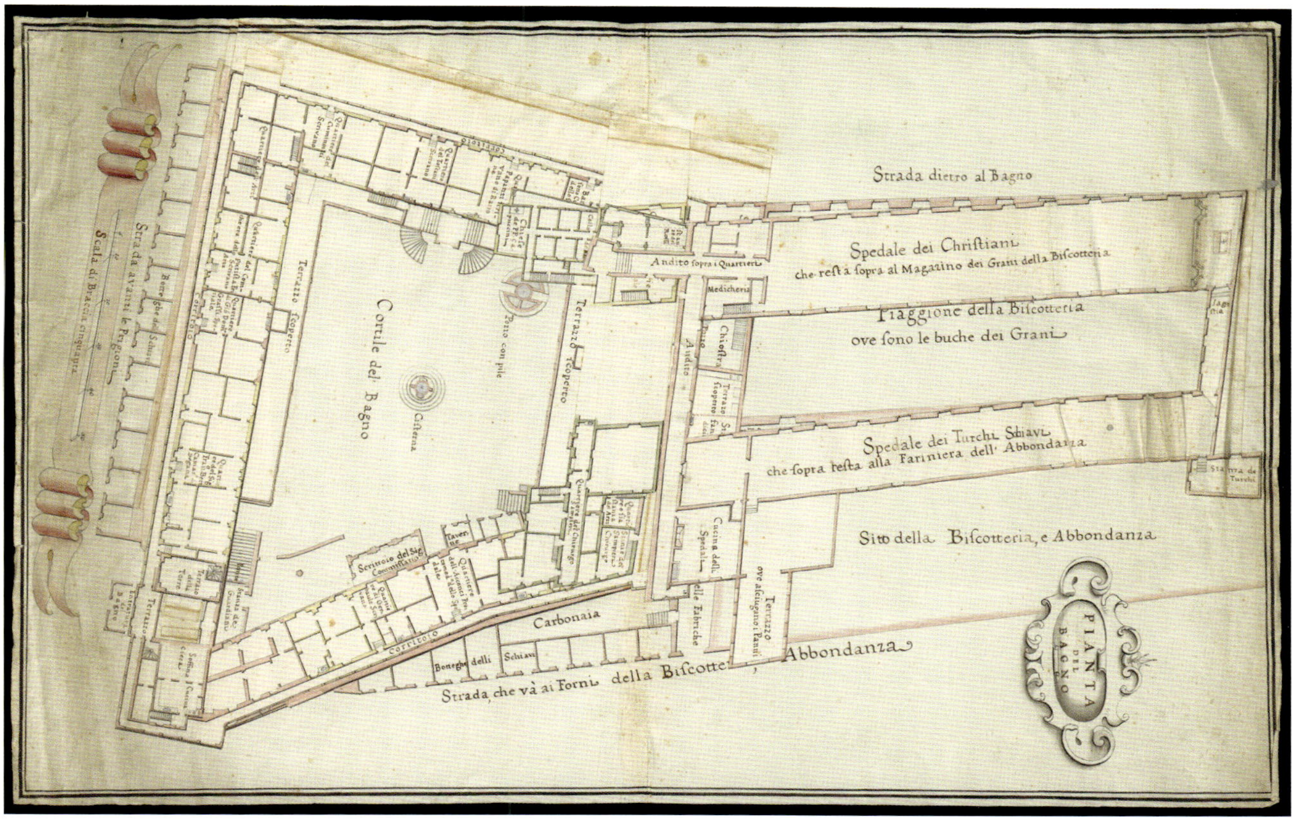

10. Map of the upper level of the Bagno showing two separate hospital wings called 'Hospital of the Turkish Slaves' (*Spedale dei Turchi Schiavi*) and 'Hospital of the Christians' (*Spedale dei Cristiani*).

of a separate 'Hospital of the Turkish Slaves' in 1697 (fig. 10).[80] However, the separation of Christian and non-Christian patients pre-dated this period and in 1691 the project of 'a new hospital of the Turks' was already under discussion.[81] In November 1693, a hospital note mentioned the galley hospitals in the plural and included a separate list of fourteen ailing captives in the 'Hospital of the Turks' in addition to the list of eighteen sick Christians.[82] And in January 1696 hospital reports referred to sick rowers in 'the Hospital of the Christians' and 'the Hospital of the Turks'.[83]

Capuchin father Ginepro da Barga (1630–1709), the chief spiritual guide of the Bagno, is usually credited for triggering such separation by complaining to Cosimo III that it was intolerable to have a priest attending to the soul of a dying Christian next to a 'Turkish minister' whispering the 'excommunicated words of the Qur'an' to an agonizing Muslim.[84] However, Bernardi's 'Relazione', where this episode is narrated, also recalls that the Grand Duke urged Barga to ensure that sick 'Turkish slaves' be allowed to have their 'Marabouts' near their bed engaging in whichever ritual was needed, because otherwise they could write to their rulers in *Barbaria* (Barbary regions) and complain, and this could negatively impact enslaved Christians there.[85] As we shall see, similar concerns also informed the management and self-representation of the galley hospital as a site where captives received proper medical care. One may add that the decision to establish a new hospital 'for the Turkish slaves' seemingly reflected existing practices and responded to different needs. In

80. APCFi, MS 282, Bernardi, 'Relazione', pp. 11–12.
81. ASFi, MP, 2087, Letter of Matteo Prini, 25 July 1691.
82. ASFi, MP, 2102, Hospital note of 20 November 1693.
83. ASFi, MP, 2103, 'Nota delli malati', 13 January 1695 [i.e., 1696].
84. APCFi, MS 282, Bernardi, 'Relazione', p. 11.
85. Ibid., p. 17.

1693, for instance, the 'sick Turks' cared for in the old hospital were moved to the '*guardarobba*' (a storage space) to make room for ailing soldiers. As the galley physician Romano Romanelli deemed this location narrow and insalubrious, it was decided to look for a better one.[86] Likewise, the creation of a separate hospital for 'Turkish slaves' likely responded to the need of monitoring ailing captives separately. Allowing for increased control over enslaved patients, it could facilitate decisions about the ransom of captives who were unable to row due to illness, injury, or disability. In fact, by separating 'Turks' and Christians, the hospital's spatial arrangement partly reflected, on a different scale, the divisions that already appeared on paper in hospital reports and other administrative records. Even before the creation of a hospital wing for 'Turkish slaves', the Bagno's hospital notes divided up sick rowers into the categories of 'slaves', 'forced laborers', and *buonavoglie*, and reported their ailments. The hospital note for 27 August 1687, for instance, accounted for fifteen 'slaves' who suffered from wounds and ailments like fever, tumors, empyema, and 'old age', and five forced laborers affected by complaints such as blindness, empyema, fistula, and pleurisy.[87] Likewise, on 9 October 1690 the hospital report recorded the presence of sixteen 'slaves' suffering from fever, scabies, diarrhea, surgical diseases, and being administered sarsaparilla, as well as seven forced laborers who had gout, empyema, and surgical diseases, and one *buonavoglia* receiving surgical treatment.[88] Creating separate hospital wings for 'Turkish slaves' and 'Christians' echoed the repartitions found in these records, allowing medical practitioners and administrators to promptly identify and assess ailing captives who were unable to row and were therefore more likely to be considered for ransom.

To be sure, the spaces of the two hospitals remained somewhat porous, reflecting, for instance, the volatility of converts' status: when a 'baptized Turk' in the Christian section of the hospital repeatedly spoke against the pope, he was relocated to the 'hospital of the Turks', again at the request of the powerful Barga.[89] Regardless, both hospitals were portrayed as sites of special care and attention to the relationship between environmental conditions and health. Bernardi's 'Relazione', for instance, highlighted how they both enjoyed great cleanliness, though the Christian hospital was especially 'airy, beautiful, and with sixty clean beds always ready for any occurrence'.[90] As historians have observed, early modern hospitals operated as privileged venues for the management of the non-naturals.[91] Over the course of the seventeenth century, Livorno's galley hospital developed as a site characterized by improved environmental conditions and special attention to non-natural factors such as air, food, and sleep.[92] Not surprisingly, just as in the case of the Bagno more generally, concerns for air quality felt particularly pressing. In July 1730, for instance, the presence of some 400 hens underneath the windows of the Bagno's hospital and apothecary shop prompted fear that in the heat of the summer the bad smell could contaminate the air and affect both the sick and their remedies.[93] The physician Romano Romanelli was then summoned to inspect the site and concluded that there was no such risk because the hospital's windows were very high and the space airy.[94]

Diet also lay at the center of hospital care. The regular diet of enslaved individuals and forced laborers was meagre, usually including bread or biscotto daily, broad bean or other legume soup three times a week, wine during navigation or in case of particularly strenuous efforts, and meat and rice at Christmas and Easter.[95] However, in the hospital the sick could count on the 'necessary things' like 'white bread, good wine, eggs', as well as mutton, and especially chicken, which was taken to have restorative properties.[96] Sleeping conditions also had to be reasonably comfortable and

86. ASFi, MP, 2102, Letter of Lepido Petrocci, 13 April 1693.
87. ASFi, MP, 2086, fol. 1270^r.
88. ASFi, MP, 2101, Hospital note of 9 October 1690 (see also Hospital notes of 17 and 26 May, 2, 9, 16, 26, and 30 June, 29 September, 22 November, and 18 December 1690).
89. ASFi, MP, 2104, Letter of Vitolino Vitolini, 9 February 1698 [i.e. 1699].
90. APCFi, MS 282, Bernardi, 'Relazione', p. 12.
91. Henderson, *The Renaissance Hospital*; Horden, 'A Non-Natural Environment'.
92. These factors continued to have wide currency into the eighteenth century; see, for instance, Donato, 'The Afterlife'.
93. ASFi, MP, 2115, Letter of Ranieri Bigani, 10 July 1730.
94. Ibid., Letter of Vincenzio Benci, 17 July 1730.
95. APCFi, MS 282, Bernardi, 'Relazione', pp. 10–11; ASLi, Governo civile e militare di Livorno, 13, fol. 73^v.
96. ASFi, Carte Strozziane, 148, fol. 155^r; ASFi, MP, 2439, fols 367^v and 372^r; ASFi, MP, 2086, fol. 98^r; APCFi, MS 282, Bernardi, 'Relazione', p. 12.

hospital patients were provided with covers and a mattress (*saccone*), which had to be turned frequently in order to remain comfortable. In short, here patients could count on improved living conditions and an organized system of care. At least, this was the message that the Bagno administration was keen to promote in response to claims of ill-treatment by enslaved groups.

In fact, the ability to showcase care for sick captives had some leverage in the regime of reciprocity that characterized Mediterranean slavery. If ailing enslaved individuals were not treated—as it were—'adequately', they could write to their rulers and voice their complaints. The fear was that, if this happened, there could be repercussions for Christian captives in Muslim Mediterranean lands. Thus, when complaints were voiced, the Bagno administration rushed to produce letters that presented the treatment of captives in the hospital as an example of the Grand Duke's magnanimous behavior. In a famous case that saw a group of enslaved individuals write to authorities in Tunis to complain about being mistreated, the Bagno administration mobilized representatives of the enslaved community through a letter written by the 'chief merchant' (an elected office within the enslaved community, probably related to captives' commercial and other activities) and countersigned by four *Coggia* (from the Turkish *HOCA*, meaning 'master' and used as an honorific title for teachers, spiritual leaders, and people of knowledge), namely, Muslim religious and intellectual authorities within the Bagno.[97] The letter highlighted the benevolent treatment of sick enslaved individuals and the respect of Muslim traditions, including burial rituals. In particular, it reiterated that, once they fell sick, enslaved individuals received adequate treatment in the hospital, where they found a proper bed with 'white sheet' covering both 'below and above', and were cared for by different practitioners, including a daily visit from a physician. They could also rely on a special diet that consisted of white bread and mutton or, in case of particularly serious illness, chicken, and received all the medicaments they needed from the apothecary shop.[98] Other letters produced in response to mistreatment allegations followed a similar pattern.[99]

Such accounts cannot, of course, be taken at face value. But they highlight the significance of health care in the dynamics of Mediterranean reciprocity and its fashioning as an object of attention and investment by the Tuscan court. In fact, things were clearly less rosy than such documents might suggest. In September 1722, for instance, the superintendent Giuseppe Prini had to reassure the court that he tried his best to ensure that, both on the galleys and in the hospital, all the various medical practitioners fulfilled their tasks and duties and ill captives received proper medical care. He also highlighted that if ailing captives complained about food scarcity, this was because the diet prescribed to them by the physician or the surgeon required avoiding excessive food that could 'harm rather than heal'.[100] Notes such as these show how the issue of the treatment of sick captives remained fraught. They also point to the flow of medical information that regularly traveled the distance between the Bagno and the Tuscan court. Reports from the Bagno kept the Grand Duke informed about the unfree workforce's state of sickness and health as well as the captives' ability or inability to row. The frequency with which we encounter such medical reports in the Tuscan slavery archive speaks to how the management of captives' health remained an object of close granducal scrutiny. It also reiterates the importance of medical practice in the life of the Bagno and the pressing need to reassure the Grand Duke that, health-wise, everything was in check. In fact, while medical practitioners were engaged in monitoring the health and fitness of the enslaved population, their activities were in turn monitored by the Tuscan court. As health management was crucial to the economy of galley slavery, medical dispatches worked as sites of negotiation of physicians' role and authority within the Bagno and their relationship with the court. For instance, they allowed physicians to showcase both therapeutic success and their ability to keep the risk of epidemics and the incidence of morbidity under control. Including information about the situation of sick and injured patients in the hospital of the Bagno, they also testify to physicians' engagement in the systematic observation of the enslaved population.

97. On the role of the 'chief merchant', see Santus, *Il 'Turco'*, p. 46.
98. ASFi, MP, 2086, fols 98^{r-v}.
99. See, for instance, ASFi, MP, 2439, fols 363^{r}, 365^{r}, and 368^{r-v}; ASFi, MP, 2106, Letter of Giuseppe Prini and attachments, 25 May 1707.
100. ASFi, MP, 2112, Letter of Giuseppe Prini, 21 September 1722.

INSPECTING THE ENSLAVED BODY

Historians have drawn attention to how observation acquired increasing significance in medical culture over the course of late sixteenth and seventeenth centuries.[101] Gianna Pomata, for instance, has reconstructed how observation was practiced by town, court, and itinerant physicians and in response to the revival of Hippocratic views.[102] The medical world of galley slavery testifies to another arena of medical practice in which observation became a feature of medical intervention. From the time of their arrival, captives were regularly subjected to medical inspection. The galley hospital, in particular, became a site of systematic observation of the ailments of unfree individuals subjected to extreme living and labor conditions. Such an approach was in line with the characterization of other early modern hospitals as sites for the observation of diseases and the investigation of their causes through dissection.[103] In the galley hospital, observation similarly extended to the post-mortems that were performed on the cadavers of unfree rowers. Sources are silent about the impact that dissections carried out on captives' bodies had in a context where the Muslim enslaved community was supposed, at least in principle, to be able to perform Islamic burial rituals.[104] But in Livorno autopsies were customarily performed as part of galley hospital practice.

In recent years, historians have started to revisit narratives that have traditionally placed the rise of 'pathological anatomy' in the late eighteenth century.[105] In particular, they have invited us to reconsider how morbid anatomy was widely pursued in different contexts of early modern medical practice. Drawing attention to galley slavery extends our understanding of the practice in a context characterized by high mortality rates and physicians' easy access to the cadavers of unfree rowers. As we have seen, as early as 1564 Orsi manifested familiarity with post-mortems and associated the symptoms shown by the enslaved individuals under his care with observations drawn from previous autopsies made in similar circumstances. In the following decades, medical practitioners continued to carry out dissections on the cadavers of unfree rowers to ascertain the causes of their deaths. In 1595, for instance, physicians dissected the body of an enslaved man who was found in agony and passed away, concluding that his death had been caused by a poisonous mushroom rather than by opium.[106] In the galley hospital, dissections took place in a setting characterized by physicians' and surgeons' regular access to large numbers of disposable bodies. In keeping with a well-established practice, autopsies were sometimes carried out in response to the fear of epidemics to detect the signs of transmissible disease.[107] Regular involvement in post-mortems also led galley physicians to investigate the causes of the diseases of unfree rowers who shared living and environmental circumstances and states of morbidity.[108]

Silvia De Renzi has shown how, in early modern Rome, physicians' cumulative evidence gathered through serial observations in post-mortems intersected with the revival of Hippocratic views that linked patterns of morbidity with given geographical and environmental circumstances. In this setting, the observation of similar symptoms and post-mortem findings in groups of patients lent itself to a quest for general knowledge in the still widely pervasive individualized context of humoral medicine.[109] In the late seventeenth century, the Bagno's physicians carried out dissections to investigate the causes of ailments affecting groups of rowers exposed to similar environmental and labor conditions and adapt treatment to what they observed

101. See *Historia*, ed. by Pomata and Siraisi; Pomata, 'Sharing Cases'; Pomata, 'Observation Rising'; Daston, 'The Empire'.
102. Pomata, 'Sharing Cases'; Pomata, 'Observation Rising'.
103. See *Pathology* ed. by De Renzi, Bresadola and Conforti.
104. On Islamic burial practices in the Bagno, see APCFi, MS 282, Bernardi, 'Relazione', p. 13. In the early eighteenth century, the artist Georg Christoph Martini observed that the 'Turks' of the Bagno were buried 'in the Turkish fashion'; see Martini, *Viaggio*, pp. 64–65. It might be worth noting that while Islamic law prohibited the mutilation of bodies, anatomy was part of pre-modern Islamic medicine; see, for instance, Fancy, 'Anatomy', pp. 42–51.
105. See *Pathology*, ed. by De Renzi, Bresadola and Conforti. See also Atkinson, 'Anomalous Bodies', Chapter 4.
106. ASFi, MP, 1209, fol. 954^r.
107. See, for instance, ASFi, MP, 2116, Letter of 9 March 1732. See also Corsini, 'Il servizio', II, p. 658. On post-mortems carried out in the context of suspicion of epidemic disease see, for instance, Park, *Secrets*, p. 79; De Renzi, 'Seats and Series', pp. 104–05; Liboni, 'Humanist Post-mortems', pp. 20, 24, 29.
108. On autopsies in the Bagno see, for instance, ASFi, MP, 2439, fol. 377^r–378^v; ASFi, MP, 2107, Notes of Romano Romanelli of 5 June 1709 and 19 October 1711.
109. De Renzi, 'Seats and Series'.

in their bodies. In November 1678, for instance, the galley physicians Clemente Cosci and Antonio Torsi were struggling to control the incidence of a long, relapsing, and lethal disease affecting rowers. They then set off to dissect the cadavers of those who had died of this bad 'influenza' hoping to shed light on its causes and 'apply the appropriate remedies'.[110] In the previous weeks, the spreading of the disease among rowers had led Cosci and Torsi to seek advice from the famous and influential court physician Francesco Redi (1626–1698), who was in regular contact with the world of Livorno's galley slavery. Redi approved of the physicians' diagnosis and noted that he had nothing to add to their observations. He also advised them to protect rowers from the cold and nourish them with good bread and wine, which in his view would be more helpful than any remedy from the apothecary.[111] Cosci proceeded then to dissect the cadavers of those who had died of the disease and sent his 'observations' to the 'Professors' in Florence.[112]

As this episode shows, dissections took place as an extension of the medical apparatus that was deployed to manage unfree rowers' fitness and health. In this setting, as we have seen, physicians operated as close observers of captives' bodies and ailments. They did so in ways that reinforced the institution of slavery, and this is worth emphasizing. In such a situation, galley physicians worked as the gatekeepers of enslaved bodies in a context in which medical observation intersected with the demands of inspection, control, and surveillance that marked the slavery apparatus. Ultimately, medical practitioners' engagement in attending to the health of captives was aimed at recovering the ability to extract labor from them and accordingly restore their place in the Tuscan slave economy. Not surprisingly, such a situation of control and uneven power relations could lead to mishandling and abuse. In his *L'armata navale*, Pantera emphasized that galley physicians had to be 'compassionate, benevolent, and patient' to avoid the risk that enslaved patients could die of 'despair' after encountering 'strict, negligent or ignorant' physicians.[113] But such a prescriptive ideal was bound to fall short of reality. In the early seventeenth century, for instance, the physician Bernardino Borromei notoriously engaged in the mistreatment of the enslaved population.[114] Archival records occasionally point to cases of mishandling and abuse even in the context of common practices like bloodletting. In 1569, for instance, a galley barber known for being 'not only negligent but also cruel' used the blood bowl to hit the mouth of the man he was bloodletting after a few drops of blood fell on him—a far cry from Pantera's recommendation that barbers be 'patient and resilient' in their cures.[115] In other cases, mismanagement could lead to death, as in the case of a galley surgeon who served in Civitavecchia, in the Papal States, and caused the death of five captives due to either 'ignorance or mistreatment'.[116] In the galley slavery archive such instances of maltreatment often remain silent. Still, it is worth reading these episodes against ordinary situations in which physicians' and surgeons' engagement in medical observation was integral to the galley slavery's system of inspection, surveillance, and control. From the outset, rules governing the life of the galleys required physicians and surgeons to report the wounds they medicated from fights among unfree rowers to help with the investigation and the administration of punishment.[117] Medical practitioners were also called to scrutinize unfree rowers' claims of sickness and disability and assess their authenticity. In fact, since ill health and 'inability' could bring about dispensation from rowing and increased the likelihood of being ransomed, medical practitioners were urged to engage in the close scrutiny of enslaved individuals' claims of infirmity.

The concern was that these claims could be nothing but '*finzioni*', fabrications.[118] If misled by such false claims, physicians ran the risk of granting healthy individuals the benefits reserved for the sick and disabled. Such apprehension was widespread across the different sites of galley slavery. Notices concerning the pontifical galleys, for instance, warned physicians about unfree laborers'

110. ASLi, Confraternite, 224, Letter of Ferdinando Bardi, 12 November 1678; ASFi, MP, 2439, fol. 362ʳ.
111. ASLi, Confraternite, 224, Letter of Francesco Redi, 5 November 1678; ASFi, MP, 2439, fol. 367ʳ.
112. ASLi, Confraternite, 224, Letter of Ferdinando Bardi, 22 November 1678; ASFi, MP, 2439, fols 376ʳ –378ᵛ.
113. Pantera, *L'armata*, p. 110.
114. Borromei also orchestrated an atrocious case of sexual violence in the Bagno; see Toaff, *La Nazione*, p. 269; Frattarelli Fischer, 'Il bagno', p. 87; Herzig, 'Slavery'; Herzig 'Enslavement'.
115. See ASFi, MP, 2077, fol. 167ʳ; Corsini, 'Il servizio', I, pp. 298–99; Pantera, *L'armata*, p. 126.
116. See ASR, Camerale II, Epistolario, 32, Captives' petition attached to the letter of 10 July 1723. See also Bono, *Schiavi musulmani*, p. 205.
117. See, for instance, ASFi, MP, 2077, fol. 578ᵛ. See also Corsini, 'Il servizio', II, p. 654.
118. Savelli, *Pratica universale*, p. 187.

'frequent inventions' aimed at receiving better treatment and exemption from rowing. They also emphasized that 'in order to look impaired or feeble', some actually became disabled, and others who pretended to be feverish became sick and even died.[119] The concern was sufficiently pressing to call for the insights of the famous papal archiater Paolo Zacchia (1584–1659), who had dealt with the issue of simulated sickness in his influential *Quaestiones medico-legales*.[120] Drawing on Zacchia, the jurist Marc'Antonio Savelli (1624–1695) provided advice about how to expose false claims of 'inability' by unfree rowers.[121] In a situation in which the body was broadly characterized by potentially ambiguous, variable, and uncertain corporeal signs, this was no easy task. And Savelli noticed that physicians had to be able to detect deception in a context in which enslaved individuals could go as far as alter their 'pulse, urine, color, and similar things'.[122] In some cases, false claims of illness could even lead to escape or mutiny. In 1684, for instance, the commissioner Lorenzo Gonieri suggested that enslaved individuals traveling from Malta to Livorno likely pretended to be sick when they carried out a mutiny after the owner of the vessel had gone ashore to buy mutton and chicken to restore their health.[123] So both the Bagno and the galleys served as special sites of medical attention, observation, and scrutiny of not only the bodies but also the health-related practices and skills of enslaved individuals. In fact, captives also actively participated in the world of healing and their practices were included in the regime of inspection and observation that local medical practitioners directed at them.

TRANSLATING VERNACULAR PRACTICE

A famous example of this dynamic involved the Livorno apothecary and savant Diacinto Cestoni, the galley physician Giovanni Cosimo Bonomo (1663–1696) and, to some extent, Francesco Redi. We have encountered Cestoni above, commenting in 1716 on the high mortality of a galley expedition. By then, Cestoni had become an important figure in Livorno's medical and intellectual life and was well connected in wider savants' networks.[124] In the previous decades, he had also befriended Redi, who regularly visited Livorno with the court and with whom Cestoni was in regular exchange. Through his apothecary shop, Cestoni equally encountered Livorno's different constituencies, including the enslaved population. In a sense, even the encounter with Bonomo took place via this space. In fact, after studying at the University of Pisa, in 1684 Bonomo returned to Livorno where he began to frequent Cestoni's apothecary shop. Cestoni then recommended him to Redi, who in turn appointed him as a galley physician and ended up describing him as 'one of the best physicians in Livorno'.[125]

Perusing the medical reports mentioned above, we can catch glimpses of Bonomo's activities as a galley physician. In 1684, for instance, he boarded a galley expedition during which he witnessed widespread disease and high mortality rates while getting himself sick twice.[126] In May 1690, he took care of his fellow galley physician Romano Romanelli, who had fallen seriously ill, and was chosen as Romanelli's possible replacement in the hospital of the Bagno.[127] In his capacity as a galley physician, Bonomo was engaged in the forms of medical practice we encountered above. Together with Cestoni, he also participated in the observation of captives' health-related practices. Cestoni regularly exchanged information with enslaved individuals, from whom he gathered information and specimens related to the natural and medical knowledge, practices, and products of the Muslim Mediterranean world. In Livorno, he engaged in the observation of how both 'women' and the Bagno's enslaved individuals treated scabies and, on this basis, together with Bonomo, developed a new account of the ailment.

The story is well known, though it has not been considered in the context of the health-related exchanges that took place in and around the Bagno, where scabies was

119. AAV, Misc., Armadio IV, 54, fol. 67ʳ.
120. Zacchia, *Quaestiones*, III, pp. 149–170.
121. Savelli *Pratica universale*, pp. 186–87.
122. Ibid., p. 187.
123. ASFi, MP, 2099, fols 998ʳ and 1000ʳ.
124. See Generali, 'Uno speziale'; Tanga, 'Giacinto Cestoni'; Dal Prete, 'Ingenuous Investigators'.
125. Redi, *Opere*, vol. 2, pp. 83–85; Redi, *Lettere*, vol. 2, p. 390.
126. ASFi, MP, 2099, Letter of Lepido Petrocci, 22 May 1684.
127. ASFi, MP, 2101, Letters of Lepido Petrocci, 10 and 15 May 1690.

widespread.[128] In keeping with the humoral tradition, some maintained that scabies was the result of melancholic humors related to an excess of black bile and had to be cured accordingly. Others suggested that it was caused by poisonous blood and irritating salts. Regardless, it had to be cured through internal remedies. However, Cestoni and Bonomo came up with a different idea altogether. In particular, Cestoni had frequently observed that 'women and their children with scabies' used a pin to pull small bubbles in their early stages out of the scabby skin and cracked them with their nails. He also noticed that in Livorno's Bagno enslaved individuals with scabies did the same 'with charitable reciprocity'.[129] Cestoni and Bonomo decided then to interview and test individuals who suffered from scabies and established that the fluid contained in their skin's small bubbles was the cause of their itching. As they observed this fluid under the microscope, they saw very small animals ('*pellicelli*' or '*bacarelli*'). After repeating the experiment numerous times, they concluded that scabies was caused by these small animals rather than by internal bodily factors. Accordingly, the cure of scabies had to focus on external medicaments such as washings and ointments based on corrosives substances like salts, mercury, and sulphur, rather than internal medicaments such as syrups, medicines, bloodletting, and 'other innumerable cheats usually prescribed by all professors in these cases, to no avail'.[130]

Cestoni successfully tried the treatment on himself and wrote to his friend and correspondent, the physician and naturalist Antonio Vallisneri (1661–1730), that 'many internal medicaments to be taken by mouth administered by physicians to individuals with scabies are of no use'.[131] On 20 June 1687, Bonomo wrote about these findings to Redi. Although Redi held a humoral view of the ailment, he published a revised version of the letter and helped to circulate the text among savants, though he softened Bonomo's criticism of professors' use of internal remedies.[132] Over the following months, Cestoni's and Bonomo's proposal triggered medical attention. On 29 July 1687, the anatomist Lorenzo Bellini (1643–1704) wrote to the famous physician Marcello Malpighi (1628–1694) that he had visited Cestoni in Livorno and learnt about his observations on the *bachi* of scabies, which he thought would be of some use for medical practice and theory.[133] However, when Bonomo sent the letter to the renowned physician and papal archiater Giovanni Maria Lancisi (1654 –1720), hoping that he would promote it in Rome, the Roman physician dismissed Bonomo's and Cestoni's suggestion and highlighted that it was based on experiments carried out only for one year, which could not counteract those made for many centuries.[134]

While Cestoni's and Bonomo's insights were dismissed by Lancisi, they found better reception among Antonio Cocchi, Antonio Vallisneri, and Giuseppe del Papa, who succeeded Redi as court physician in Florence after this latter's passing.[135] They were also adopted by galley physicians like Romano Romanelli, who, having formerly treated scabies patients with purges, in 1716 referred to the *pellicelli* in his account of scabies in the Bagno and used sulphur to treat it.[136] The Bagno came then to be identified as the venue where the new 'external' treatment of scabies was carried out (see the caption in fig. 5). In fact, well before the unfolding of these events, in the early seventeenth century a (former) captive of the Bagno, 'Isuf' from Tunis, had already cured scabies with an ointment, namely, an external remedy.[137] Discussing this case in further detail would go beyond the scope of this essay. Yet, it is worth noting that the episode involving Cestoni and Bonomo sheds light on the appropriation and re-elaboration of a vernacular practice into an experimental pursuit leading to a re-conceptualization of the ailment and new treatment. In this sense, it highlights a case of a special relationship between medical practice and medical theory in a setting marked by proximity to large numbers of enslaved individuals and systematic observation of both their bodies and their practices. As in other cases of

128. See, for instance, Generali, 'Uno speziale', pp. 101–04; Tanga, 'Giacinto Cestoni', pp. 84–115.
129. Letter of Giovanni Cosimo Bonomo to Francesco Redi of 20 June 1687, in *Scienziati*, ed. by Altieri Biagi and Basile, p. 715.
130. Ibid., pp. 715–20 (citation p. 720).
131. Cestoni, *Epistolario*, vol. 2, pp. 558–63 (citation p. 560).
132. Redi, *Osservazioni*, pp. 7–8. See also Tanga, 'Giacinto Cestoni', pp. 87–98.
133. Malpighi, *The Correspondence*, III, p. 1285.
134. 'Dissertazione apologetica', p. 12.
135. Cocchi, *Dei bagni di Pisa*, II, pp. 170–71.
136. ASFi, MP, 2102, Letter of Lepido Petrocci, 13 April 1693; ASFi, MP, 2110, Note of Romano Romanelli of 3 March 1716 [i.e., 1717].
137. ASDP, Inquisizione, 5, fol. 410^{v}; also cited in Santus, *Il 'Turco'*, p. 180n133. On 'Isuf' from Tunis, see Santus, *Il 'Turco'*, pp. 62–79.

encounter between vernacular and institutional cultures, here a vernacular practice was transformed into an articulated language of experiment that informed new medical claims. Notably, this happened in a context in which Livorno's enslaved population cured scabies and prompted interest in new approaches to it while becoming the subject of further observation and medical intervention.

CONCLUSION

Exploring the entanglements of medicine and galley slavery in Livorno brings into focus the relationship between medical practice and medical theory in a situation characterized by the convergence of violence and health management. As the foregoing account shows, medicine was central to the Tuscan slave economy. Galley slavery, in particular, demanded special medical attention. A pervasive and composite medical apparatus was then deployed to attend to the bodies of enslaved individuals from the time of their inception until after their death. In this situation, medical practitioners were called to maintain and support the institution of slavery by observing, inspecting, treating, and controlling large numbers of individuals coerced to live and labor in extreme conditions.

The fragmented nature of the slavery archive makes it hard to delve into all the details of the entangled relationship between medicine and galley slavery. But even a bird's-eye view like the one presented in this essay can add to our understanding of some of the dynamics of medical practice and medical theory in the early modern Italian lands. Notably, the period of galley slavery in Tuscany coincides with what the historiography has traditionally singled out as a time of change related to the development of new views of the body. Historians have appropriately highlighted the persistence of humoral-inspired practice in this context of change. Drawing attention to galley slavery as a special site of medical intervention can help us appreciate in turn how medical practice participated in shifting approaches to bodies and their ills. As we have seen, galley medical practitioners reflected traditional medical hierarchies and roles, and relied on the principles of humoral practice—such as diet and medicaments—in the care of unfree rowers. Yet, the hazards of galley labor also encouraged physicians to develop surgical skills. Moreover, galley medical practice required attending to numerous individuals who shared extreme living and labor conditions that impaired their health. At a time in which environmental circumstances were deemed instrumental to the health of groups, the Bagno and its hospital materialized a medical setting that catered to unfree rowers by engaging in the control and management of the non-naturals to maintain and restore their health. Its medical practitioners further engaged in the regular inspection of the bodies of both the living and the dead, as well as in the observation of captives' healing practices, to investigate the ailments that collectively affected them and identify appropriate remedies. As we trace their pursuits, we turn our attention to sites of medical practice often overlooked by the historiography of early modern medicine in Italy: vessels, slavery, and coasts. We are further led to interrogate the relationship between medical practice and medical theory in the context of the interconnected political economy of control, coercion, and care that governed health management in this setting.

WORKS CITED

Printed Primary Sources

Cestoni, Giacinto, *Epistolario ad Antonio Vallisneri*, ed. by S. Baglioni, 2 vols (Rome: Reale Accademia d'Italia, 1940–1941), II (1941).

Cocchi, Antonio, *Dei bagni di Pisa, trattato di Antonio Cocchi*, in *Opere di Antonio Cocchi*, 3 vols (Milan: Società Tipogr. De' Classici italiani, 1824), II (1824).

Davies, William, *A True Relation of the Travailes and Most Miserable Captiuitie of William Dauies, Barber-Surgion of London, under the Duke of Florence* (London: Nicholas Bourne, 1614).

'Dissertazione apologetica fra'l Sig.r Dr Gio: Cosimo Bonomo e il Sig.r Dr Gio: Maria Lancisi intorno a' vermi osservati nella Rogna', in *La polemica Bonomo-Lancisi sull' 'origine acarica della scabbia'* ed. by Ugo Faucci (Livorno: S. Belforte, 1937), pp. 3–22.

Malpighi, Marcello, *The Correspondence of Marcello Malpighi: 1684–1688*, ed. by Howard Bernhardt Adelmann, 5 vols. (Ithaca, N.Y.: Cornell University Press, 1975), III.

Martini, Georg Christoph, *Viaggio in Toscana (1725-1745)*, trans. by Oscar Trumpy (Massa: Palazzo di S. Elisabetta and Modena: Aedes Muratoriana, 1969).

Pantera, Pantero, *L'armata navale, del capitan Pantero Pantera* (Rome: Egidio Spada, 1614).

Redi, Francesco, *Lettere di Francesco Redi patrizio Aretino*, 2nd edn, 3 vols (Florence: Gaetano Cambiagi, 1779), II (1779).

Redi, Francesco, *Opere di Francesco Redi*, 3 vols (Venice: Gio. Gabbriello Ertz, 1712), II (1712).

Redi, Francesco, *Osservazioni intorno a' pellicelli del corpo umano fatte dal Dottor Gio: Cosimo Bonomo, e da lui con altre osservazioni scritte in una lettera all'illustriss. Sig. Francesco Redi* (Florence: Piero Matini, 1687).
Savelli, Marc'Antonio, *Pratica universale*, 2nd edn (Florence: Vincenzo Vangelisti Stampatore Arcivescovile, 1681).
Scienziati del Seicento, ed. by Maria Luisa Altieri Biagi and Bruno Basile (Milan: Ricciardi, 1980), pp. 713–20 (Letter of Giovanni Cosimo Bonomo to Francesco Redi of 20 June 1687).
Statuti, e costituzioni dell'Ordine de' Cavalieri di Santo Stefano (Florence: Giunti, 1577).
Vasari, Giorgio (il Giovane), *La città ideale: Piante di chiese (palazzi e ville) di Toscana e d'Italia*, ed. by Virginia Stefanelli (Rome: Officina, 1970).
Zacchia, Paolo, *Quaestiones medico-legales: In quibus eae materiae medicae, quae ad legales facultates videntur pertinere, proponuntur, pertractantur, resolvuntur*, 3rd edn (Amsterdam: J. Blaeu, 1651).

Secondary Sources

Agostini, Anna, *Istantanee dal Seicento. L'album di disegni del cavaliere pistoiese Ignazio Fabroni* (Florence: Edizioni Polistampa, 2017).
Angiolini, Franco, 'Slaves and Slavery in the Early Modern Tuscany (1500-1700)', *Italian History and Culture*, 3 (1997), pp. 67–82.
Angiolini, Franco, *I cavalieri e il principe. L'Ordine di Santo Stefano e la società toscana in età moderna* (Florence: Edifir, 1996).
Atkinson, Esther, 'Anomalous Bodies: Representations of Deformities in Children in Britain, 1740–1790' (unpublished doctoral thesis, University of Toronto, 2021).
Barker, Hannah, *That Most Precious Merchandise. The Mediterranean Trade in Black Sea Slaves, 1260-1500* (Philadelphia: University of Pennsylvania Press, 2019).
Bartels, Victoria, 'Prisoners for War: Convicts, Slaves, and the Culture of Forced Labour in Sixteenth-Century Tuscany', in *Shadow Agents of Renaissance War: Suffering, Supporting, and Supplying Conflict in Italy and Beyond*, ed. by Stephen Bowd, Sarah Cockram, and John Gagné (Amsterdam: Amsterdam University Press, 2023), pp. 71–93.
Blumenthal, Debra, *Enemies and Familiars: Slavery and Mastery in Fifteenth-Century Valencia* (Ithaca, N.Y.: Cornell University Press, 2009).
Blumenthal, Debra, 'Domestic Medicine: Slaves, Servants and Female Medical Expertise in Late Medieval Valencia', *Renaissance Studies*, 28.4 (2014), pp. 515–32.
Bonazza, Giulia, *Abolitionism and the Persistence of Slavery in Italian States, 1750–1850* (Cham, Switzerland: Palgrave Macmillan, 2019).
Bonazza, Giulia, 'Collective and Individual Experiences of Slaves in Leghorn, Pisa and Florence, 1702-1826', *Esclavages & Post-esclavages*, 8 (2023), http://journals.openedition.org/slaveries / 8676.
Bono, Salvatore, *Schiavi musulmani nell'Italia moderna. Galeotti, vu' cumprà, domestici* (Naples: Edizione Scientifiche Italiane, 1999).
Bono, Salvatore, *Schiavi: Una storia mediterranea (XVI–XIX secolo)* (Bologna: Il Mulino, 2016).
Brege, Brian, *Tuscany in the Age of Empire* (Cambridge, MA: Harvard University, 2021).
Calafat, Guillaume and Cesare Santus, 'Les avatars du "Turc". Esclaves et commerçants musulmans à Toscane (1600-1750)', in *Les Musulmans dans l'histoire de l'Europe. I. Une intégration invisible*, ed. by Jocelyne Dakhlia and Bernard Vincent (Paris: Albin Michel, 2011), pp. 471–522.
Carmichael, Ann, 'Contagion Theory and Contagion Practice in Fifteenth-Century Milan', *Renaissance Quarterly*, 44.2 (1991), pp. 213–56.
Cavallo, Sandra, 'Health, Air and Material Culture in the Early Modern Italian Domestic Environment', *Social History of Medicine*, 29.4 (2016), pp. 695–716.
Cavallo, Sandra and Tessa Storey, *Healthy Living in Late Renaissance Italy* (Oxford: Oxford University Press, 2014).
Chizzolini, Benedetta, 'Medicare, osservare, controllare: medici e galeotti a Livorno Tra XVI–XVIII secolo', in *Un mare connesso. Europa e mondo islamico nel Mediterraneo (secoli XV–XIX)*, ed. by Jake Dyble, Alessandro Lo Bartolo, and Elia Morelli (Rome: Carocci, 2024), pp. 71–91.
Cohn, Samuel K., Jr., *Cultures of Plague: Medical Thinking at the End of the Renaissance* (Oxford: Oxford University Press, 2009).
Conserving Health in Early Modern Culture: Bodies and Environments in Italy and England ed. by Sandra Cavallo and Tessa Storey (Manchester, UK: Manchester University Press, 2017).
Cooper Owens, Deirdre *Medical Bondage: Race, Gender, and the Origins of American Gynecology* (Athens: The University of Georgia Press, 2017).
Corsini, Andrea, 'Il servizio sanitario nella marina toscana', *Annali di medicina navale e coloniale,* 23 (1917), I, pp. 282–321, 438–84 and II, pp. 652–78, pp. 789–838.
Dal Prete, Ivano, 'Ingenuous Investigators: Antonio Vallisneri's Regional Network and the Making of Natural Knowledge in Eighteenth-Century Italy', in *Empires of Knowledge: Scientific Networks in the Early Modern World*, ed. by Paula Findlen (London: Routledge, 2018), pp. 181–204.
Daston, Lorraine, 'The Empire of Observation, 1600-1800', in *Histories of Scientific Observation*, ed. by Lorraine Daston and Elizabeth Lunbeck (Chicago, IL: University of Chicago Press, 2011), pp. 81–113.

De Renzi, Silvia, 'Seats and Series: Dissecting Diseases in the Seventeenth Century', in *Pathology in Practice: Diseases and Dissections in Early Modern Europe*, ed. by Silvia De Renzi, Marco Bresadola, and Maria Conforti (London and New York: Routledge, 2018), pp. 96–115.

Donato, Maria Pia, 'The Afterlife of the Non-Naturals in Early Eighteenth-Century Hippocratism: from the Healthy Individual to a Healthy Population', in *Conserving Health in Early Modern Culture: Bodies and Environments in Italy and England* ed. by Sandra Cavallo and Tessa Storey (Manchester, UK: Manchester University Press, 2017), pp. 158–82.

Dugan, Holly, *The Ephemeral History of Perfume: Scent and Sense in Early Modern England* (Baltimore, MD: Johns Hopkins University Press, 2011).

Emch–Dériaz, Antoinette, 'The Non-Naturals Made Easy', *The Popularisation of Medicine, 1650—1850* ed. by Roy Porter (London: Routledge, 1992), pp. 134–59.

Errico, Clara and Michele Montanelli, *La biscotteria* (Livorno: CTL, 2019).

Errico, Clara and Michele Montanelli, *Il bagno degli schiavi e dei forzati* (Livorno: CTL, 2019).

Fancy, Nahyan, 'Anatomy', in *1001 Cures: Contributions in Medicine & Healthcare from Muslim Civilisation*, ed. by Peter E. Pormann (Manchester, UK: Foundation for Science Technology and Civilisation, 2018), pp. 42–51.

Ferragud, Carmel, 'The Role of Doctors in the Slave Trade during the Fourteenth and Fifteenth Centuries within the Kingdom of Valencia (Crown of Aragon)', *Bulletin of the History of Medicine*, 87.2 (2013), pp. 143–69.

Fett, Sharla M., *Working Cures: Healing, Health, and Power on Southern Slave Plantations* (Chapel Hill: The University of North Carolina Press, 2002).

Fiume, Giovanna, *Schiavitù mediterranee: Corsari, rinnegati e santi di età moderna* (Milan: Bruno Mondadori, 2009).

Fogu, Claudio, *The Fishing Net and The Spider Web: Mediterranean Imaginaries and the Making of Italians* (Cham: Palgrave Macmillan, 2020).

Frattarelli Fischer, Lucia, 'Il bagno delle galere in "terra cristiana". Schiavi a Livorno fra Cinque e Seicento', *Nuovi Studi Livornesi*, 8 (2000), pp. 69–94.

Frattarelli Fischer, Lucia, *L'Arcano del mare. Un porto nella prima età globale* (Pisa: Pacini, 2018).

García-Ballester, Luis, 'On the Origin of the "Six Non-Natural Things" in Galen', in *Galen und das hellenistische Erbe*, ed. by Jutta Kollesch and Diethard Nickel (Stuttgart: Franz Steiner Verlag, 1993), pp. 105–15.

Geltner, Guy and Janna Coomans, 'The Healthscaping Approach: Toward a Global History of Early Public Health', *Historical Methods: A Journal of Quantitative and Interdisciplinary History*, 56.1 (2023), pp. 18–33.

Generali, Dario, 'Uno speziale che "superava la sua condizione". Il caso dell'invisibilità postuma di Diacinto Cestoni', in *Figure dell'invisibilità: le scienze della vita nell'Italia d'antico regime: atti delle giornate di studio, Milano-Ginevra, novembre 2002—giugno 2003*, ed. by Maria Teresa Monti and Marc J. Ratcliff (Florence: Olschki, 2004), pp. 83–118.

Guarnieri, Gino, *I Cavalieri di Santo Stefano nella storia della Marina italiana, 1562–1859* (Pisa: Nistri-Lischi, 1960).

Henderson, John, *The Renaissance Hospital: Healing the Body and Healing the Soul* (New Haven, Conn.: Yale University Press, 2006).

Henderson, John, *Florence Under Siege: Surviving Plague in an Early Modern City* (New Haven, Conn.: Yale University Press, 2019).

Hershenzon, Daniel, *The Captive Sea: Slavery, Communication, and Commerce in Early Modern Spain and the Mediterranean* (Philadelphia: University of Pennsylvania Press, 2018).

Herzig, Tamar, 'Slavery and Interethnic Sexual Violence: A Multiple Perpetrator Rape in Seventeenth-Century Livorno', *American Historical Review*, 127.1 (2022), pp. 194–222.

Herzig, Tamar, 'Enslavement, Religion, and Cultural Commemoration in Livorno', *Religions*, Special Issue 'Rethinking Catholicism in Early Modern Italy: Gender, Space, Mobility' ed. by Diego Pirillo and John Christopoulos, 14.5 (2013), 607, https://doi.org/10.3390/rel14050607.

Historia: Empiricism and Erudition in Early Modern Europe, ed. by Gianna Pomata and Nancy G. Siraisi (Cambridge, MA: MIT Press, 2005).

Horden, Peregrine, 'A Non-Natural Environment: Medicine without Doctors and the Medieval European Hospital', in *The Medieval Hospital and Medical Practice*, ed. by Barbara S. Bowers (Aldershot: Ashgate, 2007), pp. 133–45.

Imagining Contagion in Early Modern Europe, ed. by Claire L. Carlin (Basingstoke: Palgrave Macmillan, 2005).

Inì, Marina, 'Materiality, Quarantine and Contagion in the Early Modern Mediterranean', *Social History of Medicine*, 34.4 (2021), pp. 1161–84.

Liboni, Gionata, 'Humanist Post-mortems: Philology and Therapy', in *Pathology in Practice: Diseases and Dissections in Early Modern Europe*, ed. by Silvia De Renzi, Marco Bresadola, and Maria Conforti (London and New York: Routledge, 2018), pp. 20–38.

Lifestyle and Medicine in the Enlightenment: The Six Non-Naturals in the Long Eighteenth Century, ed. by James Kennaway and Rina Knoeff (New York: Routledge, 2020).

Lo Basso, Luca, *Uomini da remo. Galee e galeotti del Mediterraneo in età moderna* (Milan: Selene, 2003).

Martin, Meredith and Gillian Weiss, *The Sun King at Sea: Maritime Art and Galley Slavery in Louis XIV's France* (Los Angeles: Getty Research Institute, 2022).

Matar, Nabil, *Mediterranean Captivity through Arab Eyes, 1517–1798* (Leiden: Brill, 2021).

McVaugh, Michael R., 'Smells and the Medieval Surgeon', *Micrologus: Nature, Sciences and Medieval Societies*, 10 (2002), pp. 113–32.

Murphy, Hannah, 'Re-Writing Race in Early Modern European Medicine', *History Compass*, 19.11 (2021), e12692, https://doi.org/10.1111/hic3.12692.

Mustakeem, Sowande M., *Slavery at Sea: Terror, Sex, and Sickness in the Middle Passage* (Urbana: University of Illinois Press, 2016).

Nadalo, Stephanie, 'Negotiating Slavery in a Tolerant Frontier: Livorno's Turkish Bagno (1547–1747)', *Mediaevalia*, 32.1 (2011), pp. 275–324.

Neri, Algerina, *Uno schiavo inglese nella Livorno dei Medici* (Pisa: ETS, 2000).

Niebyl, Peter H., 'The Non–Naturals', *Bulletin of the History of Medicine*, 45.5 (1971), pp. 486–92.

Ostrow, Steven F., 'Pietro Tacca and his "Quattro Mori": The Beauty and Identity of the Slaves', *Artibus et Historiae*, 36.71 (2015), pp. 145–80.

Palmer, Richard, 'In Bad Odour: Smell and Its Significance in Medicine from Antiquity to the Seventeenth Century', in *Medicine and the Five Senses* ed. by W. F. Bynum and Roy Porter (Cambridge, UK: Cambridge University Press, 1993), pp. 61–68.

Pampalone, Antonella, 'Pier Leone Ghezzi pittore della flotta navale pontificia e altri documenti sulla sua attività per la camera apostolica', *Annali della Pontificia insigne Accademia di Belle Arti e Lettere dei Virtuosi al Pantheon*, 15 (2015), pp. 147–99.

Park, Katharine, *Secrets of Women: Gender, Generation, and the Origins of Human Dissection* (New York: Zone Books, 2006).

Pathology in Practice: Diseases and Dissections in Early Modern Europe, ed. by Silvia De Renzi, Marco Bresadola, and Maria Conforti (London and New York: Routledge, 2018).

Paugh, Katherine, *The Politics of Reproduction. Race, Medicine, and Fertility in the Age of Abolition* (Oxford: Oxford University Press, 2017).

Pomata, Gianna, 'Sharing Cases: The Observationes in Early Modern Medicine', *Early Science and Medicine*, 15.3 (2010), pp. 193–236.

Pomata, Gianna, 'Observation Rising: Birth of an Epistemic Genre, 1500–1650', in *Histories of Scientific Observation*, ed. by Lorraine Daston and Elizabeth Lunbeck (Chicago, IL: University of Chicago Press, 2011), pp. 45–80.

Pomini, Marco, 'Image Making on a Precarious Border: Ignazio Fabroni's Drawings in the Galley (1664–1688)', unpublished essay.

Poole-Jones, Katherine, 'The Medici, Maritime Empire, and the Enduring Legacy of the Cavalieri di Santo Stefano', in *Florence in the Early Modern World: New Perspectives*, ed. by Nicholas Scott Baker and Brian Jeffrey Maxson (London: Routledge, 2020), pp. 156–86.

Rawcliffe, Carole '"Delectable Sightes and Fragrant Smelles": Gardens and Health in Late Medieval and Early Modern England', *Garden History*, 36.1 (2008), pp. 3–21.

Roberts, Carolyn Elizabeth, 'To Heal and to Harm: Medicine, Knowledge, and Power in the Atlantic Slave Trade' (unpublished doctoral thesis, Harvard University, 2017).

Rombough, Julia, 'Air Quality and the Senses in Early Modern Italy', *Renaissance and Reformation / Renaissance et Réforme*, 44.2 (2021), pp. 39–60.

Rosen, Mark, 'Pietro Tacca's *Quattro Mori* and the Conditions of Slavery in Early Seicento Tuscany', *The Art Bulletin*, 97.1 (2015), pp. 34–57.

Salvadorini, Vittorio, 'Traffici con i paesi islamici e schiavi a Livorno nel XVII secolo: problemi e suggestioni', in *Atti del convengo Livorno e il Mediterraneo nell'età medicea* (Livorno: Bastogi, 1978), pp. 206–55.

Santus, Cesare, *Il 'Turco' a Livorno. Incontri con l'Islam nella Toscana del Seicento* (Milan: Officina Libraria, 2019).

Savitt, Todd L., *Medicine and Slavery: The Diseases and Health Care of Blacks in Antebellum Virginia* (Urbana: University of Illinois Press, 1978).

Schiebinger, Londa, *Secret Cures of Slaves: People, Plants, and Medicine in the Eighteenth-Century Atlantic World* (Stanford: Stanford University Press, 2017).

Shefer Mossensohn, Miri, 'Medical Treatment in the Ottoman Navy in the Early Modern Period', *Journal of the Economic and Social History of the Orient*, 50.4 (2007), pp. 542–68.

Silva, Joseph M., '"To the Victor Go the Spoils": Christian Triumphalism, Cosimo I de' Medici, and the Order of Santo Stefano in Pisa', in *Art, Mobility, and Exchange in Early Modern Tuscany and Eurasia*, ed. by Francesco Freddolini and Marco Musillo (New York: Routledge, 2020), pp. 33–47.

Tanga, Mario, 'Giacinto Cestoni, i rapporti con Redi e le scienze della vita nel XVII secolo' (unpublished doctoral thesis, University of Pisa, 2006).

Terpstra, Nicholas, 'Found and Lost: Race, Demography, and Reason of State in Early Modern Foundling Care', in *Lost and Found: Locating Foundlings in the Early Modern World*, ed. by Nicholas Terpstra (Florence: I Tatti—The Harvard University Center for Italian Renaissance Studies / Rome: Officina Libraria, 2023), pp. 315–38.

Toaff, Renzo, 'Schiavitù e schiavi nella Nazione Ebrea di Livorno nel Sei e Settecento', *La Rassegna Mensile di Israel*, 51.1 (1985), pp. 82–95.

Toaff, Renzo, *La Nazione Ebrea a Livorno e a Pisa (1591–1700)* (Florence: Olschki, 1990).

Tommasino, Pier Mattia, 'Bulghaith al-Darawi and Barthélemy d'Herbelot: Readers of the Qur'an in Seventeenth-Century Tuscany', *Journal of Qur'anic Studies*, 20.3 (2018), pp. 94–120.

Turner, Sasha, *Contested Bodies: Pregnancy, Childrearing, and Slavery in Jamaica* (Philadelphia: University of Pennsylvania Press, 2017).

Wilbourne, Emily, *Voice, Slavery, and Race in Seventeenth-Century Florence* (New York: Oxford University Press, 2023).

5

Bodies and Stones in Michele Mercati's *Metallotheca.*

The Study of Nature and the Practice of Medicine in Late-Sixteenth Century Rome[*]

Elisa Andretta

The coronation of Cosimo de' Medici as Grand Duke of Tuscany, which took place on 5 March 1570 in Rome at the hands of Pope Pius V, was a political event that aroused bitter resistance from various European powers. It was also the moment when the pontiff's health, already precarious, deteriorated sharply, greatly worrying his doctors and entourage.[1] A strong catarrh, which the physicians attributed to the cold that Pius V had stoically endured to officiate at the entire ceremony, was added to a urinary ailment that had been tormenting the pontiff for some time.[2] While the Pope's health was at its lowest, bitter controversies developed between the different medical views of the professionals at his bedside.

In the context of the health crisis of March 1570, the papal entourage began to negotiate the arrival in the city of Michele Mercati, a Tuscan doctor trained at the University of Pisa and very close to the Medici court, who had probably come to Rome with Cosimo to assist him in the important event.[3] Mercati accepted the assignment of papal doctor and in October 1570, his name was registered in the list of the members of the Apostolic family.[4] Much appreciated by the pontiff and his entourage, he treated Pius V until his death in the spring of 1572. But, unusually for the papal court, the death of the Pope did not put an end to Mercati's time at the Vatican.[5] He was appointed personal physician to the new Pope Gregory XIII, overseeing the Pope's health until his fatal illness in 1585. He was present at the Pope's final moments, following which suspicions and grievances arose against him. He defended himself from these accusations with a report in which he described his work during the last hours of Gregory XIII's life and analyzed the fatal symptoms of his illness.[6]

Mercati was an experienced practitioner. He spent more than twenty years in Rome, remaining until his death in 1593, during which time he also treated Sixtus V and Clement VIII, though he did not limit himself to working as papal physician. He also cared for several members of the Apostolic Family, princes and lords passing through Rome.[7] He practised outside the Vatican and the papal sphere. Bound to Philip Neri by a deep devotion, he continuously served as a doctor at the Oratory, treating several brothers and supervising the medical examinations to which aspiring Oratorians were subjected.[8]

The practice of medicine, however intense, was far from being Mercati's only activity. Besides serving as the court physician, he quickly took on the role of *semplicista* (expert in simples). He was in charge of two important 'sites of

---

* Many thanks to Sandra Cavallo and John Henderson for their insightful and stimulating analysis of this text.

1. Marengo, 'De Pii V. Pont. Max morbo'.
2. Ortroy, 'Le Pape Saint Pie V', pp. 200–207.
3. On Michele Mercati, see Accordi, 'Michele Mercati'; Andretta, 'Mercati, Michele'.
4. BAV, *Ruoli*, 64, 6.
5. Palmer, 'Medicine at the Papal Court'.
6. Michele Mercati, 'Relatione della morte di Papa Gregorio XIII fatta dal Signor Michele Mercati medico di Sua Santità', AAV, Misc. Arm. II, 145, 90^r–91^v.
7. Mercati, *Metallotheca*, p. XXXVIII.
8. Touber, *Law, Medicine and Engineering*, pp. 175–178, 257–258, 265–267, 272–276, 278–279; Tomassetti, *Cura corporum, ad indicem*.

knowledge'[9] that flourished within the Vatican space: the botanical garden, which had been established in a portion of land of the Giardini del Belvedere during the 15th century, and had recently begun to receive more attention;[10] and the *Metallotheca Vaticana*, a collection of stones, earths, metals and minerals, which he himself conceived and assembled.[11] From these two spaces, he also developed a publishing programme that he described in a letter addressed to the Nuremberg physician Joachim Camerarius II. It included two ambitious works dedicated to the natural world and its therapeutic qualities, one devoted to plants and the other to the mineral world.[12] But, at the end of Mercati's life, this programme still lay largely unpublished. Apart from two works celebrating the Egyptian obelisks erected by Sixtus V on Rome's main squares, in his lifetime Mercati only published a collection of short treatises that he had written at the request of various lords and addressed to Giacomo Boncompagni, one of the prominent figures at the court of Gregory XIII.[13] The central treatise contained 'instructions' on the plague, a work the physician had composed several years prior. In 1576, when a severe threat of plague loomed over the city of Rome, Mercati decided to make it accessible by having it printed in Italian translation. On this occasion, he included three additional *Instruttioni*, all in the vernacular. The second treatise, originally written for Cosimo de' Medici, was dedicated to poisons. The last two were devoted to gout and various forms of paralysis, respectively. These four texts were distinctly practical in nature. After a theoretical section dedicated to defining and explaining the causes of the respective diseases and the phenomenon of poisoning, they reviewed a series of preventive and curative remedies combining diet and pharmacopeia.

Regrettably, Mercati did not manage to publish the two treatises dedicated to the plant and mineral realms mentioned in the letter to Camerarius. There is no surviving evidence of the first, although he invested considerable time and effort in the second, entitled *Metallotheca*, the same name as his collection, and by his death he had written a substantial portion of it. Moreover, he had overseen the creation of an extensive set of illustrations intended to accompany his work. It was only in 1717, thanks to the determination of another papal physician, Giovanni Maria Lancisi, that the part of the *Metallotheca* that Mercati had completed during his lifetime and the engravings were published.[14]

In the letter to the reader that opened the *Metallotheca*, Mercati explained the general plan of the work, the method followed and his epistemological and narrative choices. Using a suggestive comparison with the creation of the world, he observed it necessary to dwell first on 'individual things' and then on their origin.[15]

He then moved into the plan of the initial work and the substantial changes he had made to it:

> Since I wanted to explain the entire history of fossils, stones and the different types of earth, I decided to divide the entire work into two parts. The first part brings together all the things of the same type, the universal parts and the different things related to each of these types. It also deals with their similarities and differences according to their faculties, dignities and known signs. In the other part, the one I have deemed worthy of publication so far, I examine things individually in as much detail as possible. I do not refrain here from translating the similarities between some of them, nor their differences, but here these same things that were previously considered in general are treated individually.[16]

Mercati's work on the third kingdom was thus initially conceived as a diptych consisting of a general exposition and an analysis that, while not entirely excluding a theoretical dimension based on comparisons, took its cue from 'things' in their individuality. In the process of

9. *Lieux de savoir*.
10. On the Vatican botanical garden, see Campitelli, *Gli horti dei Papi*, pp. 84–106.
11. Cooper, 'The Museum and the Book'.
12. Universitätsbibliothek Erlangen-Nürnberg, H62/trewbr Mercatus_Michael, 1, 1ᵛ.
13. Mercati, *Instruttione*.
14. Mercati, *Metallotheca*. The manuscript is in BAV, *Vat. Lat.*, 7211.
15. Ibid., p. LIV.
16. 'Omnem hanc, amice Lector, fossilium, lapidum, variorum terrae generum, iisque similium historiam, cum explicare constituissem; in duas Partes universum Opus dividere constitui, quarum alter ipsa rerum genera, generibusque subjectas partes universe complecteretur, & quae inter ipsas similitudo sit, quid inter se differant, natura, facultate, dignitate, notis, ac signis exponeret ; altera vero, quam nunc in lucem mihi edendam esse putavi, singularis res distincte (quantum ipse potuit) pretactaret.' Ibid.: *'Benevolo Lectori'*.

developing the work, the second part had become increasingly important, to the point of deciding to print it first, reversing the initial order of publication. No trace remains of the first part of the *Metallotheca* in which things were to be 'considered in general'. We do not even know whether Mercati had actually begun to write it.

The passage shows his conviction that the work on 'particular things' was the most successful and the one that most urgently needed to be made available to the scholarly community.[17]

Although they had very different aims, Mercati's collection of *Instruttioni* and the *Metallotheca*, allow us to examine the relationships between the theoretical study of nature, empirical research practices and concrete applications of the knowledge acquired.

In this chapter, I will examine how for Mercati the care of bodies and the study of nature interacted with each other, analyzing these two treatises and other sources documenting his activities.

I will first delve into Mercati's keen theoretical interest in the mineral world and the significance he attributed to it in relation to practice. Next, I will concentrate on his collection of inanimate natural objects at the pontifical court, examining its various functions, particularly its potential role within the court's healthcare organization. I will then turn my attention to some of the epistemological choices Mercati made when he decided that recording the knowledge he had accumulated should be an integral part of his work as a collector of nature, choices that directly linked theoretical study and practical activity, in the exercise of medicine as in the investigation of nature. Finally, I will examine a specific case: that of bezoars. I will analyze how Mercati, through his museum and in his books, produced knowledge about these natural objects, which constituted prized ingredients in pharmacopeias, were increasingly sought after by the elite, and sparked extensive debates among physicians and naturalists.

FROM PLANTS TO MINERALS

It is likely that, in addition to his qualities as a practical physician, Mercati's commitment to the study of the natural world laid the groundwork for its integration into the pontifical court. This commitment allowed him the opportunity to reside in the Vatican for more than twenty years, resisting the pressure of the Roman political system which normally led to a radical change of offices and functions after the death of each pontiff.[18]

The Hortus was entrusted to Mercati a few months after his arrival in Rome, based on skills he had developed in previous years. He had developed an interest in the study of the natural world during his training in Pisa, where he was one of the first students of Andrea Cesalpino. He also benefited from the botanical garden established by Luca Ghini with the support of Cosimo de' Medici.[19] Alongside Cesalpino, he conducted explorations of the Tuscan hills and the island of Elba.[20] After moving to Rome, Mercati focused on expanding and organizing the gardens there. His exploration of the natural environment, conducted with papal support of finance and manpower, was undertaken primarily in the lands of the Papal State, but also in other territories of the peninsula.[21] This fieldwork, combined with repeated exchanges with some of the most famous naturalists of the time, such as Ulisse Aldrovandi, Ferrante Imperato and Joachim Camerarius II, as well as the possibilities offered by the Vatican's diplomatic networks, allowed him to bring together in the Vatican gardens rare plants from distant countries.[22]

The study of the plant world, however, was only a stage in Mercati's scientific journey, for he also studied inanimate things, 'metals, gems, stones and other things that emerge from the earth'.[23] The epistemological, but also political and religious reasons for this choice, are made explicit in the paratexts of the *Metallotheca*-book. Firstly, according to Mercati, the Ancients did not pay sufficient attention to this

17. Cooper, 'The Museum and the Book', p. 5. Mercati's focus on individual objects undoubtedly refers to a more general interest in material objects that characterizes the natural history of the early modern age, on which see *Early Modern Things* and *Natural Things*.
18. On the effects on medical and naturalistic activities of the Roman political specificities, see Donato, *Sudden Death*; Andretta, *Roma medica*; Brevaglieri, *Natural desiderio di sapere*.
19. *Giardino dei Semplici*.
20. Several references to this activity can be found in Mercati, *Metallotheca*, see in particular pp. 13, 17 and 164.
21. On the fieldwork of sixteenth-century naturalists, see Egmond, 'Into the Wild'.
22. Andretta, *Le monde sous l'oeil des médecins*, pp. 157–224.
23. '[...] *a natura vegetis, vividisque, a ea processit, quae minime vegeta, metalla, gemmae, lapides, & ejusmodi alia, e terra effodiuntur*', Mercati, *Metallotheca*, p. XLIX.

aspect of the natural world: while there were descriptions of earths, stones, or minerals, along with references to their therapeutic properties in the works of important authors such as Galen, Dioscorides, or Pliny, there was no systematic work comparable to those conducted on the plant or animal world. It is likely that Mercati had in mind Aristotle's *De animalibus* or Theophrastus's *De plantarum historia*. The fragmented and incomplete nature of ancient knowledge posed numerous problems, particularly in terms of nomenclature and identification, issues that persisted into his time.[24] Secondly, Mercati expressed some apprehension about the fact that the most important contemporary contributions came from the German world. On the one hand, his admiration for Georg Agricola did not prevent him from engaging in a sort of 'battle' of words concerning mineral resources of the Italic and Germanic world.[25] On the other hand, in spite of his in-depth knowledge of the work of the Calvinist physician Conrad Gessner and his correspondence with the Lutheran Camerarius, he bitterly observed that certain works that were fundamental for the study of the mineral world were unreadable because they were tainted with heresy. It's no coincidence that Mercati adopted this categorical stance in the dedication of the *Metallotheca* addressed to Pope Clement VIII.[26] Finally, he considered that this field of study was a priority, as the therapeutic potential of the resources of the earth was not being utilized properly, which from his perspective was particularly harmful. Given the value of many of these remedies, the primary victims of such misapplications were princes, sovereigns, and other lords. And the health of these rulers not only affected their own well-being, but also had implications for the well-being of their subjects.[27] This approach to inanimate objects as central components of pharmacopeias, whose use needed to be expanded, is particularly evident in Mercati's collection of *Instruttioni*. Here Malacca stones, Armenian bole, Samos earth, coconuts from the Indies or a deer heart bone, together with unicorn powder, rhinoceros corn powder, corals, finely ground emerald and other gems are regarded as therapeutic resources available to both doctors and patients, particularly in the treatment of plagues and poisonings.[28] They could be carried on one's person, set into jewelry, or placed inside fabric pouches worn under clothing. They could be ingested in powdered form, dissolved and diluted in wine, water, or herbal infusions. The therapeutic properties attributed to these objects by the physician are diverse. Precious stones, in particular, are mentioned for their preservative function. An entire section of Chapter VIII of the *Instruttione sopra la peste* (*Del modo di preservarsi dalla peste con il reggimento della vita*) is dedicated to 'jewels, and precious stones & other things to defend from the corrupt air'. Here, Mercati also seizes the opportunity to include a list of those that were 'useful at all times': 'the true hyacinth stone worn around the neck or on the finger, the diamond fastened to the left arm, the carbuncle known as ruby, the sapphire, and the Syrian garnet'.[29] He then adds 'that stone Agate, which is as transparent as glass, the Topaz, which is marvelously praised by a renowned practitioner of his time, the coral worn around the neck or on the chest, a sachet of sulphur enclosed in a taffeta pouch, placed so that it touches the flesh on the side of the heart', of which Nicolas Monardes, 'a physician from Seville, writes of having observed remarkable experiences among the attendants in hospitals, where there were many plague victims.'[30]

In the *Instruttione sopra i veleni,* stones are accorded multiple functions. They are part of those 'things that reveal the poison and that nature has not yet failed to produce in defence of man'.[31] Meticulously quoting Pietro Andrea Mattioli's commentaries on the 6th book of

24. Ibid., p. L.
25. Ibid., p. LI.
26. Ibid., p. L.
27. Ibid., p. LI.
28. Mercati, *Instruttione*, pp. 100–101.
29. 'Il Iacinto vero, portato al collo o in dito. Il Diamante legato in su'l braccio sinistro. Il Carbonchio chiamato Rubino. Il Zaffiro. Il Granato Soriano', Mercati, *Instruttione*, p. 44.
30. ' [...] quella pietra Achate, che è trasparente come vetro. Il Topazio [che] è lodato maravigliosamente da un pratico famosissimo de' suoi tempi [...]. Il Corallo portato al collo, o in seno [...]. Un sacchetto di solimato rinchiuso in un sacchetto di taffettà, in modo che tocchi la carne dalla banda del core. Et il doctor Monardes medico di Siviglia, scrive di haverne visto bellissime sperienze in infermieri di spedali, dove erano molti appestati', ibid., pp. 44–45.
31. '[...] cose, che manifestano il veleno [che] la natura non ha mancato ancora, in difesa dell'huomo, [di] produrre', ibid., p. 93.

Dioscorides' *Materia Medica*,[32] he says that the Prassina stone (Plasma), the Bufone or Botta stone bound in a golden ring touching the flesh, the oriental diamond fastened to the left arm, as well as the Agate, Hyacinth, oriental Sapphire, Emerald, and the stone said to be found in the head of the Dragon, all break the potency of any poison.[33]

But gems, can also be dangerous poison carriers. Therefore, Mercati urges princes to be 'considerate and cautious in receiving gifts, such as unknown precious stones or other things that may, through hidden properties, affect the vital spirits.'[34] Endowed with potent qualities, the products from the subterranean and mineral world, therefore, had to be approached and handled with circumspection and expertise.

Mercati's commitment to building a reliable, correct and as comprehensive knowledge as possible about the mineral world, which was also capable of guiding medical practice, was two-sided. First, taking advantage of the many resources offered by his position as papal doctor, he assembled a collection unprecedented in its thematic scope. In the museums, cabinets, and collections of natural objects scattered across the Italian landscape, objects from the mineral world found their designated spaces, but the choice to dedicate an entire collection solely to these items was far from common.[35]

But, as we have seen, Mercati did not stop at this. While setting up his collection, the physician also worked on the treatise bearing the same name, *Metallotheca*. The book has many functions. Celebrating the sovereigns-pontiffs who had made possible the collection, it presented it to those who, far from Rome, could not visit it in person. But the book was also conceived by its author as a reference work on the mineral world that reviewed the fragmentary knowledge of the Ancients and encapsulated the new information he had accumulated both as a collector and as a physician.

As Lancisi pointed out at the beginning of the eighteenth century and as Alix Cooper suggested in a study on Mercati's two *Metallothecae*—the book and the museum—the physician understood the act of collecting objects and describing them in a treatise as complementary.[36] In the museum, as in his book, Mercati constructs a natural history of the subterranean natural world deeply intertwined with the value that the various categories of natural products could contribute to the preservation or restoration of human health. This history engages therapeutic practice and the understanding of the natural world in a meaningful dialogue. Let us first dwell on the collection of natural objects assembled by Mercati in the Vatican.

A 'MUSEUM OF MEDICINE'?

It is difficult to reconstruct the exact appearance of the *Metallotheca*-museum. At first, it was kept in a room of a building near the *Hortus*. During the pontificate of Gregory XIII, it was moved to one room in the Belvedere Palace,[37] the centre of the Vatican's architectural complex that also housed the Library and underwent significant transformations during Mercati's tenure. The indications found in Mercati's works[38] together with some other contemporary testimonies, reveal that the collection was open to visitors: doctors and scholars, Roman and non-Roman, students of the faculty of medicine of the *Studium urbis,* ambassadors and diplomatic agents, princes and sovereigns from different states, passed through the cabinets of the museum, under the expert guidance of Mercati.[39] The *Metallotheca* could also host technical and scientific demonstrations. It was here, in fact, that the engineer Camillo Agrippa presented to Gregory XIII the model of a device for lifting and moving the Egyptian obelisk that stood beside St. Peter's Basilica.[40]

32. Mattioli, *Il Dioscoride*. Book 6, although recognized as spurious, continued to be published with the rest of the *Materia medica* throughout the sixteenth century and remained a reference for physicians dealing with the issue of poison.
33. Mercati, *Instruttione*, p. 93.
34. '[...] considerati, e cauti nel ricevere presenti, come pietre pretiose non conosciute, o altre cose, che possono qualche volta per occulta proprietà risolvere li spiriti vitali', ibid., p. 93.
35. Lugli, *Naturalia et mirabilia* ; Falguière, *La chambre des merveilles*; *La licorne et le bézoard*.
36. Giovanni Maria Lancisi, 'In Metallotheca praefatio', in Mercati, *Metallotheca*, p. XV and Cooper, 'The Museum and the Book', pp. 1–8.
37. Accordi, 'Michele Mercati', p. 6.
38. See, for example, the account of the museum visit by Istoma Schewrigin, ambassador of the Muscovite king, in Mercati, *Metallotheca*, p. 156.
39. See, among others, the testimonies of Ulisse Aldrovandi (BUBo, Fondo Aldrovandi, vol. 21, pt. IV, c. 169^r (29-08-1595), Durante, *Herbario Nuovo*, p. 8); Pansa, *Della Libreria Vaticana* p. 274 or Baronio, *Annales ecclesiastici*, I, p. 174).
40. Mercati, *Obelischi*, pp. 377–78. On this episode, see also Curran, Grafton, Long, *Obelisk*, p. 107.

The famous engraving that opens the *Metallotheca*-book depicts a large room within which two long rows of cupboards containing the different categories of objects assembled by Mercati are distributed.

Such a representation is idealized and aims to give the reader an immediate overview of both the museum's content and the book's content at a glance.[41] With its two sets of cabinets, and above all in the cartouche inserted at the bottom of the print, the engraving illustrates the different categories of objects stored. On the one hand, there were the *OPYKTA* ('objects emerging from the earth') and on the other the *METAΛΛ EYTA* (metals). Among the former, there were earths, salts and saltpetre, alums, sulphites, sulphurs, marine products, earth-like stones, stones produced by animals, idiomorphic stones, rocks and marbles; among the latter, golds and silvers, bronzes, lead and antimony, ferrous products and steels, metal-like objects of spontaneous formation derived from castings.[42]

Within these categories we find various objects that constituted indispensable components of the therapeutic arsenal since antiquity, as testified by Hippocrates, Galen and Theophrastus, but also in the Arabic and medieval tradition in authors such as Mesue, Albertus Magnus, Serapion, Matteo Silvatico.[43] Lapidaries, a widespread genre in medieval and early modern Europe, as noted by Thorndike,[44] were often found in the libraries of physicians and scholars interested in the natural world and its therapeutic properties.[45] Even in the most celebrated pharmacopoeia of Antiquity, studied and commented on in later centuries, the *Materia medica* of Dioscorides, we find in fact many of those *ORYKTA* and *METAΛΛ EYTA* mentioned by Mercati. Earths, gems, bezoards, gold, antimony, are considered by Dioscorides as powerful ingredients of compound medicines, made to combat a wide range of diseases or to counteract the effects of intentional or accidental poisoning. In the numerous sixteenth-century editions of *Materia medica*, the chapters of the work devoted to these objects are often abundantly commented on and illustrated.[46] In the works that embodied the encounter between European medical traditions and medical conceptions and cultures developed in other worlds, such as the *Colóquios* of the Portuguese doctor resident in Goa, Garcia da Orta,[47] specific attention is paid to the variety of therapeutic uses of some of these elements, such as bezoars, or gems, made available by the development of long-distance trade.[48]

Mercati emphasized the therapeutic value of the objects preserved in his collection in the dedication to his treatise. While addressing the pontiff, he expressed his hope that foreigners and learned men visiting Rome from various parts of the world—having explored the sacred places of the city and observed the plant specimens preserved in the popes' gardens—would extend their visit to the Metallotheca. There, they could appreciate not only the beauty and diversity of the natural objects reflecting the richness of Creation, but also recognize their 'numerous and significant properties, largely unknown to many, useful for the preservation and recovery of human health'.[49] Gathering natural objects that could be effectively employed in healthcare practices, the *Metallotheca* aligned with collections widespread in Europe at the time, which Paula Findlen classified as 'Museums of Medicine', places where 'the possession of nature was predicated upon the idea of medical utility'.[50] According to Findlen, the main aim of many sixteenth-century nature collectors, including the naturalist physician Ulisse Aldrovandi, was 'the reform of materia medica, the formal study of nature as a medical entity prescribed by Galen, Dioscorides, and medieval

41. Bredekamp, *Machines et cabinets de curiosité*, pp. 22–27. Actually, Mercati's unfinished manuscript and its iconography concern only ten of the *ORYKTA*'s cabinets. The section on *METAΛΛEYTA* was probably not even begun.
42. Accordi, 'Michele Mercati', p. 14.
43. Reinbacher, *Healing earths*.
44. Thorndike, *A History of Magic and Experimental*, vol. 7, pp. 298–324. On lapidaries, also in non-European tradition, see the contributions of Bycroft, Dupré, Hendriksen, Viens in *Gems in the Early Modern World*, pp. 1–32; 197–220; 259–79.
45. Andretta and Pardo-Tomás, 'La naturaleza en la biblioteca'.
46. See for example the case of gems studied by Galech Amillano, 'Las piedras preciosas'.
47. Orta, *Colóquios dos simples*.
48. Loureiro, 'Enter the Milanese lapidary'; Cooley, 'Bezoar'.
49. 'Neque etiam illud ei ingratum, peregrinos, & doctos viros, qui Romam ex omnibus terrarum partibus conveniunt, post religiosa loca a se frequentata, post plantarum in Vaticanis hortis spectatam seriem, habere in eodem Vaticano, ubi tot res tam varias, novas, admirabiles, in unum tanto labore a me collectas spectare possint: quae non solum oculos forma, & varietate, & admirabili parentis Naturae artificio pascant; sed multas, & magnas suppeditent, usque huc non a multis cognitas in hominum valetudine vel tuenda, vel recuperanda utilitates', Mercati, *Metallotheca*, LI.
50. Findlen, *Possessing Nature*, p. 241.

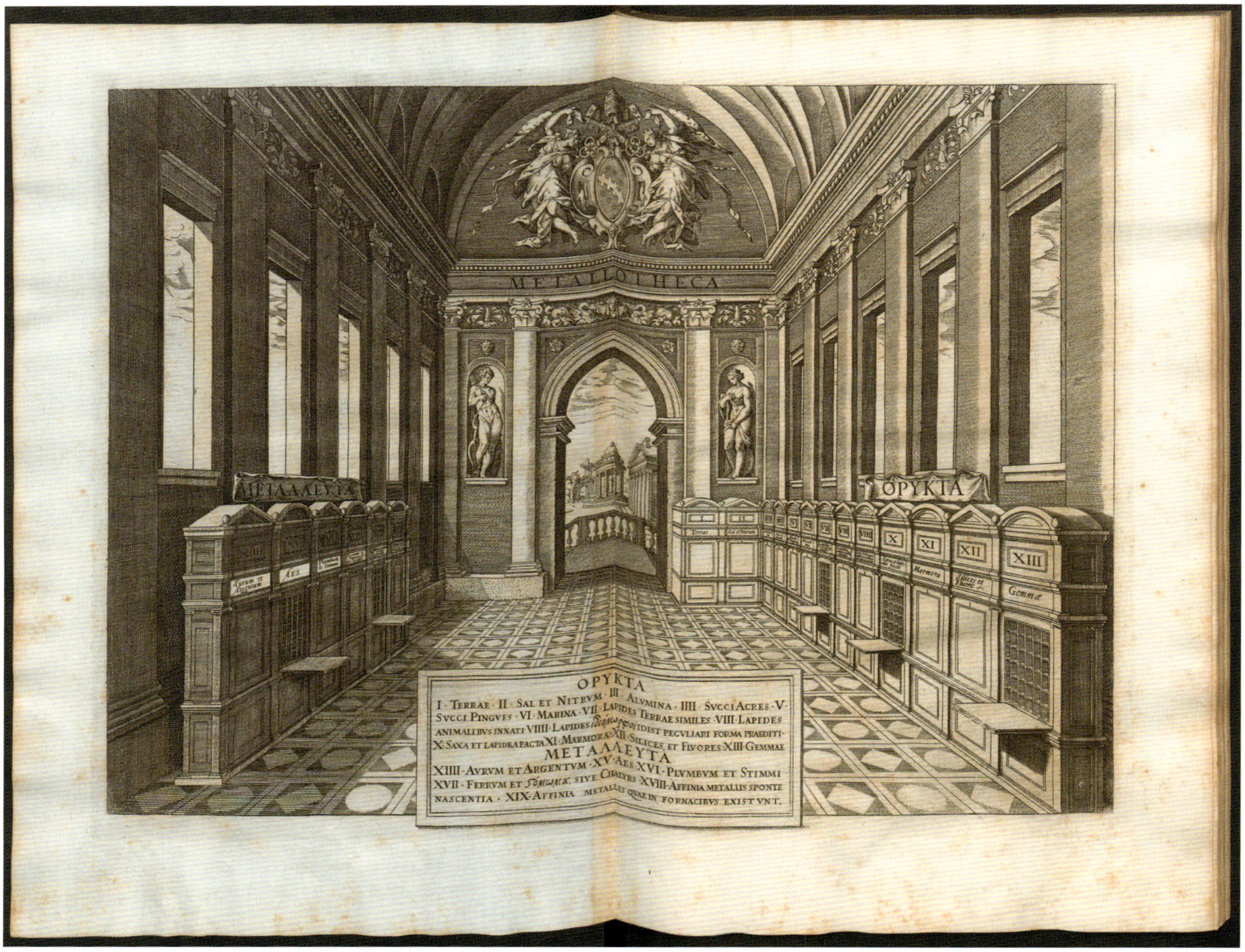

11. Overview of Mercati's Methalloteca-museum, in Michele Mercati's *Metallotheca* (Rome, I. Salvioni, 1719).

commentators such as Avicenna'.[51] Alongside the introduction of specific university chairs dedicated to pharmacopeia, the establishment of the first botanical gardens, and the reform of the *antidotarii* in major cities on the peninsula, naturalistic collections played a crucial role in the renewal of medical knowledge and practices, as well as in defining the status and ethos of the sixteenth-century physician. What made the Metallotheca particularly important was its 'specialization' in the inanimate world.

While the therapeutic purpose of the Metallotheca is evident from Mercati's words and the type of specimens it contained, understanding how these objects were effectively used is more difficult. It remains unclear whether the collection played a role in the organization of healthcare in the Apostolic Palace and, consequently, how Mercati's daily activities as the pontifical physician and collector were linked. The sources provide extremely limited information on the therapeutic uses that the pontiffs and their entourage might have made of these precious objects. As in other courtly contexts, the almost constant presence of physicians at the side of their patients and the predominantly oral nature of doctor-patient communication in the Vatican considerably limits the evidence available for reconstructing daily therapeutic practices.

The dedication to the collection of *Instuttioni* provides some interesting insights. Here, the physician, fearing that the pestilential fevers might also spread to Rome, insisted that princes should stock up on 'remedies':

51. Olmi, *L'inventario del mondo*, p. 271; Cook, 'Physicians and natural history'.

> And because it is necessary for such remedies to be available in times of need, it seems commendable that every great Prince keeps them [...] in his own storehouses and gardens, than relying on books and public apothecaries. This enables the saving of lives in sudden situations of necessity. Moreover, they prove beneficial during epidemics and for many other malignant illnesses.[52]

Is it conceivable that Mercati was referring to his own experience here? Was he contemplating the acquisition of natural specimens that, with the backing of his patrons, he was undertaking in the same years to enhance the *Hortus* and the *Metallotheca* of the popes? When he alluded to remedies '*in cassa*,' stored in a protected space, could he have been referring to those housed in the cabinets of his museum?

The absence of detailed information about the papal apothecary workshop prevents us from understanding the relationships such a place might have had with the garden and the museum under Mercati's direct responsibility. While the presence of apothecaries and their names are recorded in the Palace's account books, we lack detailed information about pharmaceutical activities and medicines produced and stored in the Vatican.[53] By analogy with other contemporary courts, however, it is probable that Mercati, as the chief physician and *simplicista*, supplied some of the simples required for the production of distillations and medicines from his garden and the *Metallotheca*.[54]

Given the value of some of the natural objects that Mercati had assembled, his collection would also have constituted an important resource in the gift economy of Roman, Italian and European courts.[55] The Metallotheca could have been a partial realization of a project conceived a few years before Mercati's arrival in the Vatican, as recorded by another physician and naturalist active in Rome, Andrea Bacci. In a *Discorso sull'Alicorno*, he recalled how Pope Julius III, following the model of the Roman emperors, had begun to assemble precious natural objects with the aim of creating a '*Spezieria di cose preciose*' in the Vatican, a complementary place to the ordinary apothecary's workshop.[56]

The precious natural specimens collected by Mercati must have been used beyond the Vatican and the exchange networks that linked European courts. Marc'Antonio Ciappi, an apothecary of Gregory XIII and one of his first biographers, states that the pontiff

> also instructed his Wardrobe not to be sparing in providing for the sick, not only in the Palace but also outside, of Bezoars, quintessences, sealed earths, Laserpitium, balms, Unicorn horns, etc. In short, everything that was available in rare and precious antidotes when requested.[57]

The therapeutic objects mentioned by the court apothecary correspond exactly to those categories of natural products that we have seen being preserved in the Metallotheca and detailed in Mercati's writings.

This passage is part of a celebration of the welfare policy of Gregory XIII, which includes direct references to 'Michele Mercati *semplicista*,' mentioned among those papal doctors sent outside the Vatican gates to assist the population in distress and provide them with the necessary medicines.[58]

Mercati's commitment to the care of the Roman population, also ascribable to his relationship with the Oratorians,[59] was celebrated in the paratext of his collection

52. 'E perché è necessario che tali rimedii sieno presentanei ne i bisogni; parmi da lodare ogni Principe grande che gli tiene preparati, e provisti più tosto in cassa, e ne i loro giardini, che su per i libri, e nelle spezierie pubbliche; perché nelle subite occasioni si può dare la vita à chi ne ha di bisogno; oltre che servono anco nel tempo della peste, et a molte maligne infirmità', Mercati, *Instruttione*, p. 102.
53. At the beginning of the pontificate of Pius V, the position of 'speziale palatino' (Palace apothecary) was held by Costantino Pietrasanta. In 1570, Antonio Mannini was appointed alongside him. Under Gregory XIII, the presence of Marc'Antonio Ciappi is documented. During the pontificate of Sixtus V, the papal apothecaries were Antonio Pasquino Ganassi and Jacopo Baldi. See BAV, *Ruoli*, 58, 64, 65, 99 and Moroni, *Dizionario di erudizione storico-ecclesiastica*, vol. 68, pp. 266–69.
54. See the Spanish *Reales boticas*, which were laboratories for the production of compound medicines prepared using plants from the gardens of royal sites, as demonstrated by Rey Bueno, *Los señores del fuego*.
55. On the use of nature in this system of exchange, see Pérez de Tuleda, and Jordan Geschwend, 'Renaissance Manageries'.
56. Bacci, *Le XII pietre pretiose*, p. 109.
57. ' [...] diceva anco al suo Guardarobba che non fosse parco nel dare a gl'infermi, non solo di Palazzo ma anco Bezzuarri, quinte essenzie, terre sigillate, Laserpitii, Balsami Alicorni etc. in somma tutto quello che vi era di antidoti rari e preziosi, quando ne veniva richiesto', Ciappi, *Compendio delle heroiche et gloriose attioni*, p. 63.
58. Ibid., p. 62.
59. Tomassetti, *Cura corporum*.

of *Instruttioni*, within a poem dedicated to him by the Spanish scholar Arias Montano, who had visited him and his collections during one of his stays in Rome. After praising the garden and the *Metallotheca*, Montano emphasized how Mercati had not limited himself to collecting and studying the wonders of nature, but had put these, as well as his art, at the service of the poor.[60] Arias Montano's words echoed those of the dedication of the work that Mercati himself had addressed to Giacomo Boncompagni, in which the doctor recalled that by publishing works in Italian, he had wished to place his knowledge and 'an ample number of undisclosed and partly new remedies' ('*copia delli rimedi non divulgati e in parte nuovi*') at the service of the health of his lords and of the Roman population, driven by the 'nature of the times' ('*qualità de' tempi*') and stimulated by the desire for 'the common good to which His Holiness is above all devoted' ('*bene universale al quale [è] soprattutto intenta la Santità Sua*').[61]

These various testimonies also reflected courtly rhetoric in celebration of Gregory XIII's charity. It is unlikely (to imagine) that the Vatican's natural history collections were opened to the population at large, especially given the exceptional and precious nature of the objects preserved in them. But, considered as a whole, they show how the *Metallotheca*, was a 'museum of medicine' in more ways than one: a place that referred to the collections assembled by doctors and apothecaries, who investigated the natural worlds, and also for its role in the preservation and restoration of human health; a reserve of precious medical ingredients to draw upon in time of need; and, at least under Gregory XIII, an institution that played an important role in papal health care policies as well as in their celebration.

MINERAL AND MEDICAL HISTORIAE

We have observed how, already in the collection of *Instruttioni*, Mercati demonstrated a pronounced interest in the therapeutic value of the natural objects preserved in his museum, along with a comprehensive understanding of their medicinal virtues and the diverse applications in treating and preventing various diseases. The *Metallotheca*-book further emphasizes how the physician perceived his role as a collector to be intricately connected to his medical practice. His in-depth knowledge of the realm of stones, metals, and minerals underscores the potential of these natural objects in therapeutic applications.

Mercati's work, as we know it from the unfinished manuscript he had begun to prepare for printing and its posthumous publication by Lancisi, is a complex work that combines different approaches to nature and its description within a narrative framework shaped by the collection and partly echoing the emerging genre of the catalog.[62]

After visually introducing the reader to his collection, through the sumptuous engraving that serves as a general summary, Mercati inserts four chapters of a more general nature in which, following the Aristotelian tradition, he discusses the place of inanimate objects within the order of nature, their internal subdivisions and introduces the various theories on their formation.[63] This is followed by ten chapters, much more detailed, significantly titled *Armaria* and devoted to the different categories of natural objects. Introduced by an engraving that physically represents the cabinet and followed by a list of the objects that Mercati kept in his museum, they once again seal the link between writing and place. For each category of objects described in an *Armarium,* he provides and discusses nomenclature, physical characteristics, origins, properties and therapeutic as well as artistic, artisanal and domestic uses.[64]

In these more general sections, the emphasis on the therapeutic aspect of various object categories becomes noticeably clear. For instance, at the beginning of the section dedicated to soils in general, Mercati, after outlining their uses in painting, ceramics, and sculpture, underscores their value in protecting against various diseases.[65]

60. Mercati, *Instruttione*, [4r].
61. Ibid., Dedication. This theme also returns in the *privilegium* of the work, which recalls how the remedies presented in the work were the most selected and appropriate and were accompanied by new and powerful 'secrets' both preservative and curative.
62. Marrache-Gouraud, *La légende des objets*, pp. 45–131.
63. On Mercati's relationship to Aristotle and the Peripatetic tradition, see Findlen, *Possessing Nature*, p. 61. On the different criteria for classifying the mineral world in the sixteenth century, see Morello, 'Alle radici della geologia sistematica'.
64. Mercati, *Metallotheca*, p. LIV.
65. Ibid., p. 8.

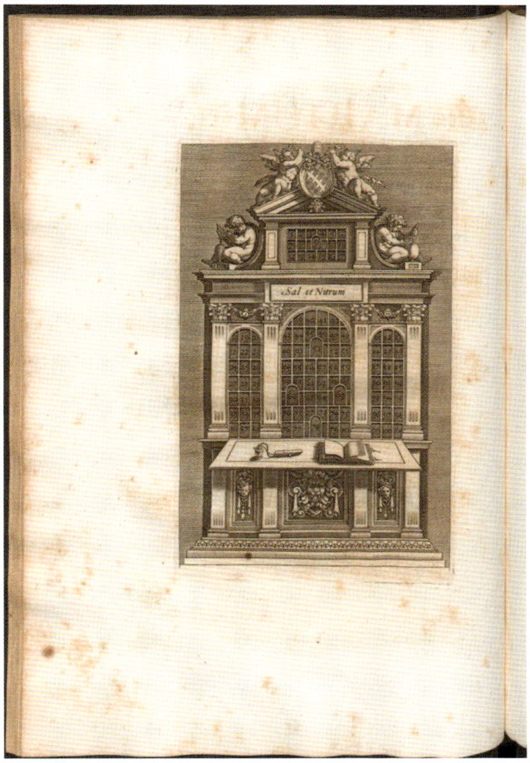

12. Cabinet II of the Methalloteca-museum containing salts and niter, in Michele Mercati's *Metallotheca* (Rome, I. Salvioni, 1719).

In Chapter VII of the second *Armarium* dedicated to the properties and uses of salts in general, all the information pertains to the medical field. Initially, he highlights the power of salt in 'warming, dispersing, contracting, drying, compacting, and densifying the substance of the bodies to which it is applied'.[66] Then, he references a passage from Pliny's *Naturalis Historia* in which the Roman author reviews instances where this element could be profitably used in the medical field—such as for bites from venomous animals, ulcers, pustules, warts, eye diseases, toothaches, and more. Finally, the focus shifts to the use of two specific types of salt, naphtenic salt and Indian salt, in the preparation of compound remedies.[67]

This emphasis on the potential health benefits of natural objects from the mineral world becomes even more pronounced as he shifts his focus to specific subcategories or specimens that he had gathered within his collection or that he had been able to observe during his visits to other collections and on his naturalistic travels. These meticulous descriptions are accompanied by extremely precise engravings in which both text and image contribute to the construction of true *historiae* of inanimate objects.[68]

This is evident right from the start in the decision to allocate so much space to the description of individual specimens. This choice echoes certain 'epistemic genres', notably *Curationes, Consultationes, Observationes medicinales*, which emphasized the individuality of the patient and the singularity of the clinical case and which gained popularity in the medical milieus of the time.[69] Some fellow papal doctors of Mercati, such as Alessandro Petroni and Angelo Vittori, were actively involved in this process of renewing medical practice, based on the examination of individual cases and their interconnection.[70] Through their publishing projects, these doctors intended to claim the exceptional value of experience and clinical observation. At the same time, by bringing together and writing about treatments of illustrious patients, they were charting social and professional paths of excellence and showcasing their diagnostic and therapeutic skills. Similarly, for Mercati, describing the individual history of objects was simultaneously a way of completing and renewing knowledge about the third realm through the new information gained from observing specimens and their uses, and a way of giving value to the particularly rare and precious objects in his museum.[71]

In describing the specimens of stones, soils, and minerals in his collection, Mercati calls upon a rich array of authorities from ancient and Arabic medicine, as well as contemporary authors. Among the ancients, two imperial physicians hold a particular place within his library: Galen (especially his *De simplicium facultatibus*) and, above all, Dioscorides. Dioscorides's vision of the natural world, based on its therapeutic potential, profoundly influenced the way nature was thought about and described from the middle of the century. The increasingly lengthy

66. 'Sal omnis calefacit, discutit astringit, siccat, cogit, ac densat substantiam corporum, quibus adhibetur', ibid., p. 40.
67. Ibid.
68. On *historia* as an intellectual tool and practice of writing in the sixteenth century, see '*Historia*'. *Empiricism and Erudition*.
69. Siraisi, 'L'individuale nella medicina'; Pomata, '*Praxis historialis*'; Pomata, 'Sharing Cases'.
70. Siraisi, *History, Medicine, and the Traditions of Renaissance Learning*, pp. 168–93.
71. On the role of rare, precious, and extravagant pieces in sixteenth-century collections, see Olmi, *L'inventario del mondo*, p. 275–76; Marrache-Gouraud, *La légende des objets*, pp. 14–15.

commentaries that accompanied the Dioscoridean text in editions that were published in different parts of Europe were the place chosen by many naturalists to describe their naturalistic observations and their therapeutic experiments. The Dioscoridean model also allowed European physicians to interact with ways of understanding the relationship between nature and human health that were often very distant from each other, and to incorporate new knowledge into a known intellectual framework.[72] In 1580, when Philip II entrusted the Neapolitan physician Nardo Antonio Recchi with the task of reorganizing and making intelligible and accessible the materials resulting from the royal physician Francisco Hernández's intensive description of American nature, he turned to the model of the Dioscoridean *materia medica*.[73] The Dioscoridean model is also fundamental to the *Colóquios* of the Portuguese physician Garcia de Orta printed in Goa in 1563, which for European physicians constituted the main gateway to the nature of the East Indies and its therapeutic use.[74]

Like many of his contemporaries, Mercati largely adopts Dioscorides's focus on the description of numerous earths and stones. Yet, by concentrating on the third realm and its therapeutic properties, he breaks the unity of a Dioscoridean model that moved seamlessly from plants to animals to minerals. However, the considerable space devoted to the description of the medical qualities of natural objects is completely embedded in the *Materia medica* and the uses that physicians such as Andrés Laguna, Pietro Andrea Mattioli or Amatus Lusitanus had made of them a few years earlier. Taking up and expanding on the injunction in Dioscorides's preface to start from certain information and especially from their own experience, all these authors include references in their commentaries to specific specimens observed in gardens, collections or *curationes*.[75] In his book, he goes beyond merely gathering and systematizing the knowledge of the ancients, particularly Dioscorides, on inanimate objects. He actively corrects and expands their understanding. Mercati assesses their properties by weighing their efficacy against various diseases, adjusting dosages, adding new recipes, refuting improper uses, and proposing innovations.

The process of scrutinizing and broadening the knowledge of the ancients regarding the therapeutic virtues of the mineral world takes several paths. One of these involves the written or spoken word of fellow physicians, whom he deems keepers of reliable knowledge, especially when grounded in direct experiences.

For instance, he relies on the therapeutic experience of the physician Guillaume Rondelet, who a few years earlier had published two important ichthyological works describing the properties of stones produced by fish in the treatment of nephritis.[76] If Mercati had become acquainted with Rondelet's experiments by reading his writings, other sections of the *Metallotheca* allude directly to verbal exchanges that occurred in the Roman medical environment he frequented.[77] This is particularly evident in the description of the therapeutic properties of the Armenian red bole, where Mercati displays considerable skepticism, not so much regarding the properties of the Armenian bole itself, but rather concerning the authenticity of the product available on the market.

Since ancient times, the identification of Armenian bole had posed significant challenges due to its resemblance to other substances such as Earth of Lemnos or Eastern Bolus. According to numerous sixteenth-century physicians, including Mattioli and Mercati himself, these difficulties were exacerbated by the alleged illicit trade practices of Turkish merchants, who sold the common Eastern bole as if it were the prized and much rarer Armenian bole.[78] Mercati enters this lengthy debate, first reiterating its terms and then adding a specific and particularly compelling piece of evidence: a medical case of which he had precise information, that allowed a comparison of clinical data with observations made during the post-mortem examination.[79] Mercati claims to have 'personally known' ('ipse novi') some renowned physicians who administered daily the Levant Bole to a patient suffering from pestilential fever, as if it possessed the same

72. *Dioscórides ante el mundo*.
73. Recchi, *De Materia Medica Novae Hispaniae*.
74. Pimentel and Soler, 'Dioscórides en Goa'.
75. Mattioli, *Il Dioscoride*, p. 1.
76. Mercati, *Metallotheca*, p. 187.
77. Regarding the role of orality in scientific exchanges during the early modern period, Azzolini, 'Marvellous Natural Particulars'.
78. References to these practices can be found not only in Mercati but also in the Mattioli, *Il Dioscoride*, V, pp. 639–40.
79. On the relationship between anatomical observations and medical practice in the early modern period, see *Pathology in Practice*.

properties as the authentic Armenian bole. The therapy had no effect, and after a few days, the patient died. During the post-mortem examination of his cadaver, the physicians were astonished ('obstupescentes') to observe that the same amount of bole administered had obstructed both the stomach and the intestines. Not only had the bole failed to overcome the 'malignancy of the disease' ('morbi malignitas'), but its side effects had proven lethal.[80]

Elsewhere in the Metallotheca, the therapeutic efficacy of natural products is assessed by Mercati through his own personal experience, as in the case of *Tophum Juvencarum*. He had been able to directly experiment how this stony concretion found in ruminants 'consumed through infusion' ('cum aqua e lapidis infusione') was effective in reducing bladder stones. The anti-venom properties of the *Malacca stone*, another concretion found this time in the viscera of the porcupine, are analyzed based on examinations and tests conducted on a specific specimen, whose image also appears in Mercati's book. This specimen had been brought back to Rome by the powerful Cardinal Alessandrino, Michele Bonelli, one of the physicians' main patrons, after a diplomatic mission to Portugal. Thanks to his closeness to this prominent figure in the Curia, praised several times in his writings, Mercati had not only been able to observe this extraordinary specimen, but also verify its therapeutic properties, both as an antidote and in 'strengthening a cold stomach' ('frigido ventriculo firmando').

Mercati also presents experimental evidence at the bedside of his patients to refute certain beliefs that led to improper medical uses of inanimate objects. He strongly criticizes, for example, those who attributed the power of relieving the pain of kidney stones and nephritis to fish stones worn around the neck. His criticism is particularly strong, as he had experienced the ineffectiveness of this remedy not only as a physician but also as a suffering patient.[81]

A certain skepticism towards beliefs regarding the properties of specific stones is evident throughout the pages of the *Metallotheca*. Nevertheless, the physician does not hesitate to describe them, sometimes in great detail. For instance, he mentions the widespread practice among the inhabitants of Sardinia to wear toadstones set in silver rings or bound together to form a small crown, purportedly to alleviate migraines. This custom had been reported to Mercati by a group of Jesuits returning from a mission to Sardinia.[82] Other uses and beliefs that Mercati scrutinizes refer to geographical areas much farther away. Just as the numerous diplomatic, commercial, and missionary networks that traversed papal Rome had granted him direct access to stones and minerals from extremely distant regions such as India or Peru, the chronicles reaching the city or the encounters with direct witnesses offer relatively precise information about their uses in different contexts.

THE BEZOAR BETWEEN MUSEUM AND PATIENT BEDSIDE

In the pages of the *Metallotheca*, East and West India are compared to objects such as bezoars, a stony concretion that can form in the stomachs of ruminants. Bezoars are the first in the long line of objects—deer tears, Malacca stones, heifer tuff, pearls, cockscombs, and so forth—contained in the chapter-cabinet dedicated to stones produced by animals. This section, in addition to being the most open to new and distant worlds, is undoubtedly the one in which Mercati's experience is especially mobilized, not only in terms of the origin and physical characteristics of the objects, but also in terms of their medicinal properties, both preservative and curative. This was above all the case with bezoars, which were considered particularly effective against poisoning and diseases such as pestilential fevers, melancholia and epilepsy.[83] However, they also aroused bitter scientific controversy due to their commercial value.[84] In dealing with these objects, as precious as they were thorny, the knowledge of physicians and their ability to assess therapeutic properties proved crucial. Here more than ever, the Mercati collector and the physician went hand in hand. Bezoars occupy a special place for Mercati, especially given the fragmentary information available on these objects and, above all, their misuse. The objectives of Mercati's work are multiple: to select the information available on these stones and on the

80. Mercati, *Metallotheca*, p. 11.
81. Ibid., p. 187.
82. Ibid., p. 338.
83. Cooley, 'Bezoar', pp. 53–86.
84. Pardo-Tomás, 'Bezoar', p. 196.

animals that produced them; to compare the eastern ones with the western ones that had begun to flow into Europe from Peru a few years earlier; to provide elements to verify their authenticity; and to denounce and rectify their improper uses.[85] In his description of the eastern bezoars, he adopts the recommendations of Garcia de Orta, whom he considers a reliable author. He supplements them with some recipes that he had personally composed and experimented with. He prescribes twelve bezoars for poisonings and seven for malignant fevers to be dissolved in white wine, myrtle, or also in water.[86]

This recipe is also found in the *Instruttione sopra la peste*. In a chapter devoted to the '*Modo di preservarsi con quelli rimedij, che fanno resistenza alla peste, & alla sua cagione*' (Methods of preserving oneself with remedies that resist the plague and its cause), Mercati recommends a series of medicines distributed over a 13-day cycle that must be repeated for the duration of the plague. Some of the recipes indicated are very complex and involve the mixing of different vegetable, mineral and animal ingredients, according to well-defined quantities. On the ninth day, Mercati invites the reader to take 12 grains of bezoar stone, exactly the same quantity prescribed in the *Metallotheca*, without the addition of any other ingredient, thus considered effective in itself.[87] In the *Instruttione sopra il veleno,* on the other hand, the bezoar is listed among the 'medicamenti che per loro spetiale qualità faccino resistenza al veleno' (remedies that, due to their special qualities, offer resistance to poison). In this case, Mercati suggests that 'the Bezoar stone be taken in a dosage of eight grains with very strong wine.'[88]

For such remedies to be effective, however, it is essential not only that they are administered correctly, but also that the stones come from the East and are not counterfeit.[89] The *Metallotheca* therefore contains indications on how to unmask false bezoars. The Portuguese doctor, Garcia da Orta's recommendations are supplemented by Mercati's own method, developed thanks to the abundance of bezoars in Rome. It combines physical interventions on the stone and the study of their effects. On the one hand, the doctor suggests trying to introduce hot liquid into the heart of the stone with a needle and observing the effect produced. If the liquid manages to enter the stone and its internal matter melts, the bezoar must be considered false. This technique consisting of manipulating and observing the substance of which the stones are composed was also supplemented by another 'entirely true and legitimate' proof, the administration of bezoar powder to animals and prisoners sentenced to death who had previously been poisoned.[90] This reflects Mercati's total trust in the ability of real bezoar to neutralize poison.

For Mercati the problem was not only counterfeiting. Like other physicians of his time, he also speaks out against the use of Western bezoars, which in his opinion were completely ineffective. His stance is based on naturalistic and medical considerations: Western bezoars, derived from animals other than those of the East, were not considered medicinal 'by the peoples of that [American] World', before the arrival of the Spanish.[91] On this basis, Mercati sharply criticized Nicolas Monardes, the Spanish physician, who had paved the way for the introduction of Peruvian stones into European medical practice.[92] But this comparison between bezoars from the two Indies is also based on the description of some specimens that he had been able to observe closely in Rome. While Rome was certainly not the only European marketplace for the circulation of bezoars and probably not even the main one, the presence of missionaries from India and Portuguese merchants certainly guaranteed a considerable supply.[93] The quantity and quality of the bezoars to which he had access allowed him to claim a precise expertise both in distinguishing the authentic from the fake and in their use. Eleven of the bezoars he was able to observe at close quarters in the city are depicted in a beautiful collective portrait. The first of them, a bezoar judged extraordinary for its whiteness and brilliance, is also the subject of a very detailed textual description of its

85. Mercati, *Metallotheca*, pp. 171–76.
86. Ibid., p. 173.
87. Mercati, *Instruttione*, p. 135.
88. 'la pietra Bezear presa al peso di otto grani con vino potente', ibid., p. 100.
89. Mercati, *Metallotheca*, p. 173.
90. Ibid.
91. Ibid., p. 173.
92. Stephenson, 'From Marvelous Antidote to the Poison of Idolatry', pp. 8–15.
93. Nelson Novoa, 'El horizonte oriental de los mercaderes portugueses'.

weight, color and composition. Here, the circumstances in which the doctor was able to observe the precious object and the routes that led it to Rome are also evoked.[94] The shiny bezoar was given by the king of Portugal to Cardinal Alessandrino in 1571, who had allowed the doctor to study it closely. The other bezoar to which Mercati devotes special attention was placed in his museum after it had been brought to Rome in 1583 by a delegation of Peruvian Jesuits. As he points out with some satisfaction, it was an exceptional stone not only for its extraordinary weight of 59 ounces, but also for its spiritual significance: it had been recovered during a fire caused by the Jesuits in an anti-idolatry campaign. The fire had altered its crust, making its different layers visible. After celebrating the exceptional itinerary and spiritual value of the stone, Mercati dwells on its characteristics - size, shape, color.[95] He then launches into a harsh indictment against his unscrupulous colleagues who recommended the use of Western bezoars, thus sacrificing the health of their patients to their own gain. The main person to be accused was Nicolas Monardes. Mercati explicitly states that, in order to prevent any misunderstanding, he will not even mention any therapeutic properties of Peruvian stones and instead lists their harmful effects, in particular the formation of tumors and the blockage of the digestive process. He concludes with the description of a clinical case he had witnessed: a Spaniard who had arrived in Rome had fallen ill with fevers. To cure himself, he had decided to repeatedly take the powder of some American bezoars he had brought with him. After a few days, he had developed a fulminating liver tumor that led to his death.[96] Evidence from medical practice was seen as decisive in putting an end to the debate.

CONCLUSION

Then, at the end of a very short chapter devoted to deer tears, three stones are described and depicted that, as Mercati recalls, were found inside Pius V's bladder during the autopsy that followed his death.[97] We do not know if they were kept in the museum until Sixtus V decided to move them to the Sistine Chapel, but the three stones find their place in the *Metallotheca*-book by virtue of their resemblance to bezoars and other stones generated by living beings. In addition to giving these hard-to-define objects a precise place within a specific organization of the natural world, the description takes on numerous other meanings. It undoubtedly allows the physician to celebrate his proximity to the vicar of Christ, and once again the exceptional nature that his position as apostolic physician conferred on his collections. Moreover, according to Jetze Touber, 'Mercati's notion of idiomorphous stones lent itself particularly well for potential miracles'.[98] By tracing Pius V's stones back to bezoars and other idiomorphic stones, generated by external factors, *praeter natura*, Mercati provides a cautious contribution to the construction of an aura of sanctity around the pope-inquisitor.

The decision to include the three stones in the book probably also refers to Mercati's activity at the bedside of the pontiff who had wanted him in Rome.

The description of the stones includes some elements of the reports written by various papal physicians[99] after the death of their illustrious patients, including that of Gian Francesco Marengo on the death of Pope Ghislieri, and that of Mercati himself on the infirmity and death of Gregory XIII. These reports scrutinized all clinical or autopsy data to prevent or dismantle possible accusations against the medical profession.[100]

The death of Pius V, as we have seen, ended a long period of the pontiff's sufferings and of doubts and dissensions within the medical profession. The ekphrasis of the *Metallotheca* allows Mercati to reaffirm the devotion with which day and night he had followed his patient through his illnesses. But above all, it highlights the fundamental value of the autopsy in ascertaining the causes of the Pope's death and thus to retrospectively judge the medical choices made. Mercati is certain that the three stones inevitably led to death. This conviction is also based on certain physical characteristics of the stones—their shape and color—which here, as with the other

94. Mercati, *Metallotheca*, p. 173.
95. Ibid., p. 175.
96. Ibid.
97. Ibid., p. 177.
98. Touber, 'Stones of Passions', p. 40.
99. De Renzi, 'Tales from Cardinals Deathbeds'.
100. See Marengo, 'De Pii V. Pont. Max morbo', p. 321, which also contains an accurate account of the stones of Pious V.

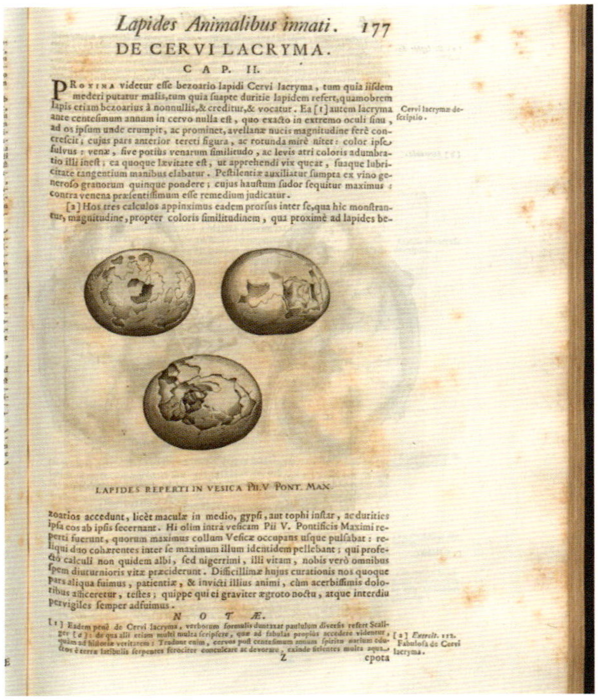

Lapides Animalibus innati. 177

DE CERVI LACRYMA.

CAP. II.

PROXIMA videtur esse bezoario lapidi Cervi lacryma, tum quia iisdem mederi putatur malis, tum quia suapte duritie lapidem refert, quamobrem lapis etiam bezoarius à nonnullis, & creditur, & vocatur. Ea [1] autem lacryma ante centesimum annum in cervo nulla est, quo exacto in extremo oculi sinu, ad os ipsum unde erumpit, ac prominet, avellanæ nucis magnitudine ferè concrescit; cujus pars anterior tereti figura, ac rotunda mirè nitet: color ipse fulvus: venæ, sive potiùs venarum similitudo, ac levis atri coloris adumbratio illi inest; ea quoque lævitate est, ut apprehendi vix queat, suaque lubricitate tangentium manibus elabatur. Pestilentiæ auxiliatur sumpta ex vino generoso granorum quinque pondere; cujus haustum sudor sequitur maximus: contra venena præsentissimum esse remedium judicatur.

Cervi lacrymæ descriptio.

[2] Hos tres calculos appinximus eadem prorsus inter se, qua hic monstrantur, magnitudine, propter coloris similitudinem, qua proximè ad lapides be-

LAPIDES REPERTI IN VESICA PII V PONT. MAX.

zoarios accedunt, licèt maculæ in medio, gypsi, aut tophi instar, ac durities ipsa eos ab ipsis secernant. Hi olim intrà vesicam Pii V. Pontificis Maximi reperti fuerunt, quorum maximus collum Vesicæ occupans usque pulsabat: reliqui duo cohærentes inter se maximum illum identidem pellebant; qui profectò calculi non quidem albi, sed nigerrimi, illi vitam, nobis verò omnibus spem diuturnioris vitæ præciderunt. Difficillimæ hujus curationis nos quoque pars aliqua fuimus, patientiæ, & invicti illius animi, cùm acerbissimis doloribus afficeretur, testes; quippe qui ei graviter ægroto noctu, atque interdiu pervigiles semper adfuimus.

NOTÆ.

[1] Eadem penè de Cervi lacryma, verborum formulis duntaxat paulùm diversis refert Scaliger [a]: de qua alii etiam multi multa scripsere, quæ ad fabulas propiùs accedere videntur, quàm ad historiæ veritatem: Tradunt enim, cervos post centesimum annum spiritu narium eductos è terræ latibulis serpentes ferociter conculcare ac devorare, exinde sitientes multa aqua

[a] *Exercit.* 112.

Fabulosâ de Cervi lacryma.

Z epota

13. Depiction of the stones found in Pope Sixtus V's bladder after his death, in Michele Mercati's *Metallotheca* (Rome, I. Salvioni, 1719).

objects in the *Metallotheca*, are described in detail. These elements together with another observed during the autopsy - their position inside the bladder - left no doubt that the stones not only caused the Pope great suffering but were also what 'cut off his life' and 'the hope of seeing him live a long time'.[101]

Elsewhere in the *Metallotheca,* the qualities of natural objects are explained and proven by medical practice. In this short and dense *historia of* the stones of Pius V, it is the physical-natural characteristics of the objects themselves that, carefully observed, make it possible to judge the correctness of the therapeutic decisions made.

These stones, depicted and detailed in the *Metallotheca* alongside the bezoars, encapsulate the multifaceted nature of the activities of the *Semplicista* and papal physician. They serve as a telling example of the intrinsic correlation between medical practice and the study of nature that defined Mercati's professional and intellectual pursuits, evident in his collections and writings. During his regular attendance of his esteemed patient, the three accretions obstructing the Pope's bladder became a diagnostic challenge, relying on a thorough understanding of the patient's medical history and careful observation of specific symptoms. In the subsequent autopsy, in which Mercati directly participated, these stones emerged as crucial evidence, elucidating the underlying causes of suffering and death, and confirming the validity of the treatment. Thus, both in the Museum and in his written works, they become pivotal objects of knowledge, contributing to define a category of stones that continued to intrigue for their position on the boundary between animate and inanimate, and their therapeutic potential, also exemplified by bezoars or Malacca stones.

This exploration of Mercati's world, culminating in the examination of Pious V's stones, underscores the essential interconnection between the theoretical study of nature and active medical practice in the sixteenth century. Mercati's case highlights how the significance of stones, earths, metals, and minerals within the pharmacopeia of the time not only was acknowledged but also shaped the priorities and methodologies in understanding the natural world.

WORKS CITED

Printed Primary Sources

Bacci, Andrea, *Le XII pietre pretiose le quali per ordine di Dio nella santa legge adornavano i vestimenti del sommo sacerdote [...]* (Rome: G. Martinelli, 1587).

Baronio, Cesare, *Annales ecclesiastici* (Rome: Tipografia Vaticana, 1588-1607).

Ciappi, Marc'Antonio, *Compendio delle heroiche et gloriose attioni, et santa vita di Papa Gregorio XIII* (Rome: Stamperia degli Accolti, 1596).

Durante, Castore, *Herbario Nuovo con figure che rappresentano le vive piante che nascono in tutta Europa e nelle Indie Orientali, & Occidentali* (Rome: B. Bonfadini, 1585).

Marengo, Giovan Francesco, 'De Pii V. Pont. Max morbo, quo obiit', published in Gaetano Marini, *Degli Archiatri pontifici vol. I. nel quale sono i supplementi e correzioni all'opera del Mandosio – vol. II. il quale contiene l'appendice de' monumenti e gl'indici a tutta l'opera*, (Rome: V. Pagliarini, 1784), II, pp. 318–23.

Marini, Gaetano, *Degli Archiatri pontifici vol. I. nel quale sono i supplementi e correzioni all'opera del Mandosio – vol. II. il quale contiene l'appendice de' monumenti e gl'indici a tutta l'opera*, 2 vols., (Rome: V. Pagliarini, 1784).

101. '[...] illi vitam, nobis vero omnibus spem diuturnioris vitae praeciderunt', Mercati, *Metallotheca*, p. 177.

Mattioli, Pietro Andrea, *Il Dioscoride* [...] *con i suoi discorsi* [...] *la seconda volta illustrati, & diligentemente ampliati: con l'agiunta del sesto libro de i rimedi di tutti i veleni, da lui nuovamente tradotto, & con dottissimi discorsi per tutto commentato,* [...] (Venice: Valgrisi, 1548).

Mercati, Michele, *Considerationi [...] sopra gli avvertimenti di Latino Latini intorno ad alcune cose scritte nel libro de gli Obelischi di Roma* (Rome: D. Basa, 1590).

Mercati, Michele, *Degli obelischi di Roma* (Rome: Domenico Basa, 1589)

Mercati, Michele, *Instruttione sopra la Peste, nella quale si contengono i più eletti et approvati rimedij, con molti nuovi et potenti secreti così da preservarsi come da curarsi. Aggiuntevi tre altre instruttioni sopra i veleni occultamente ministrati, podagra, & paralisi* (Rome: Vincenzo Accolti, 1576).

Mercati, Michele, *Metallotheca opus posthumum, auctoritate, & munificentia Clementis undecimi pontificis maximi e tenebris in lucem eductum; opera autem, & studio Ioannis Mariae Lancisii archiatri pontificii illustratum* (Rome: Giovanni Maria Salvioni, 1717).

Moroni, Gaetano, *Dizionario di erudizione storico-ecclesiastica*, vol. 68 (Venice: Tipografia Emiliana, 1854).

Orta, Garcia da, *Colóquios dos simples e drogas he cousas medicinais da Índia* (Goa: J. de Endem, 1563).

Pansa, Muzio, *Della Libreria Vaticana* (Rome, G. Martinelli, 1590).

Recchi, Nardo Antonio, *De Materia Medica Novae Hispaniae. Manuscrito de Recchi*, ed. by Raquel Álvarez Peláez and Florentino Fernández González (Madrid and Valladolid: Ediciones Doce Calles et Junta de Castilla y León, 1998).

Secondary Sources

Accordi, Bruno, 'Michele Mercati (1541-1593) and the Metallotheca', *Geologica romana*, 19 (1980), 1–50.

Andretta, Elisa and José Pardo-Tomás, 'La naturaleza en la biblioteca: los Herbarios de El Escorial y las colecciones de Diego Hurtado de Mendoza', *Cuadernos de Historia Moderna*, 48.1 (2023), 37–56.

Andretta, Elisa, 'Mercati, Michele', *Dizionario Biografico degli Italiani*, (Rome: Istituto dell'Enciclopedia Italiana Treccani, 2009), pp. 606–11.

Andretta, Elisa, *Le monde sous l'oeil des médecins. Nature et politique à l'Escorial et au Vatican (XVIme siècle)* (Paris: Classiques Garnier, 2024).

Andretta, Elisa, *Roma medica. Anatomie d'un système médical au XVIe* siècle (Rome: École française de Rome, 2011).

Azzolini, Monica, 'Marvellous Natural Particulars: Testimony, Rumour, and Proof in Ulisse Aldrovandi's Work', in *'Dicitur'. Hearsay in Science, Memory and Poetry*, special issue of 'Micrologus', ed. by Agostino Paravicini Bagliani and Francesco Santi (vol. XXXII, 2024), pp. 567–91.

Bredekamp, Horst, *Machines et cabinets de curiosité* (Paris: Diderot, 1997).

Brevaglieri, Sabina, *Natural desiderio di sapere. Roma barocca fra vecchi e nuovi mondi* (Rome: Viella, 2019).

Bueno, Mar Rey, *Los señores del fuego: destiladores y espagíricos en la corte de los Austrias* (Madrid: Corona Borealis, 2002).

Campitelli, Alberta, *Gli horti dei Papi: i giardini vaticani dal Medioevo al Novecento* (Milan: Jaca Book, 2009).

Cook, Harold, 'Physicians and natural history', in *Cultures of Natural History*, ed. by Nicolas Jardine, James Secord, and Emma Spary (Cambridge: Cambridge University Press, 1996), pp. 91–105.

Cooley, Mackenzie, 'Bezoar: Medicine in the Belly of the Beast', in *Natural Things in Early Modern Worlds*, ed. by Mackenzie Cooley, Anna Toledano, and Duygu Yıldırım (London-New York: Routledge, Taylor & Francis Group, 2023), pp. 53–86.

Cooper, Alix, 'The Museum and the Book. The Metallotheca and the history of an encyclopaedic natural history in early modern Italy', *Journal of the History of Collections*, 7.1 (1995), 1–23.

Curran, Brian, Anthony Grafton, and Pamela Long, *Obelisk: A History* (Cambridge: Burndy Library, 2009).

De Renzi, Silvia, 'Tales from Cardinals' Deathbeds: Medical Hierarchy, Court Etiquette and Authority in the Counter Reformation', in *Être médecin à la cour (Italie, France et Espagne, XIII-XVIII s.)*, ed. by Elisa Andretta and Marillyn Nicoud (Florence: Sismel, 2013), pp. 235–58.

Dioscórides ante el mundo. Usos plurales de un 'libro-laboratorio' en la edad moderna, ed. by Elisa Andretta and José Pardo-Tomás (Madrid: CSIC, 2025).

Donato, Maria Pia, *Sudden Death: Medicine and Religion in Eighteenth-Century Rome* (Farnham: Ashgate, 2014, ed. it. 2010).

Early Modern Things: Objects and their Histories, 1500-1800 ed. by Paula Findlen (London-New York: Routledge, 2013).

Egmond, Florike, 'Into the Wild: Botanical Fieldwork in the Sixteenth Century', in *Naturalists in the Field. Collecting, Recording and Preserving the Natural World from the Fifteenth to the Twenty-First Century*, ed. by Arthur MacGregor (Leiden: Brill, 2018), pp.166–211.

Falguière, Patricia, *La chambre des merveilles* (Paris: Bayard, 2003).

Findlen, Paula, *Possessing Nature. Museums, Collecting and Scientific Culture in Early Modern Italy* (Berkley-London: University of California Press, 1994).

Galech Amillano, Jesús María, 'Las piedras preciosas en la materia médica renacentista', in *Dioscórides ante el mundo*. pp. 187–215.

Gems in the Early Modern World. Materials, Knowledge and Global Trade, 1450-1800, ed. by Michael Bycroft and Sven Dupré (Cham: Palgrave Macmillan, 2019).

Giardino dei Semplici. L'Orto botanico di Pisa dal XVI al XX secolo, ed. Fabio Garbari, Lucia Tongiorgi Tomasi, and Alessandro Tosi (Pisa: Cassa di Risparmio di Pisa, Pacini, 1991).

'Historia'. Empiricism and Erudition in Early Modern Europe, ed. by Gianna Pomata and Nancy Siraisi (Cambridge Mass.: The MIT Presse, 2005).
La licorne et le bézoard. Une histoire des cabinets de curiosités (Montreuil: Gorcuff Gradenigo, 2013).
Lieux de savoir, ed. by Christian Jacob (Paris: Albin Michel, 2007-2011).
Loureiro, Rui Manuel, 'Enter the Milanese Lapidary: Precious Stones in Garcia de Orta's *Coloquios dos simples, e drogas he cousas mediçinais da India* (Goa, 1563)', *Journal of History of Science and Technology*, 8 (2013), 29–47.
Lugli, Adalgisa, *Naturalia et mirabilia: il collezionismo enciclopedico nelle Wunderkammern d'Europa* (Milan, Mazzotta, 1983).
Marrache-Gouraud, Myriam, *La légende des objets. Le cabinet des curiosités réfléchi par son catalogue: Europe, XVIe-XVIIe siècles* (Geneva: Droz, 2020).
Menghini, Alessandro and Felicita Menghini Di Biagio, *Paolo III. Pillole e Profezie. Astrologia e medicina alla corte papale del Cinquecento* (Città di Castello: Petruzzi Editore, 2004).
Morello, Nicoletta, 'Alle radici della geologia sistematica: il XVI secolo', *Geologica romana*, 29 (1993), 567–82.
Natural Things in Early Modern Worlds, ed. by Mackenzie Cooley, Anna Toledano, Duygu Yildirim (Abingdon-New York: Routledge, Taylor & Francis Group, 2023).
Nelson Novoa, James, 'El horizonte oriental de los mercaderes portugueses en Roma (1555-1655)', *Cuadernos de historia moderna*, 48.2 (2023), 539–61.
Olmi, Giuseppe, *L'inventario del mondo. Catalogazione della natura e luoghi del sapere nella prima età moderna* (Bologna: Il Mulino, 1992).
Ortroy, François van, 'Le Pape Saint Pie V', *Analecta Bollandiana*, 33 (1914), 187–215.
Palmer, Richard, 'Medicine at the Papal Court in the XVI century', in *Medicine at the Courts of Europe 1500-1837*, ed. by Vivian Nutton (London-New York: Routledge, 1990), pp. 49–78.
Pardo-Tomás, José, 'Bezoar', in *New World Objects of Knowledge: A Cabinet of Curiosities*, ed. by Mark Thurner and Juan Pimentel (London: University of London Press, 2021), pp. 195–200.
Pathology in Practice: Diseases and Dissections in Early Modern Europe, ed. by Marco Bresadola, Maria Conforti, and Silvia De Renzi (London-New York: Routledge, 2018).
Pérez de Tuleda, Almudena and Anne-Marie Jordan Geschwend, 'Renaissance Menageries. Exotic Animals and Pets at the Habsburg Courts in Iberia and Central Europe', in *Early Modern Zoology: the Construction of Animals in Science, Literature and the Visual Arts*, ed. by Karl A. Enenkel and Paul Smith (Leiden: Brill, 2007), pp. 419–47.
Pimentel, Juan and Isabel Soler, 'Dioscórides en Goa. Garcia de Orta, Davo y las tramas orientales de la materia medica renacentista', in *Dioscorides ante el mundo*, pp. 147–183.
Pomata, Gianna, '*Praxis historialis*. The uses of Historia in early modern medicine', in *Historia*, pp. 105–46.
Pomata, Gianna, 'Sharing Cases: the *Observationes* in Early Modern Medicine', *Early Science and Medicine*, 15.3 (2010), 193–236.
Reinbacher, Rudolph, *Healing Earths. The Third Leg of Medicine: A History of Minerals in Medicine with Rare Illustrations from 300 to 1000 Years Ago* (Bloomington, IN: 1st Book Library, 2003).
Siraisi, Nancy, 'L'individuale nella medicina tra medioevo e umanesimo: i casi clinici', in *Umanesimo e medicina. Il problema dell'individuale*, ed. by. Roberto Cardini and Mario Regoliosi (Rome: Bulzoni, 1996), pp. 33–62.
Siraisi, Nancy, *History, Medicine, and the Traditions of Renaissance Learning* (Ann Arbor: University of Michigan Press, 2007).
Stephenson, Marcia, 'From Marvelous Antidote to the Poison of Idolatry: The Transatlantic Role of Andean Bezoar Stones during the Late Sixteenth and Early Seventeenth Centuries', *Hispanic American Historical Review*, 90.1 (2009), 3–39.
Thorndike, Lynn, *A History of Magic and Experimental Science* (New York: Columbia University Press, 1923-1958).
Tomassetti, Stefano, *Cura corporum. Carità, medicina e religione nell'Oratorio filippino (secoli XVI–XVII)* (Rome: Viella, in print).
Touber, Jetze, 'Stones of Passions: Stones in the Internal Organs as Liminal Phenomena between Medical and Religious Knowledge in Renaissance Italy', *Journal of the History of Ideas*, 74.1 (2013), 23–44.
Touber, Jetze, *Law, Medicine and Engineering in the Cult of the Saints in Counter-Reformation Rome: The Hagiographical Works of Antonio Gallonio, 1556-1605* (Leiden-Boston: Brill, 2014).

6
Translating New World Drugs in Late Renaissance Italy:
The Case of Indies Balsam

Sharon Strocchia (ORCID 0000-0002-0315-7543)

This essay asks how an indigenous drug called Indies balsam moved from the fields of Hispaniola in the 1520s to the authorized pages of the Florentine pharmacopeia forty years later. Recent studies have shown that medicinal substances played a significant role in the commercial motives and political justification for colonial projects in the Americas from the sixteenth through the eighteenth centuries.[1] Yet many questions remain about how New World drugs were 'translated' for everyday use in European medical practice. Translating medicinals was not simply a matter of introducing unfamiliar substances into new areas: it involved complex discursive and material transformations of medical knowledge, healing objects, and embodied practices for new purposes and audiences. At the heart of this process were movement across geographic, cultural, and linguistic boundaries, alterations in the goods and knowledge being exchanged, and intentionality on the part of historical actors in making texts, practices, and products usable in different settings.[2] Although the translation of New World drugs shared common traits with the cultural reframing of food plants—physical identification, hands-on experience, information exchange—it prompted a higher degree of analogizing between Old and New World *naturalia* to identify similar curative properties and map new meanings onto them.[3]

Among the many forces at work in this multilayered process were commercial initiatives and innovative marketing strategies that generated knowledge about New World drugs while promoting their acceptance. The market played an outsized role in translating unfamiliar medicinals for European consumption not simply in terms of volume or price point, but in catalyzing empirical practices that underpinned coveted licensing privileges and inclusion in official pharmacopeia. Both the Spanish Crown and Italian states were at the forefront of these developments, despite asymmetries in geopolitical power. For instance, Italian states pioneered the award of patent privileges as a commercial stimulus following the passage of the first general patent law in Venice (1474); the Spanish Crown later made extensive use of these types of temporary monopolies in exploiting the natural resources of the Americas.[4] Italian states also led the way in developing drug formularies with the 1499 publication of the Florentine civic pharmacopeia—a standardized listing of the ingredients, recipes, and procedures that guild-licensed apothecaries had to follow when compounding remedies. This pathbreaking volume underwent several revisions over the next two centuries, during which time similar compilations sprang up across Europe.[5] The inclusion of certain medicaments in civic formularies gave them tremendous staying power as well as real competitive

1. Key studies include Schiebinger, *Plants and Empire*; Schiebinger and Swan, eds, *Colonial Botany*; Norton, *Sacred Gifts;* Boumediene, *La colonisation du savoir.*
2. Alberts, Fransen, and Leong, 'Translating Medicine'; Barrera-Osorio, 'Translating Facts'; Wintroub, Translations'.
3. Gentilcore, 'Impact of New World Plants'; Podgorny, 'The Elk, the Ass'. See also the essays in *Knowledge in Translation.*
4. Mandich, 'Privative industriali veneziane'; Barrera-Osorio, 'Local Herbs, Global Medicines'.
5. Corradi, *Le prime farmacopee italiane;* Huguet Termes, 'Standardising Drug Therapy'. Italian states that developed their own formularies included Mantua (1547), Bologna (1574), Siena (1577), Bergamo (1580), Rome (1583), Naples (1642), and Milan (1668). Other cities that created their own

advantage. To maintain much-needed elasticity, approved substitutes could be used to replace missing or unavailable ingredients.[6]

The case of Indies balsam studied here offers several important perspectives on the role of the market in translating New World drugs for Iberian and Italian consumers in the first half of the sixteenth century. First, it connects a fragmented global history of *materia medica* in ways that highlight contingency, nodes of convergence, and the agency of historical actors who are often hidden in the textual record.[7] Second, it foregrounds how commercial considerations spurred the development of empirical testing on both sides of the Atlantic. Although testing drugs on humans and animals had a long history in Western and Islamic medicine, these practical investigations assumed new probative importance after 1500 as the number and volume of imported drugs increased, and as experimentation became a more powerful tool for scientific inquiry.[8] The most spectacular of these demonstrations were so-called 'poison trials' that used human and animal subjects to test the efficacy of both foreign and familiar antidotes.[9] Although these high-stakes trials raised unique ethical issues due to their potentially fatal outcomes, hundreds of less dramatic trials involving ordinary medicaments like Indies balsam took place in hospitals, prisons, and princely courts across the Italian peninsula after 1550. Ranging in scale from a handful of subjects to upwards of a thousand people, these everyday experiments were prompted less by princely curiosity than by burgeoning commercial demands, such as the pursuit of marketing licenses and patent privileges by small-scale vendors, family businesses, itinerant healers, and established medical practitioners.[10]

Finally, understanding the role of the market in translating Indies balsam complicates conventional dichotomies between early modern medical theory and practice. Trials of imported substances created both a practical framework and an intellectual space in which the respective knowledge claims of authoritative classical texts and hands-on empirical practices could be hammered out. Because New World medicaments had little textual history compared to the ancient drugs noted by Pliny and Dioscorides, European practitioners relied more heavily on empirical sources of information such as testing and clinical observation to understand their therapeutic value. Yet many early clinical trials had inconclusive outcomes or otherwise failed to establish reliable knowledge. These forays showcased the probative limits of early modern experimentation and opened questions about who was authorized to interpret results.[11]

The essay begins by introducing the history of balsam as a medicinal substance and surveying the methods early modern Europeans used to evaluate medicaments. Part Two turns to the indigenous origins of this substance and the initial acts of translation in Hispaniola and Spain that led to its commercial success. These included a robust promotional campaign involving multiple field tests in Spanish hospitals, the production of eyewitness testimonies by well-placed physicians, and the publication of a vernacular treatise explaining the balsam's therapeutic uses. The third part probes the comprehensive trial of Indies balsam held at the Medici court in 1561. Because that investigation was linked to the award of monopoly privileges, it generated an exceptionally detailed account by top health officials; it also impacted the decision whether to include this

---

pharmacopeia were Barcelona (1535), Saragoza (1546), Nuremberg (1546), Cologne (1565), London (1618), Amsterdam (1633), and Paris (1638); Minuzzi, *Sul filo dei segreti*, pp. 45-46. See also the essays in *Drugs on the Page*.

6. Boumediene and Pugliano, 'La route des succédanés'.
7. Recent scholars have pointed to the value of 'itineraries' as an analytical framework for understanding both knowledge production and commodity exchange. See Leong, 'When the Tallamys Met John French'; Safier, 'Global Knowledge on the Move'; Smith, 'Itineraries of Materials and Knowledge'.
8. McVaugh, 'Determining a Drug's Properties'. For accounts of early testing practices and protocols, see Guerrini, *Experimenting with Humans and Animals*, who observes that animals have historically borne the brunt of drug testing. Other studies include Álvarez Millán, 'Drug Testing'; and Maehle, *Drugs on Trial*.
9. Rankin, *Poison Trials*, p. 3, notes that over a dozen documented poison trials on condemned criminals took place in Italy, France, and the Holy Roman Empire between 1524 and 1600. Other poison trials using animal subjects add to that total. The Spanish king Philip II, for instance, first trialed tobacco on a small dog to verify reports that it could counteract poison; Norton, *Sacred Gifts*, p. 117.
10. Rankin and Rivest, 'Medicine, Monopoly, and the Premodern State', sketch some of the important connections between empirical testing and marketing privileges in the early modern period. Minuzzi, *Sul filo dei segreti*, emphasizes the social diversity of applicants for early modern Venetian marketing licenses, dismantling the idea of a competitive divide between charlatans and university-trained physicians as an explanation for increased testing.
11. Rankin and Leong, 'Testing Drugs and Trying Cures'.

medicament in the revised civic formulary a few years later. By stressing the role of the market throughout this process, the essay shows that commercial considerations stimulated the frequency of early clinical trials, highlighted their limitations, and jeopardized the reliability of their results.

BALSAM AS MATERIA MEDICA AND GLOBAL COMMODITY

Known since the days of Pliny, 'Old World' balsam was a resinous plant extract harvested in Egypt and Judea that was used to treat wounds, eye ailments, and other conditions.[12] Balsam had been a staple in the Mediterranean medicine chest for centuries, but its economic value soared after 1400 partly due to its inclusion in theriac, an ancient poison antidote also used as a prophylactic against plague. As the number of published plague tracts increased in the sixteenth century, theriac gained greater visibility as both a preventive and curative remedy in the Renaissance armamentarium.[13] Given the intense demand for theriac in these plague-ridden centuries as well as balsam's use as a stand-alone remedy, this precious extract was literally worth its weight in gold when marketed for distribution around the Mediterranean. By the 1550s, however, a combination of privateering, dwindling supplies, and rising geopolitical tensions in the eastern Mediterranean jeopardized its availability throughout Europe. Imports of this substance declined rapidly in the second half of the century; by 1615, Mediterranean balsam had become so scarce that the Medici Grand Duke Cosimo II reportedly paid a rich Egyptian merchant in Livorno a pound of silver for one ounce.[14]

These pressing supply-side problems were offset by the almost providential appearance of a similar substance from the other side of the globe. Commonly called Indies balsam, this cultivar, which flourished in the West Indies, Colombia, and Peru, became one of the most commercially valuable exports from the Americas by 1600. Spanish colonial agents touted its medicinal 'virtues' or healing powers as early as the 1520s, when the Crown began ceding monopoly interests to interested bioprospectors like the entrepreneur Antonio Villasante discussed below. Some Italian princes and prelates who had been gifted specimens of New World balsam for its curiosity value tried unsuccessfully to grow this cultivar locally in hopes of launching native industries.[15] In the seventeenth century, Jesuit missionaries facilitated the transmission of this plant from Spanish America to China and Japan, where the resin was highly prized not only for its aromatic and medicinal properties but also for its use in embalming the dead.[16] Thus Indies balsam simultaneously represented an 'exotic' medicinal plant to Renaissance Italians and a welcome substitute for a familiar but endangered bioresource.

Given the tight connections between body, place, and health in Hippocratic theory, new *materia medica* like Indies balsam provoked great debate among sixteenth-century European medical professionals. On the one hand, the exotic nature of unfamiliar plants held real allure for a society fascinated by the new and the marvelous; on the other, botanicals not mentioned by revered ancient writers aroused deep suspicion.[17] Complicating these issues even further was the question of whether wonder drugs from the New World were suitable for treating European bodies.[18] Even the Spanish physician Nicolás Monardes, who played an outsized role in classifying New World medicaments, initially hesitated to use substances about which 'there was nothing written nor knowne', preferring instead to rely on 'the Medicines that we had heere, of which there was so greate experience and knowledge, in written Authors'.[19]

In view of these cautions, the first step in translating New World drugs centered on assigning specific Galenic qualities so that learned practitioners could determine their therapeutic uses. For example, Monardes considered

12. Milwright, 'Balsam in the Mediaeval Mediterranean'; Milwright, 'Balsam of Matariyya'. See also Barrera-Osorio, 'Local Herbs, Global Medicines'.
13. Di Gennaro Splendore, 'The Triumph of Theriac', 433, states that '[e]arly modern authors wrote about theriac more often and more regularly than about any other drug'.
14. BNCF, TARG. 211. 12, #12, unpaginated.
15. Dal Canto, 'I fratelli Campi'.
16. Schottenhammer, '"Peruvian balsam"'.
17. Pugliano, 'Non-colonial Botany'.
18. Rankin, 'Empirics, Physicians, and Wonder Drugs', summarizes some of the debates surrounding the use of indigenous Eurasian and foreign drugs.
19. Monardes, *Joyfull Newes*, I, fol. 25.

tobacco to be hot and dry in the second degree.[20] In the humoral understanding of the time, these properties could counteract excessive cold or moist humors that caused afflictions like epilepsy and catarrh. In other words, tobacco's hot and dry qualities provided the necessary heat to restore a healthy humoral balance.[21] Using Galen's *De complexionibus* as a starting point, European physicians followed two time-honored paths to determine the properties of drugs: reasoning through sensory attributes like taste, color, and odor (*via rationis*); and hands-on experimentation (*via experimentis*). Around 1300 university medical faculties began to develop a more systematic program for determining a drug's properties, supplementing Galen's insights with ideas advanced by the medieval Arabic physician Ibn Sīnā.[22] Information obtained through sensory reasoning and direct experimentation allowed medical practitioners to locate unfamiliar drugs within a known theoretical universe while confirming their physiological effects in practice. These assessments helped to Europeanize foreign medicaments, first by making them theoretically intelligible and then by showing that they were clinically effective.

Once practitioners had determined a drug's properties, medicaments still had to be calibrated to suit individual health needs, which were conditioned by age, gender, birthplace, humoral complexion, climate, and the season. In 1563 the Portuguese physician Garcia da Orta, active in Goa, explained that he took these factors into account when using guaiacum and china root as syphilis remedies in his own clinical practice. Da Orta noted that a remedy should be given 'with reference to the quality and character of the patient, then to the nature of the illness, the season, the country, the heat, the cold, the sex and age of the person who takes it' to ensure its effectiveness as well as the correct dosage.[23] As physicians, apothecaries, and other knowledgeable persons gauged imported medicaments over time, some botanicals were judged to be unsuitable for certain European complexions. An itinerant vendor in Florence, for instance, was heavily fined in 1617 for selling 'certain seeds' from the Indies called 'Turkish beans'. This remedy, known to possess exceptionally hot therapeutic properties, was considered to be dangerous to the health of local inhabitants, who lacked the 'right complexion' to take such a strong purgative.[24] Thus even when New World drugs had been assigned specific properties, variations in humoral complexions and environmental conditions meant that they had to be tested multiple times on multiple subjects to establish their efficacy and resulting commercial value.

VILLASANTE'S BALSAM

The story of Indies balsam began in the Spanish town of Burgos, when sixteen-year-old Antonio Villasante sought his fortune in the Indies as a crew member on the second Columbian voyage. In 1496, he took up permanent residence in Santo Domingo, where he expanded his landholdings and consolidated his social position. Over the next two decades, Villasante developed amicable relations with local Amerindians; his marriage to Catalina de Ayahibex, a high-born Taino woman who converted to Catholicism, proved instrumental to his success in the medicines trade. Building on the practical knowledge she and her family had accumulated as well as his own botanizing experience, Villasante vigorously promoted the commercial cultivation of this plant, variously known as *guaconax*, *boni*, or *canaguey* depending on locale. He began the long process of translation by calling its resinous extract 'balsam,' thereby connecting it to a familiar European substance. The act of transferring this name across continents brought with it a layered set of medical meanings and practices that encouraged the remedy's acceptance on both sides of the Atlantic.[25] Common extraction methods further strengthened analogies between old and new varieties. Native peoples slit the bark of this plant to yield a thick exudation akin to the Mediterranean substance called *opobalsamum*, which they used as an antiseptic, styptic, and general wound remedy. Villasante argued that this common method of harvesting balsam provided persuasive proof of likeness between old and new. Yet his balsam was not a raw material obtained

20. Norton, *Sacred Gifts*, pp. 114–17. On Monardes's role in classifying medicaments, see Bleichmar, 'Books, Bodies, and Fields'; and Rankin, 'New World Drugs'.
21. On the theoretical classifications and therapeutic actions of New World drugs, see Estes, 'European Reception of the First Drugs'.
22. McVaugh, 'Determining a Drug's Properties'.
23. Da Orta, *Colloquies*, p. 380.
24. ASFi, OSMN, Vol. 199, fols 347ʳ–348ʳ, dated 6 May 1617: 'in questi paesi sono pericolissimi non (es)sendo le complessioni atte.'
25. Podgorny, 'The Elk, the Ass', p. 66.

directly from the plant but a manufactured product involving complex mechanical processing—grinding, maceration, evaporation, sieving, bottling—that set it apart from indigenous production methods.[26] A lesser-grade product could be obtained by decocting the leaves and wood (called *xilobalsamum* in ancient texts); both could be mixed with other liquids to increase their volume. In addition, the plant exuded a vinegar-like substance that could be combined with the sap and some wax to make a topical ointment, further emphasizing resemblances with the ancient medicament. Early European chroniclers of the Indies like Pietro Martire d'Anghiera (1530) and Gonzalo Fernández de Oviedo (1535), who were familiar with the original Mediterranean remedy, praised the curative powers of these processed indigenous substances as their use spread throughout the Caribbean.[27]

Villasante offered a detailed, point-by-point recitation of the drug's curative powers when petitioning the Spanish Crown for marketing privileges in 1526, touting it as a near panacea for treating cuts, wounds, and swellings, as well as gout, nerve pain, toothaches, and digestive problems. He emphasized that these healing properties had either been 'proven by experience' through repeated empirical demonstrations *(esperiencias)* or related by reputable physicians.[28] Two years later, he sought more lucrative patent privileges, backed by a Genoese trading firm headquartered in Seville.[29] To obtain the patent, he was required to submit a comprehensive report detailing the plant's physical appearance, habitat, and production methods. This account drew extensively on indigenous knowledge but reframed it for an Iberian bureaucratic and commercial audience. As a businessman, Villasante never tried to explain the physiological processes by which his product achieved such good results. What mattered for his audience was its proven practical value that would translate into profits.[30]

Patent in hand, Villasante and his trading partners launched an innovative, three-pronged business strategy to promote the balsam in Iberian markets.[31] In 1530 the firm recruited prominent Spanish physicians to provide endorsements, encouraged adoption by large-scale consumers like hospitals and monasteries, and commissioned a vernacular treatise that certified the balsam's therapeutic value. Their goal was to create convincing medical knowledge about this product through a combination of authoritative texts and empirical trials in order to develop robust markets for it throughout Spain and satellite areas. Iberian medical consumers reportedly were quick to adopt New World remedies, although that eagerness may be less a sign of cultural receptivity than a reflection of massive promotional campaigns conducted under the guise of empiricism.[32]

Central to the firm's tactics was the use of eyewitness testimonies by medical professionals. Scholars have noted the importance of witnesses in producing and legitimizing medical knowledge but have disagreed about the significance of social status in determining the perceived value of their information.[33] The consortium immediately turned to well-recognized Spanish practitioners to validate the balsam, making only perfunctory use of first-hand reports offered by soldiers, merchants, and indigenous peoples. Although physicians and surgeons in the Crown of Aragon had been called upon to testify as expert witnesses in judicial proceedings since the late fourteenth century, their public responsibilities had never extended to endorsing products for commercial purposes.[34]

To seed the balsam's commercial reputation, the firm asked twenty-nine carefully chosen practitioners working in virtually every corner of Spain to trial it on local

26. Schäfer, 'Antonio de Villasante', includes detailed information about how this medicinal was prepared. Pereda López, 'Antonio de Villasante', p. 8, stresses Villasante's personal familiarity with the plant, reflected in his extensive description of its height, bark, leaves, fruit, and habitat. A full transcription of his report is published in *Santo Domingo en los Manuscritos de Juan Bautista Muñoz*, pp. 449–53.
27. Fernández de Oviedo, *Historia general y natural de las Indias*, Bk. X, Cap. III; Pardo Tomás and López Terrada, *Las primeras noticias sobre plantas americanas*, pp. 216–18.
28. *Santo Domingo en los Manuscritos de Juan Bautista Muñoz*, pp. 451–52.
29. The Genoese firm was headed by Franco Leardo and Pedro Benito de Basiniana; Pereda López, 'Antonio de Villasante', pp. 10–11, details their financial arrangements.
30. The royal physician on Hispaniola noted important qualitative differences between this substance and the Old-World variety, but nevertheless confirmed the remedy's healing powers; Barrera-Osorio, 'Local Herbs, Global Medicines', pp. 166–72.
31. González Bueno, Cueli Trelle, and Ramos Carrillo, '"Cierta merced en el bálsamo…"'.
32. Norton, *Sacred Gifts*, pp. 109–14.
33. Shapin, *Social History of Truth*, stresses the importance of social status in persuasive acts of witnessing; by contrast, Barrera-Osorio, 'Translating Facts', p. 325n, argues that, in an Atlantic World context, direct experience carried 'more weight than the social status of the informant'.
34. García-Ballester, McVaugh, and Rubio-Vela, *Medical Licensing and Learning*, pp. 16–17.

hospital patients and private clients in April 1530, using precious samples they distributed *gratis*.[35] The men, who were handsomely compensated for their efforts, were asked to certify the balsam as a stand-alone remedy as a first step toward market penetration; they left aside its suitability as a substitute in theriac, where its full commercial potential could be realized. Other physicians and surgeons were recruited for this same task a few months later.[36] The resulting reports did not describe trial protocols in any detail, but they did praise the balsam's curative powers without reservation. Their unanimity suggests that these field tests were not thorough or unbiased investigations but rather were intended to reach predetermined results. Certainly, their experiments had a disproportionate impact on commercializing Indies balsam in Iberia, since these practitioners recommended large-scale purchases of medicaments in their roles as hospital visitors, court physicians, and public health consultants.

Similar promotional efforts were scaled up at charitable institutions across Spain to encourage product placement among large-volume consumers. In the spring and summer of 1530, generous samples of the balsam were donated *gratis* to principal hospitals in Toledo, Seville, Galicia, Burgos, Granada, and Santo Domingo de la Calzada, which collectively treated thousands of patients annually. A few months later, the consortium sent a supply to the royal monastery of Santa Maria de Guadalupe, renowned for its medical and botanical activities, to trial in its infirmary. Once again, hospital wardens and monastic officials were asked to issue written reports certifying the balsam's healing powers; once again, the results were uniformly positive. In fact, the effusive testimonial penned by the prior of Guadalupe functioned as an extended advertisement that was later appended to the printed treatise on balsam discussed below to enhance its promotional value.[37]

The crown jewel in this novel business strategy was the commission of a printed treatise describing the balsam's medicinal virtues. Written by the Sevillian physician García Pérez de Morales, the tract, published in September 1530 and titled *Tractado del Balsamo y de sus utilidades para las enfermedades del cuerpo humano,* became the definitive text on Indies balsam as well as the standard means for advertising it.[38] Pérez Morales held a chair in the medical faculty at the Colegio de Santa María de Jesús (later the University of Seville) and eventually became Monardes's mentor and father-in-law. He personally consulted with Villasante about promising indigenous medicaments for European markets when the latter visited Seville in 1529.[39] The Habsburg emperor Charles V, who commissioned the treatise, reportedly asked him 'to observe and experiment' with the balsam on local patients and issue the results in book form—a task for which he received 200 ducats.[40] Like other Iberian colleagues, Pérez Morales focused on the balsam as a stand-alone remedy, not as a potential substitute in theriac. This approach allowed him to sidestep thorny intellectual issues regarding drug substitutes as well as local differences in theriac recipes, which were closely guarded secrets; it also suggests the gradual, step-by-step approach to market penetration adopted by Iberian merchants and monarchs. The resulting publication was distributed with balsam samples sent to hospitals, monasteries, and court physicians to explain the remedy's medicinal virtues and uses. Although the choice of the vernacular meant that the book lacked the intellectual authority of Latin, it conversely gave the work crossover appeal to apothecaries, barber-surgeons, bath masters, and other practice-based healers.

What made this tract such an effective promotional vehicle was its skillful blend of clinical observation and textual authority. Organized in ten chapters that moved from head to toe like a vernacular health regimen, the book intermingled the everyday language of illness with frequent citations to Galen, Mesue, and other canonical writers. As the author tacked back and forth between vernacular and learned registers, he turned the usual methods of determining pharmacological properties on

35. The physicians practiced in Seville, Toledo, Segovia, Madrid, Granada, Cadiz, Baeza, S. Domingo de la Calzada, and at the court itself; Alegre Pérez, 'El balsamo descubierto por Antonio Villasante'.
36. Most members of this group received 50 ducats in exchange for their endorsement; González Bueno, Cueli Trelle, and Ramos Carrillo, '"Çierta merced en el bálsamo…,"' pp. 24–25.
37. Ibid., p. 24.
38. Pérez de Morales, *Tractado del Balsamo*.
39. González Bueno, Cueli Trelle, and Ramos Carrillo, '"Çierta merced en el bálsamo…,"' p. 34; Pereda López, 'Antonio de Villasante', p. 13.
40. Pérez Morales, *Tractado del Balsamo,* Prologue: 'para que y lo viesse e experimentasse;' Pereda López, 'Antonio de Villasante', pp. 13–14, provides additional details about his compensation.

their head. Rather than starting with sensory reasoning to understand the drug's theoretical qualities (later judged to be hot and dry in the second degree), he extrapolated them from extensive testing on patients; in other words, he used empirical practice as the basis for theorizing about the medicament, not the other way around. Most of his observations came from managing wounds inflicted by military weapons, starting with head wounds in classic Hippocratic fashion before moving down the body to the chest, abdomen, and limbs. In some instances, he mixed the imported balsam with other medicaments like rose honey and myrrh to create tailor-made ointments, for which he supplied the recipes.[41] Most often, Pérez Morales conducted these trials himself but included no names, places, or stories in his account, giving it a generic quality that contrasted sharply with the specificity of physicians' casebooks and practice journals.[42] In the closing chapters, he reported using the remedy successfully to treat internal ailments such as headaches, vertigo, melancholy, and dropsy in both hospital patients and private clients. After the balsam had been 'much proven and tested by me,' Pérez Morales concluded that it was indeed 'quite marvelous' as both an external and internal remedy.[43]

With the publication of this treatise, the firm had achieved its goals of certifying Indies balsam for Iberian medical professionals while boosting sales in Mediterranean distribution hubs. The imported product initially commanded high prices on par with its Old-World counterpart; when Indies balsam was first brought to Spain in 1526, it fetched ten to twenty ducats per ounce, while in Rome an ounce reportedly sold for 100 ducats.[44] Even though balsam trees yielded relatively small volumes, roughly 475 liters (29.5 *arrobas*) of this product entered Seville in 1532 alone due to increased cultivation and production on Hispaniola.[45] However, a cascade of events soon loosened Villasante's iron grip on the balsam trade. Charles V licensed German traders working in Venezuela to explore that region for other cultivars; Villasante died circa 1536, and the lawsuit brought by his heirs to maintain the monopoly was denied in 1539. Within a few decades, the product lost its trade name and became simply known as Indies balsam.[46]

BALSAM ON TRIAL IN MEDICI FLORENCE

As supplies of Indies balsam grew more plentiful by the mid-sixteenth century, Italian physicians, surgeons, and apothecaries hotly debated the equivalence of old and new varieties, comparing details of morphology and exudations in ways that advanced botanical and scientific knowledge across the peninsula.[47] These medical professionals, who sometimes doubled as botanists and naturalists, acted as commercial knowledge brokers for secondary markets and distribution hubs. What complicated their assessment of Indies balsam was the abundance of different Caribbean cultivars, the absence of standard nomenclature to describe them, and the fragmented or adulterated state of specimens and products upon arrival in Italian ports. At least eight different New World balsams were marketed in sixteenth-century Europe, each bearing a distinct (if generic) name and selling at different price points.[48]

Italian medical guilds responded to this rapidly shifting situation in different ways. Some Venetian pharmacies already stocked New World balsams in the 1560s, but their practices were not standardized because the city lacked an official pharmacopeia until 1617.[49] Indies balsam was mentioned among approved substitutes in theriac in the 1550 Florentine *ricettario,* which acknowledged that 'time has revealed new sorts of medicine'. However, this update—the first since the original compilation of 1499—was a cursory reworking by guild representatives, rather than a systematic overhaul like the third edition issued in 1567.[50] Nevertheless, Florence was in the vanguard of incorporating new drugs into its formulary

41. Pérez Morales, *Tractado del Balsamo,* Chap. 2.
42. On these genres of medical writing, see Stolberg, 'A Sixteenth-Century Physician and His Patients', and Pomata, 'Medical Case Narrative'.
43. Pérez Morales, *Tractado del Balsamo*, Chap. 7: 'muy maravilloso y pormi muy aprovado el dicho liquoro Balsamo y muy experimentado'.
44. Monardes, *Joyfull Newes,* I, fol. 8.
45. González Bueno, Cueli Trelle, and Ramos Carillo, '"Çierta merced en el bálsamo...,"' p. 32.
46. Pereda López, 'Antonio de Villasante', pp. 18–19.
47. Pugliano, 'Natural History in the Apothecary's Shop'.
48. López Piñero and López Terrada, *La influencia Española*, p. 144; see also Estes, 'European Reception of the First Drugs'.
49. Parrish, 'Marketing Nature', p. 258; Minuzzi, *Sul filo dei segreti,* p. 48.
50. *El ricettario dell'arte, et universita de medici, et spetiali della città di Firenze*, p. 3: 'il tempo mostrato nuove sorti di medicina'. On the 1550 edition, see Sonnedecker, 'Florentine Pharmacopeia'.

compared to its neighbors. The balsam was not listed in Bologna's 1574 pharmacopeia, which drew heavily on the botanical expertise of Ulisse Aldrovandi. Despite the heady circulation of information about New World plants in these decades, it took time to integrate this inchoate body of information into official European formularies.[51]

The opportunity to generate more secure knowledge about this wonder drug presented itself to the Medici court in mid-March 1561, when the Spanish physician Giovanni Sanchez petitioned Duke Cosimo for exclusive privileges to market 'balsam of the Indies' ('balsamo dell'Indie') throughout the Medici state.[52] The duchy represented a promising venue in which to secure a short-term monopoly, normally granted for a period of ten years. Even though Italy figured among the earliest outlets for Spanish colonial *materia medica,* the product known as Indies balsam had not yet gained a firm foothold by the time of his arrival, leaving an opening in the local market for this privilege.[53] Moreover, connections between Spain and Tuscany were exceptionally strong at this time; the marriage of Cosimo to Eleonora of Toledo two decades earlier and the significant capital investments Italian merchants had made in Iberian business ventures since the late fifteenth century cemented commercial relations. These ties were further strengthened in the early 1550s when the transplanted Florentine banker Raffaele Acciaiuoli and other partners in Lisbon, Seville, and the court city of Valladolid joined the Genoese trading firm as distributors of indigenous medicaments.[54]

Whether Sanchez was working for the firm or acting on his own, he appeared at guild headquarters carrying small-scale models of his distillation equipment, along with a copy of the balsam tract published thirty years earlier. This enterprising physician, a native of Granada who had spent seven years in the West Indies, reportedly wanted to recoup some of his investment in learning how to distill this precious liquor by obtaining exclusive rights to its distribution. A year earlier (1560), Roman medical officials had awarded him a sales license valid in perpetuity 'to market a balsam or liquor from the west [...] similar to and with the same medicinal virtues as eastern balsam, which can be substituted in the composition of theriac'.[55] His Florentine patent application was supported by a now-lost affidavit sworn by the apothecary Stefano Rosselli, one of the main pharmaceutical suppliers to the ducal court, who asserted that this liquor was 'a noble thing'. Apparently, Rosselli had already received a complimentary sample, which he eagerly forwarded to the duke and guild officials. In fact, it was Rosselli who pressed for approval so that local apothecaries would have a reliable source of a rapidly diminishing commodity. His interest was not purely altruistic, however, since he had already contracted to buy four ounces of the balsam from Sanchez and was eager to purchase more when available.[56]

Despite Rosselli's backing, the Medici duke opted to follow standard practice for patent awards by gathering as much preliminary information as possible. To satisfy his longstanding interests in medical botany, Cosimo decided to send a practiced botanist 'to the Indies to bring back some simples from those regions in order to prove if they have the same virtue, or if there are other types that have greater virtues than ours'.[57] In the meantime, he instructed the local College of Physicians to issue a thorough report about the theoretical properties of Indies balsam, the ailments it could treat, and the medicinal compounds in which it could be used.

The ensuing report, written in an elegant humanist hand, offers one of the most comprehensive accounts of drug testing anywhere in Renaissance Europe. Although the detailed nature of the report is unusual, the practice of

51. Rotelli, 'Exotic Plants'.
52. ASFi, OSMN, Vol. 193, fasc. 113-117. I am using the Italianized version of the physician's surname, which is used interchangeably with the Spanish (Sances) in the dossier.
53. Pardo Tomás, 'Obras Españolas'.
54. González Bueno, Cueli Trelle, and Ramos Carrillo, '"Çierta merced en el bálsamo...,"' pp. 28, 30. Raffaele Acciaiuoli, who belonged to one of the oldest Florentine families, maintained robust credit relations with the Medici court. In 1552, he covered the huge debt of 3,000 ducats incurred by Don Luis de Toledo, brother of the Medici Duchess Eleonora of Toledo, on her behalf; Hernando Sánchez, 'Naples and Florence in Charles V's Italy', p. 173.
55. Bertolotti, 'La medicina, chirurgia e farmacia in Roma', p. 230: 'Perpetua a Maestro Giov. Sancies naturale di Granata, mercante di droghe occidentali, per vendere un balsamo o liquore occidentale, estratto da albero, vegetante nelle Indie occidentali, simile e con le stesse virtù del balsamo orientale, al quale poteva esser sostituito nella composizione della Teriaca'.
56. ASFi, OSMN, Vol. 193, fasc. 117, dated 12 March 1561. For Rosselli's experimental activities and collections of secrets, see Strocchia, *Forgotten Healers*, under index.
57. 'Relazione di Firenze di Messer Vincenzo Fedeli', p. 356: '...lo voleva mandare nell'Indie per riportare delli semplici di quelle parti, per farne prova se sono dell'istessa virtù, o se ve ne sono d'altre sorti di maggiore che non sono dalle nostre bande'.

trying out remedies on hospital patients was commonplace by this time. Public health officials in Venice and Padua had already begun conducting large-scale trials of plague remedies in local plague hospitals *(lazaretti)* in the 1550s, many for commercial reasons.[58] Closer to home, guild reforms enacted in Florence in 1560 required that anyone wishing to practice medicine or sell remedies in the Medici state had to be licensed in one of two ways: either they could pass an oral examination based on canonical texts; or they could conduct a small-scale empirical trial *(prova)* under guild supervision to demonstrate a drug's efficacy.[59] This reform, reportedly proposed by Cosimo himself, marked a pivotal moment in the history of Italian medical practice, since it placed practice-based and text-based knowledge on a similar footing for credentialing purposes.

As the number of imported remedies and proprietary 'secrets' blossomed across the peninsula after 1560, dozens of clinical trials, mainly in the form of field tests conducted on hospital patients, took place in Medici Florence alone. Similar market-driven trials were staged in Venice, Mantua, Siena, Bologna, Genoa, Naples, and other major Italian cities after 1550 to evaluate medicaments ranging from vermifuges and medicinal oils to plague treatments and cancer cures.[60] Each locale set its own threshold for the required scale and demonstration of efficacy; in Florence, a small-scale field trial involving two to four subjects was set as the bare minimum, although some 'proof tests' could involve a thousand subjects or more. Because Sanchez had requested exclusive marketing privileges on the sales of Indies balsam, the standard of proof was especially high, with the exact level of efficacy to be determined by the duke in concert with the College of Physicians.

Conducting the Medici balsam trial were the court apothecary Rosselli along with three eminent practitioners, all members of the College of Physicians: the city's chief health officer Baccio Baldini, who headed the group; the salaried convent doctor Francesco da Gamberaia; and the respected rural practitioner Francesco da Montevarchi.[61] The group's mixed composition, with each member bringing a different background and skill-set, underscores the collaborative nature of early modern knowledge production. Baldini himself experimented with pharmaceutical remedies and became an active member of Medici experimental circles at the Casino di San Marco in the 1570s; his proprietary recipe for a topical ointment found its way into the 1597 edition of the Florentine *ricettario*.[62] The team reported the progress of the investigation to guild members every other week, which opened a space for licensed apothecaries, physicians, and surgeons to debate the relative medicinal virtues of old and new varieties; archival records indicate that some guild members had already formed strong opinions about their merits. Duke Cosimo wanted the inquiry to be conducted with all due speed in view of the pending patent application and the temporary suspension of theriac production until the question was resolved. However, proceedings were slowed by an insufficient supply of Indies balsam for testing. Only some crystallized residue remained in Sanchez' distillation equipment, so the guild sent to Rome for a large sample weighing two to three pounds.[63]

Following Galenic convention, the team began by reasoning from sensory information, using their well-schooled senses to determine the balsam's properties from its taste and smell. Italian apothecaries used these same methods to evaluate whether medicaments were fraudulent or had been adulterated.[64] To some team members, the substance tasted astringent, to others, more bitter. Despite these differences of opinion, they agreed that the balsam had a 'pleasing' odor, although it evaporated quickly. However, the Medici court physician Andrea Pasquali cast doubt on their conclusions by claiming that, in his prior experience with Indies balsam some years before, the product had been devoid of any smell. Frustrated by this disagreement, Baldini acknowledged that the senses could give rise to false or misleading information. Although scholars have argued for the complementarity of textual knowledge and experimentalism among Italian court physicians in

58. Stevens Crawshaw, *Plague Hospitals*, p. 153.
59. ASFi, Arte dei Medici e Speziali. Vol. 269, fol. 38^{r-v}.
60. I take up these and related issues in a forthcoming book.
61. The following discussion is based on ASFi, OSMN, Vol. 193, fasc. 113–17.
62. Marinozzi, Giuffra, and Kieffer, 'Baccio Baldini'.
63. ASFi, OSMN, Vol. 193, fasc. 117: 'egli ha qualche secreto in se stesso di fornelli et stillamenti et forma del cristallo con modelli di furnace da lavorarlo'.
64. Rotelli, 'Exotic Plants', pp. 834–35.

everyday practice, the trial to this point highlighted their inherent tensions.[65] In the end, the team was unable to derive definitive sensory evidence about its properties, but reached the provisional conclusion that Indies balsam was hot and dry in the second degree. These qualities presumably made it useful for an assortment of 'cold and humid' afflictions; at the same time, the practitioners sternly warned that the balsam should be administered only 'by learned and prudent persons' who were mindful that this was 'a new medicament' with unstudied effects on the body.[66]

To augment their understanding, the group turned next to textual authorities for guidance, but not surprisingly discovered no mention of this substance by ancient writers. Among modern authors, the only information came from the 1530 Spanish treatise by Pérez Morales. Here Baldini and his associates sharply reproached the Spanish physician for not describing his clinical and experimental methods more precisely. For instance, they chided him for his failure to report the exact dosage used or the length of treatment required before achieving results. In a similar vein, the Medici team noted that Pérez Morales often mixed balsam with other ingredients in his clinical applications; as a result, it was difficult to judge its intrinsic benefits. In their view, deficiencies in both the protocols and the written reporting of the Sevillian field trials undercut the utility of their evidence. Based on the information gathered to this point, the team expressed its initial preference for medicaments that had been 'approved' by the test of time to those that were still 'unknown'—a refrain repeated by Monardes a decade later. In the meantime, Cosimo solicited additional input from the city's apothecaries, who also expressed a strong preference for proven ingredients like clove oil or nutmeg oil as substitutes; Indies balsam remained their last choice.[67] Their conservative position should not be read as stiff-necked resistance to all new medicaments, however, but more as an expression of respect for hallowed pharmacy traditions.[68]

Having reached an impasse, the group concluded that only empirical testing could provide definitive evidence about the balsam's nature and worth. They first tried a physical experiment noted by Pliny, who observed that 'true' balsam solidified in hot water and sank to the bottom of a vessel, whereas falsified or adulterated versions floated to the top like oil mixed with water.[69] When the team tried it, the results proved inconclusive. Hence the only remaining pathway was to try the cure directly on the sick. Thus, in May 1561, the group administered it to four hospital patients suffering from conditions commonly treated with balsam. Involving hospital patients in early clinical trials proved advantageous for several reasons. These charitable institutions cared for the most vulnerable members of society—financially strapped, socially dislocated, and poor in relational resources. Once admitted to hospital, patients could be closely observed, their diet and medications monitored, their physical responses recorded. In addition, their subjective descriptions of bodily sensations generally were thought to be more reliable than the testimony of convicted criminals, at least in German-speaking lands.[70] Most importantly, these sick poor presented significant corporeal differences that were essential for gauging efficacy across variations in humoral complexion, age, gender, and length of illness. As Baldini himself noted, it was necessary to test a remedy on multiple subjects multiple times to obtain accurate results.[71]

The first patient treated was an unnamed man recovering from a head wound at the civic hospital of Santa Maria Nuova. Italian medical professionals considered head wounds to be among the most serious conditions they encountered; in fact, it was customary for Renaissance hospitals to have dedicated spaces for their care.[72] The man's injury provided a reasonable test case since it was severe but not life-threatening; although the

65. Marinozzi, Giuffra, and Kieffer, 'Baccio Baldini', pp. 355–56.
66. ASFi, OSMN, Vol. 193, fasc. 116: 'persone dotte e prudenti... considerino quello che importa usare un medicamento nuovo nel corpo nostro'.
67. Ibid.
68. Pugliano, 'Pharmacy, Testing, and the Language of Truth' argues that sixteenth-century Venetian apothecaries were inclined toward 'tweaking' or making incremental changes in recipes in order to preserve pharmacy traditions.
69. Schottenhammer, '"Peruvian balsam"', p. 3.
70. Heinrichs, 'Live Chicken Treatment'.
71. ASFi, OSMN, Vol. 193, fasc. 116: 'E non credere alla prima o seconda sperienza perchè e per la ragion detta e per la varietà de subbietti e mille altre occorrenze facilmente può ingannarne'. Schickore stresses the epistemic role of multiple repetitions in 'Trying Again and Again'.
72. Savoia, '*Book of the Sick*'.

wound was quite painful, 'it did not expose the bone'.[73] The team reportedly made every effort to avoid inflicting needless pain on their subjects, but applying Indies balsam inflamed his wound until it became filled with pus. Galen had considered the development of 'laudable pus' (*pus bonum et laudabile)* to be an important stage in the healing process, but this view had been repeatedly challenged by surgeons since the thirteenth century.[74] Since the Medici physicians were unsure how to interpret this sign, they suspended use and resumed treatment with a well-known resinous oil (*olio d'abezzo*), which cured the man in a few days.

Moving on to the second subject, the team then applied the remedy multiple times to relieve heavy discharge in the eyes of a young woman. Unfortunately, the Indies balsam caused her considerable pain with no benefit whatsoever, leading the physicians to stop the test.[75] To avoid another inconclusive outcome, however, the physicians trialed the remedy on another young female patient whose eyes 'were red and rather inflamed.' Like the previous subject, she too experienced intense pain with no perceptible benefit, so the therapy was discontinued.[76] Finally, the team shifted venue from Santa Maria Nuova to the smaller hospital of San Paolo, where they tested the balsam as a topical ointment on a man who had recently been castrated for unknown reasons. Here the results were more positive, with some improvement in his condition.[77] With three patients experiencing little benefit and one showing only minor gains, this field trial not only failed to demonstrate the balsam's curative powers but instead highlighted its negative side effects.

To fulfill their charge, however, the group also needed to establish whether Indies balsam could be substituted for the Mediterranean variety in theriac. In fact, most American botanicals were used as substitutes for Old World ingredients in compound medical remedies.[78] Here the physicians expedited their evaluation by using testing protocols developed in earlier poison trials. From the 1520s onwards, Renaissance popes and princes tested possible poison antidotes on dogs, birds, and condemned criminals. Most of these high-stakes experiments took place in court settings, although some Italian civic governments also conducted trials on persons sentenced to capital punishment.[79] These demonstrations were the first to develop a clear-cut methodology because poison could artificially induce identical symptoms in otherwise healthy subjects, thereby providing a more consistent baseline for evaluation.[80] Members of the Medici family had shown interest in these spectacles since the papacy of Clement VII. Cosimo himself had solicited a recipe for a poison antidote from Duke Ferrante Gonzaga in 1548, which he planned to test 'on someone destined to die'. Five years after the balsam trial, the duke ordered that another potential antidote should be tried on a condemned prisoner—a gruesome experiment for which Baldini kept a meticulous, step-by-step record.[81]

Using these evolving protocols, the Medici team selected three dogs to be used as test subjects in this portion of the balsam trial. All three animals were intentionally bitten by vipers; the balsam was then applied topically to the bite and also administered by mouth. Two of the dogs died shortly afterward but the third one survived, creating additional uncertainty about the remedy's effectiveness. In the absence of clear-cut evidence, the physicians stepped in to interpret the results. They speculated that the lucky dog might have survived because 'a great quantity of blood gushed out' from the snakebite, possibly releasing some of the venom before it

73. ASFi, OSMN, Vol. 193, fasc. 116: 'in S. Maria Nuova applicatolo sopra una ferita del capo senza scopertura dell'osso oltra il dargli dolore, et non piccolo lo riscaldo di sorte, che attraendovi materia cominciava piu tosto a infiammarsi che altramente onde lasciatolo stare e tornando a l'olio d'abezzo in pochi giorni fu guarita'.
74. For example, Henri de Mondeville, professor of surgery at Montpellier, viewed pus formation as a surgical complication, rather than a normal stage of healing.
75. ASFi, OSMN, Vol. 193, fasc. 116: 'Posto poi sopra gli occhi d'una giovane la quale vi haveva in panno da materia fredda con alquanto dolore, e senza benefitio alcuno dopo molte volte haverlo operato si abbandonò'.
76. Ibid.: 'Sopra gli occhi poi d'una altra, i quali erano rossi e alquanto infiammati messolo con dolore intensissimo non ne riportò frutto alcuno'.
77. Ibid.: 'Nello spedale poi di S. Pagolo s'unse uno il quale essendo stato castrato si convelleva e in costui certo si vedde qualche giovamento'.
78. Boumediene and Pugliano, 'La route des succédanés'.
79. Rankin, *Poison Trials;* Pastore, 'Médicine légale et investigation judiciaire'; Barker, 'Poisons and the Prince'. Bolognese officials tested a poison antidote on a condemned prisoner in 1540. The man died as a result, but his corpse was nevertheless hanged afterward to serve the cause of justice; Savoia, *'Book of the Sick'*, p. 180.
80. Gibbs, 'Poisonous Properties'.
81. Rankin, *Poison Trials,* pp. 2-3, 7-8. ASFi, MdP, Vol. 9, fols. 329r–330r, dated 11 January 1548: 'in qualcuno destinato a morte'. Marinozzi, Giuffra, and Kieffer, 'Baccio Baldini', provide a detailed account and full transcription of the 1566 poison trial.

could take effect.[82] Given these mixed results with both human and animal subjects, team members agreed that Indies balsam did not confer significant advantages in treating 'malignant, pestilential, or poisonous maladies' beyond the medicaments already available.[83] Without persuasive empirical proof or a rousing endorsement from prestigious local practitioners, Sanchez's petition to market his product throughout the Medici state languished at court.

Regardless, the failed trial did little to alleviate mounting pressures on local balsam supplies. Continued demand, along with steady exposure to imported medicaments, prompted Cosimo to update the civic formulary again under the direction of twelve appointed 'reformers.' This edition, issued in 1567, added fifty-eight new recipes and medicaments to the original sixty-nine, almost doubling the number of original listings.[84] Despite the concerns that had surfaced six years earlier, Baldini bowed to necessity and approved Indies balsam as a substitute for 'true' balsam in theriac, since it was one of the medicines 'which are impossible to provision at present'. This was a purely pragmatic decision and his approval remained guarded; the list of recommended substitutes echoed his original judgment that time-tested medicaments such as clove oil or distilled nutmeg oil could be used just as effectively in theriac and in fact were to be preferred.[85] Enhancing his argument was the view that traditional drugs were not only safer but also less expensive than imported balsam. Despite his grudging approval, Baldini must have wondered whether it was worth investing in an expensive import whose efficacy remained unclear. In light of these reservations, it is not surprising that only three other New World medicaments (guaiacum, sarsaparilla, china root) besides balsam were approved for inclusion in the 1567 Florentine pharmacopeia. All three were treatments for 'the pox' thought to have originated in the New World, which probably accelerated their adoption; contemporaries commonly argued that a beneficent God had placed a cure in the same areas where the disease had flourished.[86]

Over the next few years, Indies balsam remained a point of contention, despite growing support among some physicians, pharmacists, botanists, and traders. The Sienese physician Pietro Andrea Mattioli mentioned this substance in the 1568 edition of his best-selling commentary on Dioscorides's *materia medica*, where he noted that he had heard about it from the physician Luca Ghini, founder of the Pisan botanical garden. Still, he preferred to use his own recipe for an 'artificial' balsam that he had tried 'time and time again' to treat 'many, many' different kinds of ailments.[87] In fact, some Florentine apothecaries refused to use Indies balsam as a substitute in theriac, despite its approval in the formulary. Although the exact nature of their objections is unclear, in January 1573 Cosimo reported to his son Francesco—an avid experimenter in his own right—that the quarrel had grown quite heated. The duke hoped the controversy would be resolved once the absent Baldini returned to the city but emphasized that Indies balsam was here to stay 'because it has been approved by these physicians.'[88]

The publications of the Sevillian physician Monardes marked an important turning point in accepting the balsam's value while acknowledging its differences from the Old-World variety. Despite his initial reluctance to recommend unproven medicaments to a European audience, Monardes changed course with his first publication—a slender volume titled *Dos libros* issued in 1565—that trumpeted the healing powers of assorted New World drugs.[89] Over the next decade, he added two more tracts that melded practical indigenous knowledge,

82. ASFi, OSMN, Vol. 193, fasc. 116: 'Sonsi da vipere stirrite fatti mordere tre cani, due de quali con i strani accidenti ancho che unti con questo liquore e datognene per bocca finalmente non dopo molto spazio di tempo si morirono rattrappati, il terzo campò forse perchè subito che la vipera cavo il dente si vide scirrar fuori gran quantità di sangue col quale potette per avventura uscir anchora il veneno' (sic).
83. Ibid.: 'Il senso dunque è la sperienza ne mostrano che nell'uso della medicina egli non ne possa apportare gran giovamento havendo molti, e varii e approvati medicamenti i quali sicuramente vagliono il medesimo o più che questo, se gia da qualità occulta (hole in document) gli non conferisse nelle malattie malignie e pestilenziali e ne veleni, nelle quali indisposizioni la medicina manca di rimedi utili'.
84. Corradi, *Le prime farmacopee italiane*, p. 50.
85. *Il Ricettario medicinale*, pp. 18–19, quote at 113: 'In questo succidaneo sono notate alcune medicine semplice, le quali al presente è impossibile provedere'. The formulary also gave the balsam's indigenous name (*coagonax*), most likely for purposes of product identification.
86. Bellorini, *World of Plants*, pp. 129, 144–45, 152; Strocchia, *Forgotten Healers*, p. 46.
87. *Discorsi di M. Pietro Andrea Matthioli*, p. 67.
88. ASFi, MdP, Vol. 241, fol. 84, dated 7 January 1573: 'che per l'advenire chi fa la triaca col mitradato o altro lattovaro dove vadia l'opobalsamo, si possa in tutti mettere il balsamo del'Indie, perché pare che da questi medici sia approvato'. See also Bellorini, *World of Plants*, p. 145.
89. Monardes, *Dos libros*.

the recommendations of diverse informants, and his own extensive experience trying new medicaments on patients. The final compilation of these three texts, published in Spanish in 1574, became the definitive introduction to the medicinal riches of the Americas.[90] As Alisha Rankin has shown, it was this volume that sparked intense translation activity (in the sense of creating linguistic equivalencies) and made Monardes a household name.[91]

The 1575 Italian translation of this work, made by the Venetian printer Giordano Ziletti directly from the Spanish, openly acknowledged that Indies balsam was not identical to the Mediterranean variety but stated that it 'is no less good in medicinal virtues than the one from Egypt'.[92] Just as Villasante and Pérez Morales had done before him, Monardes and his translator Ziletti heaped praise on the remedy's prodigious healing powers. This mediated position—that the two substances were not identical, but that Indies balsam nevertheless possessed great therapeutic value—paved the way for intensive bioprospecting for balsam in Colombia, Peru, and Venezuela. Still, Italian medical professionals continued to disagree about its utility as a substitute in theriac both in their private correspondence and in a string of pamphlet wars lasting into the 1630s and 40s.[93]

CONCLUSION

Translating Indies balsam from the fields of Hispaniola to the pages of the Florentine pharmacopeia required multiple actions—some discursive, some empirical—that have larger implications for understanding the movement of *materia medica* in the first century of globalization. The process of analogizing between old and new medicinal substances brought with it the transfer of names and meanings that modified pharmaceutical practices on both sides of the Atlantic. In the case of Indies balsam, Villasante took the first step in Europeanizing this wonder drug by calling it 'balsam,' which placed it in a matrix of known referents for a bureaucratic and commercial audience. The Spanish physician Pérez Morales translated this substance for university-trained practitioners by assigning it specific Galenic properties, which helped them understand its potential uses and applications. Paradoxically, however, he arrived at these theoretical conclusions by trialing the remedy directly on patients.

Both the Iberian and Italian scenarios examined here highlight the importance of testing New World drugs on living subjects as a way to generate new medical knowledge about them. Still, it is crucial to recognize the role of the market in driving these inquiries. Conducting early clinical trials to obtain marketing licenses or patent privileges on unfamiliar wonder drugs involved significant socioeconomic investments by both medical and commercial agents as well as substantial engagement on the part of political authorities. In both cases studied here, the success or failure of these investigations was contingent upon demonstrations of perceived efficacy that were adjudicated and scaled up or down depending on the probative standards set by local political officials. What looms especially large in the Iberian example are the innovative business strategies developed by Spanish authorities and transnational trading firms to ensure the success of colonial products, including the unprecedented recruitment of medical practitioners who were paid to trial the balsam in local hospitals and monasteries and testify about it in writing. Certainly, the evaluative role they played underscores the importance of testimonials from expert witnesses both in seeding commercial reputation and in fostering product placement among large-scale consumers. Yet their uniformly positive judgments also point to the potential for biased empirical outcomes stemming from a combination of vested financial interests, heavy political pressures, competitive market forces, and reputational concerns—issues that continue to haunt pharmaceutical testing today.

The commercial stakes driving the acceptance of Indies balsam in mid-sixteenth-century Florence differed from the Spanish scenario in several ways. Forty years after the balsam's introduction to European consumers, the Medici duke could insist on a comprehensive empirical investigation before awarding patent privileges. Thanks in part to changing market conditions, this inquiry was more thorough than the Spanish field trials; intensive

90. Monardes, *Segunda parte del libro*; Monardes, *Primera y segunda y tercera partes de la historia medicinal*.
91. Rankin, 'New World Drugs', unpacks the ways that European translators appropriated, reframed, and suppressed parts of Monardes's work.
92. Monardes, *Delle cose*, Bk. I, Chap. 7: 'il quale è a mio parere non è in virtù medicinale men buono di quello d'Egitto'. Rankin, 'New World Drugs', pp. 73–75, discusses Ziletti's word-for-word approach to the translation.
93. See for example Campi, *Parere sopra il balsamo*, and Baldi, *Del vero opobalsamo orientale*.

bioprospecting in the greater Caribbean after 1530 had increased the supply of imported balsams, giving Italian practitioners greater exposure to these products as well as wider choice among them. But the careful, step-by-step approach taken by the Medici team also showcases how local pharmaceutical traditions acted as a brake on sudden innovations in official practice. Italian institutional pharmacy as codified in civic formularies was slow to change; new drugs often took many decades to become fully authorized by their inclusion in pharmacopeia. The fact that, in issuing a final decision about Indies balsam, Medici court practitioners preferred to remain safely in the realm of time-tested drugs, traditional pharmacopeias, and canonical medical authors speaks to the conservative nature of their approach, despite the seemingly innovative use of experimentation as a tool of inquiry. Ultimately, it was market forces that enabled Indies balsam to join the Florentine list of approved drugs.

While this case study highlights the growing use of testing to evaluate new drugs, it also underscores the interpretive questions these practices raised. Trying remedies on human subjects promised to provide incontrovertible evidence about their healing powers. Duke Cosimo had placed this kind of proof-making on a new footing in 1560 when he permitted small-scale clinical trials to substitute for more formal medical credentials when obtaining a sales license for various medicaments. Rather than arriving at definitive conclusions, however, the balsam trial conducted at the Medici court instead threw important evidentiary questions into sharp relief. What threshold of proof was required to establish a drug's therapeutic value? How should the results obtained from sensory reasoning be weighed against subjective patient responses and clinical observations? Who was authorized to judge conflicting outcomes? These questions highlighted growing tensions between time-honored Galenic theory and the burgeoning new knowledge produced by empirical practice—tensions and problems that continued to vex early modern clinical trials until more standardized protocols were introduced in the late eighteenth century.[94]

The field trials conducted by Spanish physicians prompted other kinds of procedural questions. Baldini and his associates harshly criticized Pérez Morales for his lack of methodological precision in reporting clinical methods and results; their criticisms indicate a rapidly developing interest outside of academic circles by 1560 in the ways that testing protocols were constructed by medical professionals and conveyed to a wider public. By challenging the value of his evidence, these Medici physicians also posed a larger question about the weight of experimentation as a common intellectual currency for validating unfamiliar medicaments across linguistic, cultural, and political spaces. As the case of Indies balsam demonstrates, translating New World drugs for European consumption was a complex, generative process whose outcomes were neither uniform nor predictable.

WORKS CITED

Printed Primary Sources

Baldi, Baldo, *Del vero opobalsamo orientale discorso apologetico* (Rome: Vitale Mascardi, 1646).

Campi, Baldassar and Michele, *Parere sopra il balsamo* (Lucca: Pellegrino Bidelli, 1639).

Da Orta, Garcia, *Colloquies on the Simples and Drugs of India*, trans. by Clements Markham (London: Henry Sotheran, 1913).

Fernández de Oviedo, Gonzalo, *Historia general y natural de las Indias* (Seville: Juan Cromberger, 1535).

Mattioli, Pietro Andrea, *I Discorsi [...] nelli sei libri di Pedacio Dioscoride Anazarbeo della materia medica* (Venice: Vincenzo Valgrisi, 1568).

Monardes, Nicolás, *Delle cose che vengono portate dall'Indie Occidentali pertinenti all'uso della medicina* (Venice: Giordano Ziletti, 1575).

Monardes, Nicolás, *Dos libros. El uno trata de todas las cosas que traen de nuestras Indias Occidentales, que sirven al uso de medicina [...] El otro libro, trata de dos medicinas maravillosas que son contra todo veneno, la Piedra Bezaar, y la yerva Escuerçonera* (Seville: n.p.,1565).

Monardes, Nicolás, *Joyfull Newes out of the newe founde worlde*, trans. by John Frampton (London: Thomas Dawson, 1577).

Monardes, Nicolás, *Primera y segunda y tercera partes de la historia medicinal de las cosas que se traen de nuestras Indias Occidentales que sirven en medicina [...]* (Seville: Alonso Escrivano, 1574)

Monardes, Nicolás, *Segunda parte del libro, de las cosas que se traen de nuestras Indias Occidentales, que sirven al uso de medicina* (Seville: Alonso Escrivano, 1571).

Pérez de Morales, García, *Tractado del Balsamo y de sus utilidades para les enfermedades del cuerpo humano* (Seville: en casa de Juan Varela, 1530).

94. Rankin and Rivest, 'Medicine, Monopoly, and the Premodern State'; Maehle, *Drugs on Trial*.

'Relazione di Firenze di Messer Vincenzo Fedeli tornato da quella corte l'anno 1561', in *Relazioni degli Ambasciatori Veneti al Senato. Raccolte, annotate ed edite da Eugenio Alberi*, Series 2, vol. 1 (Florence: Tipografia all'Insegna di Clio: 1839).

El ricettario dell'arte, et universita de medici, et spetiali della città di Firenze. Riveduto dal collegio de medici per ordine dello illustrissimo et eccellentissimo signore duca di Firenze (Florence: Lorenzo Torrentino, 1550).

Il Ricettario medicinale necessario a tutti i Medici e Speziali (Florence: Giunti, 1567).

Secondary Sources

Alberts, Tara, Sietske Fransen, and Elaine Leong, 'Translating Medicine, ca. 800-1900: Articulations and Disarticulations', *Osiris*, 37 (2022), 1–21.

Alegre Pérez, María Esther, 'El bálsamo descubierto por Antonio Villasante (s. XVI)', in *Prodigios y naufragios. Estudios sobre terapéutica farmacológica en España y América, durante el Siglo de Oro*, ed. by Javier Puerto Sarmiento, Juan Esteva de Sagrera, and María Esther Alegre Pérez (Madrid: Doce Calles, 2006), pp. 167–208.

Álvarez Millán, Cristina, 'Drug Testing, Tested Remedies and Medical-Literary Genres in Medieval Islam', *Suhayl*, 18 (2021-21), 205–73.

Barker, Sheila, 'Poisons and the Prince: Toxicology and Statecraft at the Medici Grand Ducal Court', in *Toxicology in the Middle Ages and Renaissance*, ed. by Philip Wexler (London: Elsevier, 2017), pp. 71–82.

Barrera-Osorio, Antonio, 'Local Herbs, Global Medicines: Commerce, Knowledge, and Commodities in Spanish America', in *Merchants and Marvels: Commerce, Science, and Art in Early Modern Europe*, ed. by Pamela H. Smith and Paula Findlen (New York, 2002), pp. 163–81.

Barrera-Osorio, Antonio, 'Translating Facts: From Stories to Observations in the Work of 17th Century Dutch Translators of Spanish Books', in *Translating Knowledge in the Early Modern Low Countries*, ed. by Harold J. Cook and Sven Dupré (Zurich/Münster: LIT Verlag, 2012), pp. 317–31.

Bellorini, Cristina, *The World of Plants in Renaissance Tuscany: Medicine and Botany* (Aldershot: Ashgate, 2016).

Bertolotti, Antonino, 'La medicina, chirurgia e farmacia in Roma nel secolo XVI', *Il Buonarroti* ser. 2, vol. 3 (1884-87): 187–98, 226–42.

Bleichmar, Daniela, 'Books, Bodies, and Fields: Sixteenth-Century Transatlantic Encounters with New World Materia Medica', in *Colonial Botany: Science, Commerce, and Politics in the Early Modern World*, ed. by Londa Schiebinger and Claudia Swan (Philadelphia: University of Pennsylvania Press, 2005), pp. 83–99.

Boumediene, Samir, *La colonisation du savoir. Une histoire des plantes médicinales du "Nouveau Monde" (1492-1750)*, (Vaulx-en-Velin: Éditions des Monde à Faire, 2016).

Boumediene, Samir and Valentina Pugliano, 'La route des succédanés. Les remèdes exotiques, l'innovation médicale et le marché des substituts au XVIe siècle', *Revue d'histoire moderne et contemporaine*, 66.3 (2019), 24–54.

Colonial Botany: Science, Commerce, and Politics in the Early Modern World, ed. by Londa Schiebinger and Claudia Swan (Philadelphia: University of Pennsylvania Press, 2005).

Corradi, Alfonso, *Le prime farmacopee italiane, ed in particolare Dei Ricettari Fiorentini. Memoria* (Milan: Rechiedei, 1887).

Dal Canto, Giuliana,'I fratelli Campi, aromatari lucchesi del sec. XVII e un loro parere sul balsamo', *Atti e memorie della Accademia italiana di storia della farmacia*, 15.3 (1998), 233–36.

Di Gennaro Splendore, Barbara, 'The Triumph of Theriac: Print, Apothecary Publications, and the Commodification of Ancient Antidotes (1497-1800)', *Nuncius*, 36 (2021), 431–70.

Drugs on the Page: Pharmacopeias and Healing Knowledge in the Early Modern Atlantic World, ed. by Matthew J. Crawford and Joseph M. Gabriel (Pittsburgh: University of Pittsburgh Press, 2019).

Entangled Itineraries: Materials, Practices, and Knowledges across Eurasia, ed. by Pamela H. Smith (Pittsburgh: University of Pittsburgh Press, 2019).

Estes, J. Worth, 'The European Reception of the First Drugs from the New World', *Pharmacy in History*, 37.1 (1995), 3–23.

García-Ballester, Luis, Michael R. McVaugh, and Agustín Rubio-Vela, *Medical Licensing and Learning in Fourteenth-Century Valencia* (Philadelphia: American Philosophical Society, 1989).

Gentilcore, David, 'The Impact of New World Plants, 1500-1800: The Americas in Italy', in *The New World in Early Modern Italy, 1492-1750*, ed. by Elizabeth Hodorowich and Lia Markey (Cambridge: Cambridge University Press, 2017), pp. 190–205.

Gibbs, Frederick W., 'Poisonous Properties, Bodies, and Forms in the Fifteenth Century', *Preternature*, 2 (2013), 19–46.

González Bueno, Antonio, Raquel Claudia Cueli Trelle, and Antonio Ramos Carrillo, '"Çierta merced en el bálsamo...". Sobre la introducción en el mercado europeo del Bálsamo de Villasante (1526-1532)', *Anuario de Estudios Americanos*, 79.1 (2022), 13–38.

Guerrini, Anita, *Experimenting with Humans and Animals: From Galen to Animal Rights* (Baltimore: Johns Hopkins University Press, 2003).

Heinrichs, Erik A., 'The Live Chicken Treatment for Buboes: Trying a Plague Cure in Medieval and Early Modern Europe', *Bulletin of the History of Medicine*, 91.2 (2017), 210–32.

Hernando Sánchez, Carlos José, 'Naples and Florence in Charles V's Italy: Family, Court, and Government in the Toledo-Medici Alliance', in *Spain in Italy: Politics, Society, and Religion, 1500-1700*, ed. by Thomas Dandelet and John Marino (Boston: Brill, 2006), pp. 135–80.

Huguet Termes, Teresa, 'Standardising Drug Therapy in Renaissance Europe? The Florence (1499) and Nuremberg Pharmacopeia (1546)', *Medicina e storia*, 8 (2008), 77–101.

Knowledge in Translation: Global Patterns of Scientific Exchange, 1000-1800 BCE, ed. by Patrick Manning and Abigail Owen (Pittsburgh: University of Pittsburgh Press, 2018).

Leong, Elaine, 'When the Tallamys Met John French: Translating, Printing, and Reading *The Art of Distillation*', *Osiris*, 37 (2022), 89–112.

López Piñero, José María and María Luz López Terrada, *La influencia española en la introducción en Europa de las plantas americanas (1493-1623)* (Valencia: Universitat de Valencia, 1997).

McVaugh, Michael, 'Determining a Drug's Properties: Medieval Experimental Protocols', *Bulletin of the History of Medicine*, 91.2 (2017), 183–209.

Maehle, Andreas-Holger, *Drugs on Trial: Experimental Pharmacology and Therapeutic Innovation in the Eighteenth Century* (Amsterdam: Rodopi, 1999).

Mandich, Giulio, 'Le privative industriali veneziane (1450-1550)', *Rivista del diritto commerciale e del diritto generale delle obbligazioni*, 34 (1936), 511–47.

Marinozzi, Silvia, Valentina Giuffra, and Fanny Kieffer, 'Baccio Baldini (1517-1589), protomedicus alla corte Medicea tra umanesimo e sperimentalismo', *Acta Medico Historico Adriatica*, 13.2 (2015), 345–64.

Milwright, Marcus. 'Balsam in the Mediaeval Mediterranean: A Case Study of Commodity and Information Exchange', *Journal of Mediterranean Archaeology*, 14.1 (2001), 3–23.

Milwright, Marcus, 'The Balsam of Matariyya: An Exploration of a Medieval Panacea', *Bulletin of the School of Oriental and African Studies*, 66.2 (2003), 193–209.

Minuzzi, Sabrina, *Sul filo dei segreti. Farmacopeia, libri e pratiche terapeutiche a Venezia in età moderna* (Milan: Edizioni Unicopli, 2016).

Norton, Marcy, *Sacred Gifts, Profane Pleasures: A History of Tobacco and Chocolate in the Atlantic World* (Ithaca and London: Cornell University Press, 2008).

Pardo Tomás, José, 'Obras españolas sobre historia natural y materia medica americanas en la Italia del siglo XVI', *Asclepio*, 43.1 (1991), 51–94.

Pardo Tomás, José and María Luz López Terrada, *Las primeras noticias sobre plantas americanas en las relaciones de viajes y crónicas de Indias (1493-1553)* (Valencia: Instituto de Estudios Documentales e Históricos sobre la Ciencia, 1993).

Parrish, Sean D., 'Marketing Nature: Apothecaries, Medicinal Retailing, and Scientific Culture in Early Modern Venice, 1565-1730', PhD dissertation, Duke University, 2015.

Pastore, Alessandro, 'Médicine légale et investigation judiciaire: expérimenter le poison sur les animaux en Italie à l'époque moderne', *Revue d'histoire des sciences humaines*, 22 (2010), 17–35.

Pereda López, Ángela, 'Antonio de Villasante y el bálsamo de la Española (1493-1536): una revisión historiográfica y nuevas aportaciones', *Naveg@merica. Revista eletrónica editada por la Asociación Española de Americanistas*, n. 28 (2002) online at doi .org/10.618/nav.505901

Podgorny, Irina, 'The Elk, the Ass, the Tapir, their Hooves, and the Falling Sickness: A Story of Substitution and Animal Medical Substances', *Journal of Global History*, 13 (2018), 46–68.

Pomata, Gianna, 'The Medical Case Narrative: Distant Reading of an Epistemic Genre', *Literature and Medicine*, 32 (2014), 1–23.

Pugliano, Valentina, 'Natural History in the Apothecary's Shop', in *Worlds of Natural History*, ed. by Helen Ann Curry, Nicholas Jardine, James A. Secord, and E.C. Spary (Cambridge, UK: Cambridge University Press, 2018), pp. 44–60.

Pugliano, Valentina, 'Non-colonial Botany or the Late Rise of Local Knowledge?', *Studies in History and Philosophy of Biological and Biomedical Sciences*, 40 (2009), 321–28.

Pugliano, Valentina, 'Pharmacy, Testing, and the Language of Truth in Renaissance Italy', *Bulletin of the History of Medicine*, 91.2 (2017), 233–73.

Rankin, Alisha, 'Empirics, Physicians, and Wonder Drugs in Early Modern Germany: The Case of the *Panacea Amwaldina*,' *Early Science and Medicine*, 14 (2009), 680–710.

Rankin, Alisha, 'New World Drugs and the Archive of Practice: Translating Nicolás Monardes in Early Modern Europe', *Osiris*, 37 (2022), 67–88.

Rankin, Alisha, *The Poison Trials: Wonder Drugs, Experiment, and the Battle for Authority in Renaissance Science* (Chicago and London: University of Chicago Press, 2021).

Rankin, Alisha and Elaine Leong, 'Testing Drugs and Trying Cures: Experiment and Medicine in Medieval and Early Modern Europe', *Bulletin of the History of Medicine*, 91.2 (2017), 157–82.

Rankin, Alisha and Justin Rivest, 'Medicine, Monopoly, and the Premodern State—Early Clinical Trials', *New England Journal of Medicine*, 375.2 (2016), 106–09.

Rotelli, Federica, 'Exotic Plants in Italian Pharmacopeia (16th-17th Centuries)', *Medicina nei secoli: arte e scienza*, 30.3 (2018), 827–80.

Safier, Neil, 'Global Knowledge on the Move: Itineraries, Amerindian Narratives, and Deep Histories of Science', *Isis*, 101 (2010), 133–45.

Santo Domingo en los Manuscritos de Juan Bautista Muñoz, ed. by Roberto Marte (Santo Domingo: Fundación García Arévalo, 1981).

Savoia, Paolo, 'The *Book of the Sick* of Santa Maria della Morte in Bologna and the Medical Organization of a Hospital in the Sixteenth Century', *Nuncius*, 31 (2016), 163–235.

Schäfer, Ernst, 'Antonio de Villasante, descubridor droguista en la Isla Española', *Investigación y progreso*, 9.1 (1935), 13–15.

Schickore, Jutta, 'Trying Again and Again: Multiple Repetitions in Early Modern Reports of Experiments on Snake Bites', *Early Science and Medicine*, 15 (2010), 567–617.

Schiebinger, Londa, *Plants and Empire: Colonial Bioprospecting in the Atlantic World* (Cambridge, MA and London: Harvard University Press, 2004).

Schottenhammer, Angela, '"Peruvian balsam": An Example of Transoceanic Transfer of Medicinal Knowledge,' *Journal of Ethnobiology and Ethnomedicine,* 16: 69 (2020), https://doi.org/10.1186/s13002-020-00407-y.

Shapin, Steven, *A Social History of Truth: Civility and Science in Seventeenth-Century England* (Chicago: University of Chicago Press, 1995).

Smith, Pamela H., 'Itineraries of Materials and Knowledge in the Early Modern World', in *The Global Lives of Things,* ed. by Anne Gerritsen and Giorgio Riello (London: Routledge, 2015), pp. 31–61.

Sonnedecker, Glenn, 'The Florentine Pharmacopeia', *Pharmacy in History,* 36.4 (1994), 175–77.

Stevens Crawshaw, Jane L., *Plague Hospitals: Public Health for the City in Early Modern Venice* (London and New York: Routledge, 2016).

Stolberg, Michael, 'A Sixteenth-Century Physician and His Patients: The Practice Journal of Hiob Finzel, 1565-1589', *Social History of Medicine,* 32 (2017), 221–40.

Strocchia, Sharon T., *Forgotten Healers: Women and the Pursuit of Health in Late Renaissance Italy* (Cambridge, MA: Harvard University Press, 2019).

Wintroub, Michael, 'Translations: Words, Things, Going Native, and Staying True', *American Historical Review,* 120 (2015), 1185–1217.

7

Medicinal and Cosmetic Waters:

Vernacular Experimentation in Sixteenth-Century Florentine Ricettari

Gaston J. Basile

The archives of Medici Florence offer insight into the centrality of water in the early modern period, encompassing water legislation, hydraulic engineering, and ice production, as well as the daily interactions of people from all social backgrounds with *acque* ('waters'). This included state-of-the-art health regimes, recreational and curative therapies at Tuscan thermal springs, spas, and baths, or the use of water in medical, alchemical, or cosmetic products, which often promised miraculous effects. This collection of water-related knowledge and practices has recently been termed 'early modern water culture'.[1] The epistolary correspondence of the Medici family and other elite members highlights the prominent role of mineral and thermal waters as experimental therapies prescribed by court physicians. For example, in a letter dated 2 November 1543, we learn that Duke Cosimo I began drinking 'three or four cups' ('tre o vero quattro tazze') of water from Montecatini to improve his health.[2] In another letter, it is mentioned that Eleonora's brother, Don Luis de Toledo, started a treatment involving bathing in the water ('aqua') of Bagno Vignoni.[3] Eleonora di Toledo herself was advised to take the waters of Montecatini to restore her health,[4] while Ferrante I Gonzaga, governor of Milan, received permission to travel to Alessandria to relieve sciatica pain with thermal waters.[5] But the exchange of letters also reveals another dimension of the Florentine water culture which has hitherto received little attention: the circulation of medicinal-cosmetic waters.[6]

Writing in March 1582, Virginio Orsini (II Duca di Bracciano) expressed his gratitude to Bianca Cappello for some delicate waters she had sent as a gift, confessing his relief that they arrived after the carnival celebrations:

> None but the most delicate waters could flow from Your Highness [Bianca Cappello-de' Medici]'s fountain of graces, such as the ones Your Highness sent me [...] which certainly, if they had arrived at carnival time, would have entailed the danger that I would not have been entirely prodigal, especially at certain parties here with these gentlemen and [...] which were very gratifying.[7]

1. See Gentilcore, 'From Vilest Beverage', pp. 677–78.
2. ASFi, MdP 1170, fol. 142r. Letter by Lorenzo di Andrea Pagni (2 November 1543). All references to the Mediceo del Principato cited herein are taken from the MIA database (The Medici Archive Project).
3. ASFi, MdP 6, fol. 262r. Letter by Cosimo I de Medici (30 September 1545).
4. ASFi, MdP 1176, fol. 869r. Letter by Lorenzo di Andrea Pagni (21 April 1551).
5. ASFi, MdP 3254, fol. 4r. Avviso from Milan (17 May 1553).
6. In the past decades, early modern cosmetics and beauty cultures have witnessed an increasing number of publications. See Cavallo, 'Health, Beauty and Hygiene', pp. 174–87; Cavallo and Storey, *Healthy Living in Late Renaissance Italy*; Storey, 'Face Waters, Oils, pp. 143–66. For a useful overview of the field, with emphasis on Italian recipe-books and books of secrets, see Spicer, 'A Fare Bella', pp. 1–18.
7. 'Dal fonte delle gratie di Vostra Altezza [Bianca Cappello-de' Medici] non potevano venire acque se non delicatissime come quelle che Vostra Altezza m'ha mandate [...] che certo se comparivano di carnevale portavan pericolo ch'io non ne fussi stato al tutto prodigo, massime in occasione di certi festini qui con questi signori e [proposed reading: servitore] quali sono stati molto gratiosi [...]' ASFi, MdP 5928, fol. 305r. Letter by Virginio Orsini (II Duca di Bracciano), dated 3 March 1582.

Other letters also reveal that Bianca Cappello had sent such charming gifts to Filippo di Francesco I and Virginia Medici around that time.[8] Another document mentions Camillo da Verona, a Florentine distiller, preparing 'waters', presumably for 'Nevers' [Lodovico Gonzaga].[9] Even the Grand Duke himself was keen on having waters and oils prepared and sent to him by members of his entourage.[10] Cosimo's diversion was shared by other members of his family as well. In November 1560, during the absence of the ducal couple, the grand Duke's secretary, Neri Rapucci, reported that Francesco de Medici spent 'much of the day in the foundry preparing certain precious waters'[11].

But what were exactly the waters (*acque*) that Bianca Cappello dispatched to her entourage, or the ones produced by the Medici family in the royal foundry? And what part did they play in the Florentine water culture and, more broadly, in early modern pharmaceutical experimentation? In this essay, I explore both the theoretical and practical dimensions of these manufactured waters in Renaissance Florence, examining official pharmaceutical literature alongside uncharted material evidence from the Florentine vernacular culture. I argue that it is in the tradition of manuscript recipe books and collection of secrets (*segreti*) that the prominence, diffusion, and manifold uses of early modern medicinal-cosmetic waters can be best appraised. The case of medicinal waters reveals the empirical base of pharmaceutical innovation in the sixteenth century, as well as the vernacular modes of recording, preserving, and transmitting medical knowledge.

WATERS IN THEORY: THE MEDICAL LITERATURE, PRINTED PHARMACOPEIAS, AND DISTILLATION MANUALS

Water is a fluid and equivocal category. Indeed, *acqua* could stand for drinking water from wells, springs, rainfall, and watercourses, but the plural *acque* could also metonymically designate the mineral and thermal waters used in hydrotherapies. In the medieval alchemical tradition, *acqua* was generally a blanket term for 'liquid,'[12] which could adopt assorted meanings when combined with different descriptors (e.g., *aqua ardens*, *aqua fortis*, *aqua regia*, *aqua vitae*, etc.),[13] but was not primarily associated with naturally occurring freshwater. On the other hand, *acqua* could also denote a range of aqueous preparations usually obtained by decoction and/or distillation, which were used for a variety of medicinal and cosmetic purposes. My discussion will primarily focus on 'waters' in this latter sense.

Although water is ubiquitous, and commonly used as standard vehicle in the preparation of medicines, the late fifteenth-century Italian pharmacopeias and civic formularies, which drew heavily on standard textbooks like Mesue's *Grabadin* and the Salernitan *Antidotarium Nicolai* (11th–12th c.), showed little theoretical interest in the properties of water and its uses in medicine preparation. Late fifteenth-century handbooks to pharmacy, printed in Northern Italy, such as the *Compendium aromatariorum* (Bologna, 1488), the *Lumen apothecariorum* (Turin, 1492), the *Luminare maius* (Pavia, 1494) and the *Thesaurus aromatariorum* (Milan, 1496), made only cursory references to water as a vehicle in the preparation of medicine, including decoctions and a few distillates, but offered no systematic treatment.[14] As manufactured medicinal

8. ASFi, MdP 5926, fol. 174ʳ. Letter by Fillipo di Francesco I de Medici (5 March 1582); ASFi, MdP 5928, fol. 280ʳ. Letter by Virginia de Medici-d'Este (2 March 1582).
9. ASFi, MdP 5923, fol. 223ʳ. Letter by Filippo Cavriani (12 May 1573).
10. ASFi, MdP 1172, fol. 417ʳ. Letter by Lorenzo di Andrea Pagni (27 October 1546).
11. ASFi, MdP 1687, fol. 28ʳ. Letter by Neri Rapucci (4 November 1560): 'passa una gran parte del giorno in fonderia, ci ha preso a fare certe acque pretiose.'
12. In alchemy *aqua* is defined as 'Liquid; the elemental matter from which water can always be obtained. It is not water from the clouds, but a dry mineral first substance, a catholic water, which dissolves all metals, and can be reduced to water even as ice is reduced.' Ruland, *Lexicon Alchemiae*, p. 46.
13. See Abraham, *A Dictionary of Alchemical Imagery*, pp. 8–10. For a comprehensive list of alchemical compounds designated as 'aquae', see Ruland, *Lexicon Alchemiae*, pp. 46–51.
14. Saladino da Ascoli's *Compendium aromatariorum* offers incidental advice on when and how to distill waters from herbs (p. 31) and includes a list of forty-three simple waters culled from Abulcasis's *Liber servitoris* (S. X), though indicating that apothecaries may substitute them for decoctions if they lack the time or skills in distillation (p. 61). Quiricus di Augustis's *Lumen apothecariorum* provides incidental observations on certain simple waters used in individual recipes (e.g., 'Aqua cucurbite', fol. 25ᵛ; 'aqua rosa', fol. 28ʳ; 'aqua marina', fol. 35ᵛ, etc.), and occasionally mentions distilled

products, 'waters' (in the plural) were not seen as a clearly distinct category of remedies and were therefore barely indexed as such in the first civic pharmacopeia, the 1499 *Ricettario fiorentino*.[15] However, interest in water grew in the following decades, especially in relation to distillation.[16] Throughout the sixteenth century, references to distilled waters, along with distillation methods and equipment, began to appear more frequently in pharmaceutical literature, particularly in Florence.

A more formal approach to distilled waters was catalyzed by the publication of distillation manuals. Among the most influential was Hieronymus Brunschwig's *Liber de arte distillandi de simplicibus* (known as the *Small Book of Distillation*, 1500), which systematized and disseminated through the printing-press the traditional knowledge of extracting medicinal waters from plants and other curative materials.[17] In his work, Brunschwig dealt with various forms of distillation, which he grouped into two classes: those made without fire and cheap, and those made with fire and expensive. The free distillations without fire were achieved through several methods, including filtration (*filtri distilationem*), solar heat (*per solis distilationem*), the heat of a bread oven (*per panis distilationem*), the heat of dung (*per fimi equi distilationem*), and even the heat of an anthill (*per formice distilationem*). Distillations involving fire included techniques such as using a bain-marie (*distilatio per balneum marie*), heating with ash (*distilatio per cineres*) or sand (*per arenam*), applying direct fire (*distilatio per ignem*), and utilizing a *rosenhut*—a common furnace designed to accommodate multiple cucurbits with conical *rosenhut*-type capitals.[18]

Brunschwig's work, which went through sixteen editions between 1500 and 1568, inaugurated a self-standing reflection on distillation that merged the alchemical tradition, and the established medical practice of producing simple and complex distilled waters. Though the *Liber de arte distillandi de simplicibus* was intended for the general public, it nonetheless stimulated a more analytic treatment of what had customarily been regarded as an artisan skill. Indeed, the impact of Brunschwig's handbook was strong. In Italy, distillation was explored more or less systematically, among others, by the technologist Vannoccio Biringuccio, (1480-1539?) in a section of his work *De la pirotechnia* (Venice, 1540)[19]; the polymath Gerolamo Cardano (1501-1576) in various works, but most notably in the encyclopedic *De subtilitate rerum* (1550)[20]; the physician Pietro Andrea Mattioli (1501-1578) in an appendix to his multi-volume commentary on Dioscorides (1565); and, in the next generation, by the polymath Giovanbattista della Porta (1535–1615) in his *De distillatione* (Rome, 1608).

Although hydro-distillation, a process using water (steam) as an extraction solvent to recover volatile or polar components of plant materials, had long been used in pharmacy for extracting oils and waters from aromatic and non-aromatic plants, Italian university-trained physicians tended to refer to it as a more recent or alternative procedure, which they associated with the method of alchemists.[21] For example, in one of his *Epistolae medicinales*

waters. Manlio del Bosco's *Luminare maius* makes sparse references to certain types of waters in connection with specific recipes, but offers no detailed treatment, except for a few paraphrases of Dioscorides, Mesue, and Avicenna (fol. 71ᵛ).

15. On pharmacopeias and the *Ricettario fiorentino* in particular, see Beck, 'The Ricettario Fiorentino', pp. 45–62, and additional bibliographical references cited therein.

16. For the medieval tradition of distillation, see Forbes, *A Short History of the Art of Distillation*, pp. 55–98. For the use of distillation in pharmacy, see Debus, *The Chemical Philosophy*, I, 19–25; and Bellorini, *The World of Plants*, pp. 168–76. As noted by Bellorini, even if distillation is associated with Paracelsian medicine, it had been used at least since the early thirteenth century in Europe to produce distilled waters and remedies (pp. 168–69).

17. See Taape, 'Distilling Reliable Remedies', pp. 236–56; Debus, *The Chemical Philosophy*, I, 21–23; and Hirsch, 'The Invention of Printing', pp. 115–41. An earlier oft-printed treatise on distillation, treating dozens of different herbal essences, is Michael Puff (1400-73) of Schrick's *Von den ausgebrannten Wassern*, which also went through several editions in the sixteenth century.

18. I have used the English translation: Brunschwig, *The vertuose boke of distyllacyon of all maner of herbes* (1527).

19. See Forbes, *History of Distillation*, pp. 132–33. In Book 9, chapter 2: 'Dell'arte distillatoria in generale con li modi da cavar le acque, ogli, e fare sublimationi', Biringuccio discusses distillation (fols 260ᵛ–275ʳ). He argues that through distillation one obtains the airy and watery parts, the composition of which depends on the base material (pp. 260ᵛ–261ʳ). I cite from Biringuccio, *Pirotechnia*, 1559.

20. On Cardano see Forbes, *History of Distillation*, p. 132. In *De subtilitate*, published in 1550, Cardano mentions different kinds of distillation, such as the bain-marie, putrefaction in horse manure, and that which takes place by means of ashes and the heat of olive husks. See Cardano, 'De subtilitate', II, 383–84. Cardano's views on distillation are also cited by Gessner, *Thesaurus Euonymi Philiatri*, pp. 29–30.

21. On the rise of alchemical interest in the Renaissance despite its criticism and lack of institutional protection, see Long, *Openness, Secrecy, Authorship*, pp. 143–74. On the general reluctance of university-educated physicians to accept distillation, which was viewed predominantly as 'an artisan activity', see Moran, *Distilling Knowledge*, pp. 37–66, esp. 55. However, in practice many physicians 'showed a readiness to study with, and

(Medical Epistles) written in 1535, the physician Giovanni Manardo (1462–1536) distinguished between the traditional remedies 'handed down to us from the ancients' ('haec ab antiquis quasi per manus nobis tradita remedia') from 'more recent ones' ('recentiores') obtained by distillation.[22] In a similar vein, Pietro Andrea Mattioli, in a short treatise on distillation appended to his lofty commentary to Dioscorides, differentiated between decoction ('decoctio'), as the traditional and prevalent method of extraction by boiling herbal material, and an alternative procedure, distillation ('distillatio'), which he associated with chemists or alchemists.[23] He noted that distillations were less effective in retaining the properties and fragrances of herbs, but could be used instead of decoctions, as they were subtler and therefore better tolerated by some patients.[24] Although distillation was a long-standing method for obtaining herbal remedies, and learned physicians were largely open to experimentation with distillation procedures,[25] distilled waters were barely recorded in the first printed pharmacopeias, and were only gradually incorporated during the sixteenth century.

The early *Ricettario fiorentino*, published by the Florentine College of Physicians in 1499, only explicitly recorded three distilled waters in a few magisterial recipes,[26] and the action of distilling (*distillare/stillare*) occurred fewer than twenty times in the whole work.[27] A sensible development can be observed, nonetheless, in the 1574 edition of the *Riccetario fiorentino*. While the remedies explicitly indexed as 'waters' continued to be limited (12 recipes), the updated pharmacopeia showed a notable attempt to incorporate some theoretical knowledge about distillation, distilled waters, and the use of water in medicine more generally. In the first part, when discussing the characteristics of simple medicines, the authors distinguished between natural waters, on the one hand, and artificial waters or distillates, on the other:

> Medicines simple to the sense are waters and earths: waters are either natural or artificial: natural waters are the rainwater, which immediately falls from the sky, and that which is collected and conserved in cisterns, or those from springs, or wells, or rivers, or from the sea, or from baths containing minerals. Artificial waters are all distillates in whatever way they are distilled.[28]

In other sections, the authors provided a definition of distilled waters (pp. 6–7), explained detailed procedures involving waters (pp. 80–100),[29] and described the various methods of distillation with accompanying images in the last section of the first part (pp. 100–108d) (fig. 14).

Close analysis reveals that the word stem—still—(including *stillare*, *destillare* and their cognates) occurs in at least fifty-nine passages of the pharmacopeia; seven recipes explicitly mention distillation in the corresponding procedures; and eight recipes of compound waters (*acque composte*) are included in the inventory of remedies.[30]

As a comparison of the 1499 and 1574 edition of the Florentine pharmacopeia demonstrates, distilled waters

learn from, contemporary alchemists.' cf. Palmer, 'Pharmacy in the Republic of Venice', p.115. On alchemy as a 'vernacular science of matter', see Smith, *The Body of the Artisan*, pp. 129–51.

22. Manardo, *Epistolarum medicinalium*, p. 372 (lib. 19, ep. 1).
23. The treatise on distillation attributed to Mattioli is titled 'De ratione distillandi aquas ex omnibus plantis, et quomodo genuini odores in ipsis aquis conservare possint'. See Mattioli, *Commentarii*, pp. 1460^r–1465^r.
24. Ibid., p.1461^r.
25. On Mattioli's personal experimentation with distillates, see Stolberg, *Learned Physicians*, pp. 368–70.
26. BNCF, Palatino MS, E.6.27: 'Nuovo Receptario composto dal famosissimo chollegio degli eximii doctori della arte et medicina della inclita ciptà di Firenze.' (Florence Compagnia del Dragho, 1499). See: *aqua distillate*: chapters I. V. 42, and III. III; *aqua stillata*: chapter I. V. 17.
27. The action of 'distillare' (eleven occurrences): I. V. 27; I. V. 39; I. V. 40; I. V. 42; I. V. 46; I. V. 47; I. V. 50; II. XVI. 2. 33; II. XVI. 2 .35; II. XVI. 2. 41; II. III; and 'stillare' (six occurrences): I. III. 12; I. V. 1; I. V. 50; II. XIII. 2; II. XVI. 2. 37; II. XVI. 2. 40.
28. 'I medicamenti semplici al senso sono l'acque, e le terre: l'acque sono ò naturali, ò artificiali: le naturali sono la piovana, che subito cade dal cielo: e quella, che si raccoglie, e si conserva nelle citerne: ò quelle de fonti, ò de pozzi, ò de fiumi, ò di mare, ò di bagni partecipi di minerali. L'acque artificiali sono tutte le stillate in qualunche modo si stillino.' Chollegio della Arte et Medicina di Firenze, *Ricettario Fiorentino* (Florence: Stamperia dei Giunti, 1574), pp. 2–3.
29. Procedures involving waters in the 1574 edition: 'Dissolvere et stemperare', pp. 80–1; 'struggere et liquefare', p. 81; 'ammorbidire', p. 81; 'scaldare', p. 82; 'tenere al sol, sotto il letame, le vinaccie, la sansa, la rena, la terra', p. 82; 'cuocere', p. 83; 'stillare', pp. 100–108. On the differences between the 1567 and 1574 editions concerning distillation, see Corradi, *Le prime farmacopee*, p. 34.
30. Preparations explicitly involving distillation in the 1574 edition: 'Conserva di foglie di bettonica', pp. 128–9; 'Sciroppo d'aceto di limoni magistrale', p. 145; 'Precipitato di Giovanni di Vico', p. 202; 'Un altro magistrale', p. 203; 'Olio balsamino magistrale', p. 245; 'Olio magistrale di Pietro d'Abano', p. 245; 'Unguento della Contessa di Guglielmo da Varignana', p. 256; 'Acque Composte', pp. 234–36 (eight recipes).

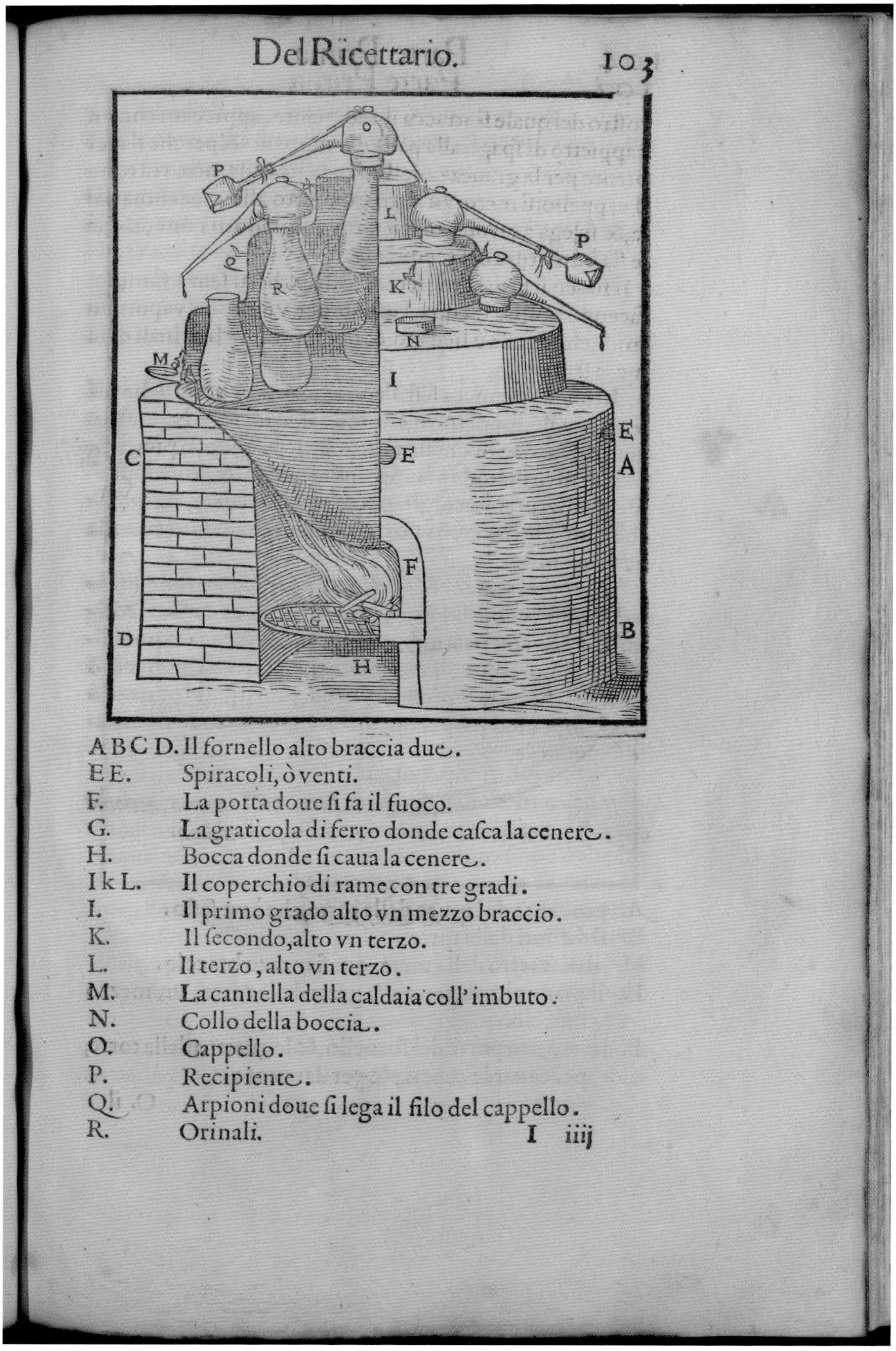

Del Ricettario. 103

A B C D. Il fornello alto braccia due.
E E. Spiracoli, ò venti.
F. La porta doue ſi fa il fuoco.
G. La graticola di ferro donde caſca la cenere.
H. Bocca donde ſi caua la cenere.
I k L. Il coperchio di rame con tre gradi.
I. Il primo grado alto vn mezzo braccio.
K. Il ſecondo, alto vn terzo.
L. Il terzo, alto vn terzo.
M. La cannella della caldaia coll' imbuto.
N. Collo della boccia.
O. Cappello.
P. Recipiente.
Q. Arpioni doue ſi lega il filo del cappello.
R. Orinali. I iiij

14. A depiction of a distilling apparatus in the 1576 edition of the *Ricettario Fiorentino.*

gradually gained prominence in the civic formularies.[31] This growing theoretical interest in medicinal waters was largely spurred by developments in the domain of practice, alongside other broader contextual factors. Continuous experimentation with distillation methods in alchemical and pharmaceutical workshops across the social spectrum, spanning the humblest domestic distilleries to the Grand Ducal foundry in Florence, played a major part. Indeed, the Medici family was personally involved in alchemical experimentation in their *fonderia,* and openly advocated the use of distillation in the preparation of remedies.[32] The expansion of distillation methods and other chemical procedures was also coeval with the rise of Paracelsian medicine and iatrochemistry in the late sixteenth century.[33] Moreover, the circulation of distillation handbooks destined to the general public may also have contributed to a greater diffusion of artisanal practices. Scientific treatises specifically dedicated to medicinal waters were, nonetheless, extremely rare. A notable exception is a monograph written by the little-known Belgian physician and naturalist Remacle Fuchs (1520–1587) entitled *Historia omnium aquarum quae in comuni hodie practicantium sunt usu, vires et recte distillandi ratio*, first published in Paris in 1542. In this work, Fuchs described the most common plants used to produce medicinal waters, the correct distillation procedures, and their medicinal properties. In the final section, the author included several useful tables that classify the different waters according to the part of the body they affect (e.g., *capitales*, *pectorales*, *cordiales*, *stomaticae*, *hepaticae*, *splenaticae*, *ureticae*, *aquae uterum respicientes*) and their quality (hot or cold).

WATERS IN PRACTICE: THE MANUSCRIPT RICETTARI, VERNACULAR KNOWLEDGE AND ARTISANAL EXPERIMENTATION

Like thermal waters and baths, manufactured waters were also at the heart of a complex social ecosystem involving various trades and occupations.[34] Two sixteenth-century publications help delineate the social dynamics of these medicinal waters in the early modern period. The Bolognese physician-surgeon, Leonardo Fioravanti, in his work *Dello specchio di scientia universale* ('On the Mirror of Universal Knowledge'), first published in Venice (1564), associated medicinal waters especially with the métier of perfumers, alchemists, and distillers.[35] Unlike the orthodox university-trained physicians of his time, the radical empiric and wanderer Fioravanti proudly extolled the art of alchemists and distillers that helped produce, among other useful items, medicinal waters. Thus, for example, he noted in a passage of his work:

> From this ingenious art (alchemy) came the art of enamels of all kinds of colors, such as solymate, cinnabar, arsenic, purple, and many other beautiful and honored inventions, as well as many kinds of oils and medicinal waters. It is not only an aid, but also a great ornament for medicine and surgery.[36]

Other writers would take a less encomiastic approach. In his encyclopedic *Piazza universale di tutte le professioni del mondo*, published in Venice in 1585, Tomaso Garzoni (1549–1589) described nearly 540 professions and

31. For a comparison of the successive sixteenth-century editions of the *Ricettario*, see Corradi, *Le prime farmacopee*, pp.1–64. The Florentine case is, nonetheless, exceptional when compared with other Italian pharmacopeias. The *Antidotarium Bononiensis* (1574) makes very few mentions of distillation or distilled waters in the individual recipes (8 records). Likewise, the *Antidotarium Mantuanum* (1558) hardly makes any reference to distillation or distilled waters (cf. pp. 88, 109, 163). The *Antidotarium Romanum* (1583) does not record any distilled water nor refers to distillation processes. Alternatively, the water-related section of the antidotary comprises eight 'collyria' (pp. 128–29), five decoctions (pp. 130–31), and one tisane (p. 132). The most frequent collocations for the noun 'aqua' are 'pluviale', 'pura', 'frigida', 'comunis', and 'rosacea', and the processes most associated with waters are cooking ('coquere' / 'decoquere'), boiling ('bullire') and macerating ('macerare'), but there is no reference to the act of distilling or distillation.
32. See, among others, Bellorini, *The World of Plants*, pp. 168–76; Perifano, *L'alchimie à la cour de Côme Ier*, pp. 46–47; Clericuzio, *Chemical Medicine*, pp. 375–76; Barker, 'Cosimo I de' Medici and the Renaissance Sciences', pp. 520–80; Conticelli, *"Guardaroba di cose rare et preziose"*; Piccardi, *La farmacia granducale*.
33. On the diffusion of Paracelsian theories and practices in Florence, see Hedesan, *Alchemy and Paracelsianism in Florence,* pp.119–43. More generally, on the expansion of Paracelsian chemical medicine in the late sixteenth century and the openness of physicians to new cures, including *chymic* remedies, see Stolberg, *Learned physicians,* pp. 363–77.
34. For a survey of sellers of medicinal-cosmetics in seventeenth-century Rome, see Storey, 'Face waters, oils', pp. 143–166, esp. 153–55.
35. See Fioravanti, *Dello specchio*: Cap. 44 'Dell'arte dell'Alchimia et delle sue inventioni', pp. 96r–97r; Cap. 50 'Dell'arte del distillare e suoi belli effetti', pp. 112r–114r; Cap. 41 'Dell'arte del profumiero, et de suoi olii odoriferi', pp. 92v–93r. On Fioravanti, see Camporesi, *Camminare il mondo*; Eamon, *Science and the Secrets of Nature*, pp. 164–93; and Gentilcore, *Medical Charlatanism,* esp. 267–68.
36. Fioravanti, *Dello specchio*, fol. 96v.

occupations of his time in 154 speeches (*discorsi*).[37] Among this panoply of skilled and manual workers, Garzoni explicitly referred to a few social actors engaged in the manufacture, marketing, and consumption of waters and their by-products in early modern Europe. Garzoni connected waters to a caste of (pseudo) intellectuals whom he described as *professori di segreti* (professors of secrets). Citing Gerolamo Cardano, Garzoni defined distillation as a science ('scientia') that aimed to extract something useful from plants and herbs ('plantarum vires'), thereby classing distillation, within an overarching typology, as a specific type of operational secret. However, Garzoni cautioned his readers against the many lies ('menzogne') preached by alchemists and distillers. He described these individuals as a mixed breed ranging from those who nobly served medicine and health to unscrupulous quacks and charlatans who peddled magical potions and produced adulterated or counterfeit preparations. In Garzoni's work, waters were also mentioned in relation to the business of apothecaries ('speciari') and perfumers ('aromatari'), alongside other artisans such as painters ('pittori') and illuminators ('miniatori'). Notably, *acque* were not only associated with the so-called professors of secrets, distillers, and alchemists—whose reputations were not always beyond reproach—but also with more marginal characters like prostitutes and ruffians, who used gifts of perfumes and waters to entice women. These licentious individuals often procured their cosmetics from perfumers ('profumieri') and ointment sellers ('unguentari').[38]

The great diversity of social actors involved in the production and circulation of medicinal waters can be also gleaned from the collection of recipe books in the Florentine libraries. In recent decades, more attention has been paid to the vernacular modes of knowledge-making and the material aspects of early modern medicine through a closer examination of documents that had previously attracted limited interest.[39] Although an exhaustive survey of the existing material is still warranted, a cursory exploration of a dozen or so recipe books confirms not only the prominence of waters in the inventory of remedies, but also their consistency in the vernacular medicinal literature across the social spectrum, from manuscript hospital pharmacopeias, and recipe books meant as court gifts, to makeshift notebooks possibly owned by surgeons, empirics or laypeople.[40] Unlike in the civic pharmacopeias, waters abound in the vernacular manuscript tradition.[41] However, *acque* could stand for a variety of medicinal products, with fluctuations in scope and meaning from one source to another.

Because water was used as the main vehicle for the preparation of medicines, water-based or fluid remedies feature prominently in pharmaceutical literature. In his typology of late-medieval pharmaceutical products, Jean-Pierre Bénézet distinguishes waters (*les eaux*) from other preparations. According to his classification, derived from a handful of sixteenth-century civic pharmacopeias and pharmaceutical works, waters strictly speaking comprised simple distilled waters and complex waters.[42] The former, he notes, were produced by placing a plant in the cucurbit/gourd part of the alembic and using vapor to extract the volatile part of the plant; the latter, in turn, consisted of aqueous solutions containing minerals (salts) and organic products (sugars, etc.) which were generally employed externally due to their toxicity. However, the Florentine *ricettari* often used the blanket term *acqua* to designate a variety of liquid preparations for oral administration that Bénézet classes separately. These include decoctions, infusions, and juices; ophthalmic remedies or collyria; and liquid medicines applied by the cutaneous-mucosal route, such as lotions, fomentations,

37. See Mocarelli, 'Attitudes to Work and Commerce', pp. 89–93.
38. Garzoni, *Piazza Universale*, fols 80ᵛ–81ᵛ (Discorso 22); fols 206ʳ–207ᵛ (Discorso 49), fols 206ᵛ; fols 287ʳ –288ᵛ (Discorso 90); fols 289ʳ –292ʳ (Discorso 91); fol. 262ᵛ, fols 267ʳ–269ʳ (Discorso 79).
39. On the shift toward the study of knowledge-making practices, see, among many others, Smith, 'Science on the Move'; on the importance of materials, see the comprehensive discussion by Klein and Spary, 'Materials and Expertise', pp. 1–24.
40. An example of a hospital recipe-book is the BNCF, Magliabechiano MS XV 92 (dated 1515); an elite gift manuscript is the Wellcome Library, Western MS 485, 'Segreti di D. Antonio de Medici... dati e donati a me Caterina Medici nel convento delle Murati di Firenze, l'anno 1598'; an example of a recipe-book attributed to a barber is the Wellcome Library, MS 174 (dated 1529). For a description of these manuscripts and those cited hereafter (S. XV-XVI), see Targioni Tozzetti, *Catalogo generale dei manoscritti Magliabechiani*, Gentile, *I codici Palatini della Biblioteca Nazionale Centrale di Firenze*, Mahmoud Salem, *Medicina e farmacologia nei manoscritti della Biblioteca Riccardiana.*
41. On recipes as a genre of technical know-how or experimentation, see Eamon, *Science and the Secrets of Nature*, pp. 126–33. On the recipe book tradition as a vernacular genre, see Stannard, 'Medieval Herbalism', p. 49; Crisciani, 'Ricette e medicina', pp. 23–25; Cifuentes, 'El receptari mèdic', pp. 103–60.
42. Bénézet, *Pharmacie et médicament*, pp. 561–66.

baths, etc.[43] In our corpus, *acque* often encompass cosmetic products not inventoried by Bénézet, such as perfumes, colognes, or toilet waters. More broadly, medicinal and cosmetic waters were often lumped together with other non-medicinal waters used for metal transmutation, assaying, dyeing, and color-making.

The *acque* recorded in the recipe-books served a variety of medical-cosmetic purposes. They were typically prescribed for treatment of the eyes, mouth and teeth, throat and face.[44] But they were also used for cosmetic or deodorant purposes,[45] and for the cure of more serious medical ailments or conditions, like wounds and lacerations, the stone, the French disease, and genital problems.[46] These preparations occur unequivocally in all forms of recipe collections, from institutional vade mecums to compilations produced by religious or secular individuals across the social spectrum. Their use, as will be discussed shortly, became especially prevalent in the late sixteenth century (fig.15, 16 and 17).

However, some *acque* were more widely used than others and were often reproduced either identically or with minor variations across different manuscripts. These variations might include differences in the recipe's name, the quantities and types of ingredients, or the instructions for preparation and administration.

The indexing of medicinal waters in the manuscript *ricettari* demonstrates a pragmatic and encyclopedic approach to pharmaceutical knowledge, which runs counter to the reductive method of civic pharmacopeias. These manuscript recipe-books relish repetition and abundance, frequently presenting similar preparations in sequence. The early sixteenth-century *Ricettario di Santa Maria Nuova* in the manuscript Magliabechiano XV 92 exemplifies this approach. Compiled in 1515 by Hectorre di Lionello di Francesco Baldovinetti, it contains over one thousand recipes sourced from 'tried and tested' remedies at the hospital of Santa Maria Nuova. As such, the collection offers valuable insights into medical practice and the cumulative knowledge of pharmaceuticals in the Florentine healthcare system. As highlighted by John Henderson's seminal study, the recipes not only draw from established Arab and classical sources, but also from contemporary practitioners, many of whom worked in Florentine hospitals.[47] Despite its institutional endorsement, likely by the College of Physicians, the *Ricettario di Santa Maria Nuova* reflects the common function of vernacular pharmaceutical collections as repositories of practical knowledge, orienting heath practitioner to treat specific patients in a variety of cases. Thus, unlike the civic pharmacopeia, it embraces repetition and employs various criteria for indexing preparations. This approach is evident in the treatment of waters as well as other remedy types. For example, recipes labeled 'acqua da occhi' in this volume are recorded at various junctures with or without modifications in the title, lacking a discernible logic.[48] On folio 113^{v}, there are two recipes for

43. Ibid., pp. 558–60, 61, 66–67, 604–06, 609–10.
44. Eyes: e.g., BNCF, Magliabechiano XV 92, 'Acqua da occhi fine', fol. 56^{r}, and also fols 58^{r}, 76^{r}, 79^{r}, 113^{v}, 139^{r}, and 143^{v}; BR, Riccardiano MS 3057, fols 72^{v}–73^{r}; Wellcome Library MS 174, fol. 12^{v}, fol. 11^{v}; BNCF, Palatino MS 543, fol. 96^{r}; BNCF, Palatino MS 941, fol. 22^{v}; BNCF, Magliabechiano MS XV 118, fol. 4^{v}. Teeth: e.g., BNCF, Magliabechiano MS XV 92: 'Acqua de denti', fol. 142^{r-v}; BR, Riccardiano MS 3056, fol. 70^{r}; BR, Riccardiano MS 3063, fols 23^{v}–24^{r}; BNCF, Magliabechiano MS XV 140, fol. 13^{r}; BR, Riccardiano MS 2376, fols 13^{r-v}. Mouth: e.g., BNCF, Magliabechiano MS XV 92: 'Affare acqua forte da boccha', fol. 34^{v}; BNCF, Magliabechiano MS XV 136, fol. 31^{r}. Face: e.g., BR, Riccardiano MS 3063: 'A fare aqua da viso dignissima', fol 30^{r}; Wellcome Library, MS 485: 'Acque per far bella la faccia', fols 50^{v}–75^{v} (multiple recipes); BNCF, Magliabechiano MS XV 136: 'Acqua da viso', fols 24^{r}–27^{v} (seven diferent recipes); BR, Riccardiano MS 3068, fol. 30^{r-v}, fol. 31^{r-v}; BR, Riccardiano MS 3058, fol. 5^{r}.
45. Cosmetic: e.g., BR, Riccardiano MS 3063: 'Aqua odorifera' fol. 27^{v}; BNCF, Palatino MS 1026: 'Per far l'acqua muscata', fol. 14^{r}, 'per fare acqua d'angioli perfettissima', fols 4^{r-v}; BNCF, Magliabechiano MS XV 136: 'Acqua di lavanda', 'acqua di belzui /storacie et oldano', 'Acqua di gielsomino', 'acqua optima di piu cose', 'Acqua rosa muscata', fols 4^{r}–5^{v}; BR, Riccardiano MS 3068: 'aqua odorifera', fol. 27^{v}.
46. Wound-healing: e.g., BR, Riccardiano MS 3056, fol. 73^{v} and fol. 75^{r}; BR, Riccardiano MS 3057, fol. 143^{v}; Wellcome Library, MS 174, fols 63^{r-v}. The stone: BNCF, Magliabechiano MS XV 92, fol. 144^{r}; BR, Riccardiano MS 2376, fol. 14^{v}. The French disease: e.g., Wellcome Library, MS 174: 'Aqua da guarire el membro zoe el mal francoso', fol. 4^{v}. Male genitals: e.g., BNCF, Magliabechiano XV 92, fol. 142^{r}; BR, Riccardiano MS 3057, fol. 46^{v}; BNCF, Magliabechiano MS XV 118, fol. 4^{r}.
47. For an in-depth examination of this recipe collection, see Henderson, *The Renaissance Hospital*, pp. 297–335. This study shows how recipes are organized based on specific symptoms and bodily regions, particularly focusing on the head, abdomen, urogenital tract, and overall bodily ailments. Henderson notes the elastic terminology and classification of symptoms, diseases, and remedies in this hospital collection. In my view, this phenomenon can be also explained by the miscellaneous sources and the encyclopedic nature of the practical-oriented vernacular medical tradition more largely.
48. 'Acqua da occhi et diemmi laricietta frate biacio la quale lebbe lui da uno valentissimo huomo doctore per li occhi', fol. 45^{r}; 'acqua da occhi fine', fols 56^{r} and 58^{r}; 'acqua daocchi fina', 'acqua comune daocchi fine', fol. 113^{v}; 'acqua daocchi', fols 123^{v} and 124^{v}; 'acqua daocchi fina auta da ghualtieri biliotti', 'acqua daocchi che susa infirençe', fol. 143^{r}; 'acqua da occhi dicholore açurro', 'acqua da occhi da rossore et dapiççichore', 'acqua daocchi da rallegrare et allarghare il vedere et mandare via la lagrime', fol. 143^{v}.

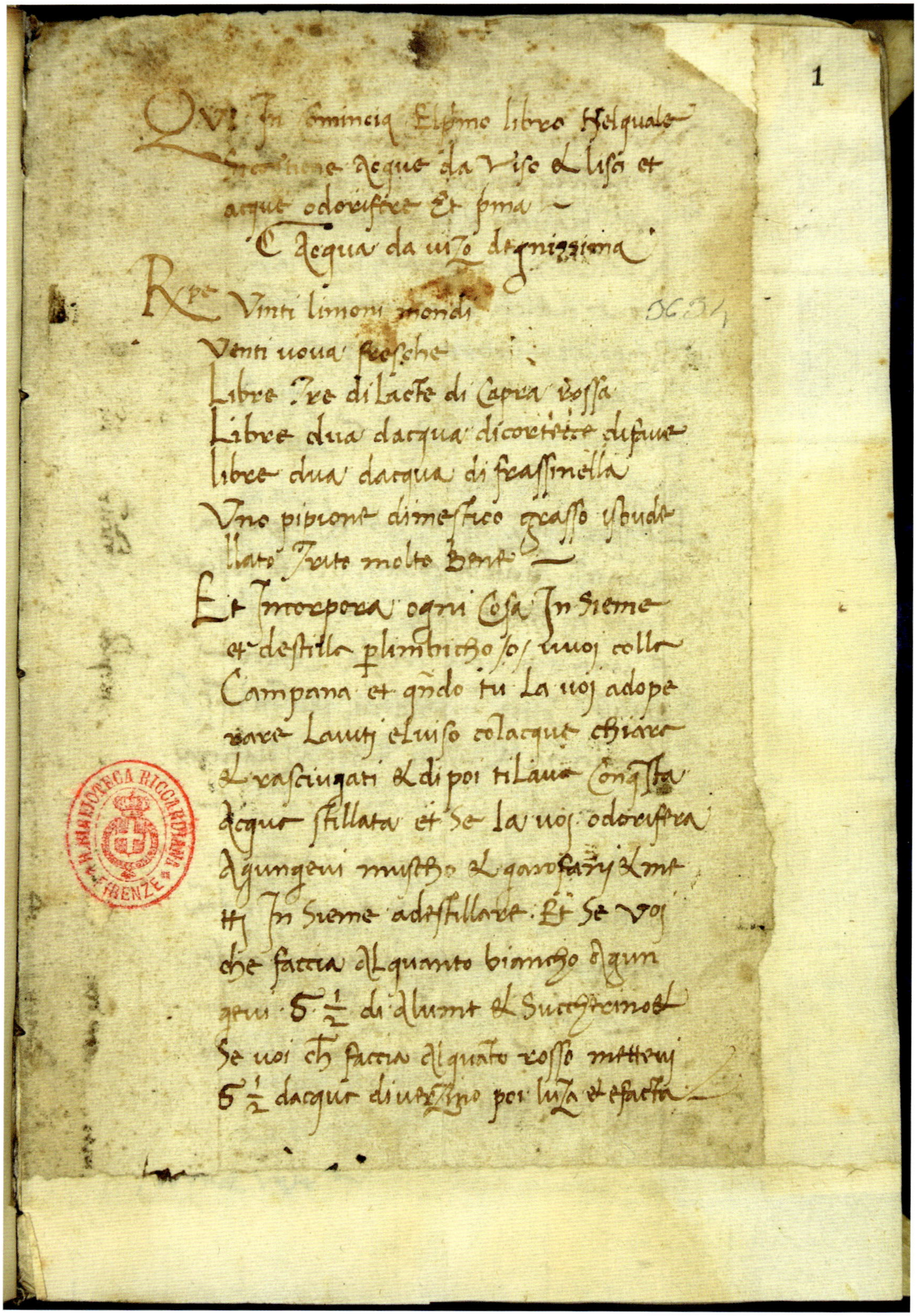

15. This is the initial page of a sixteenth-century cosmetics manual, containing an array of beauty recipes organized into separate sections. Penned in a refined humanist cursive script with minimal abbreviations, generous interlinear spaces and margins, the manuscript offers meticulous guidance on the preparation and application of various formulations.

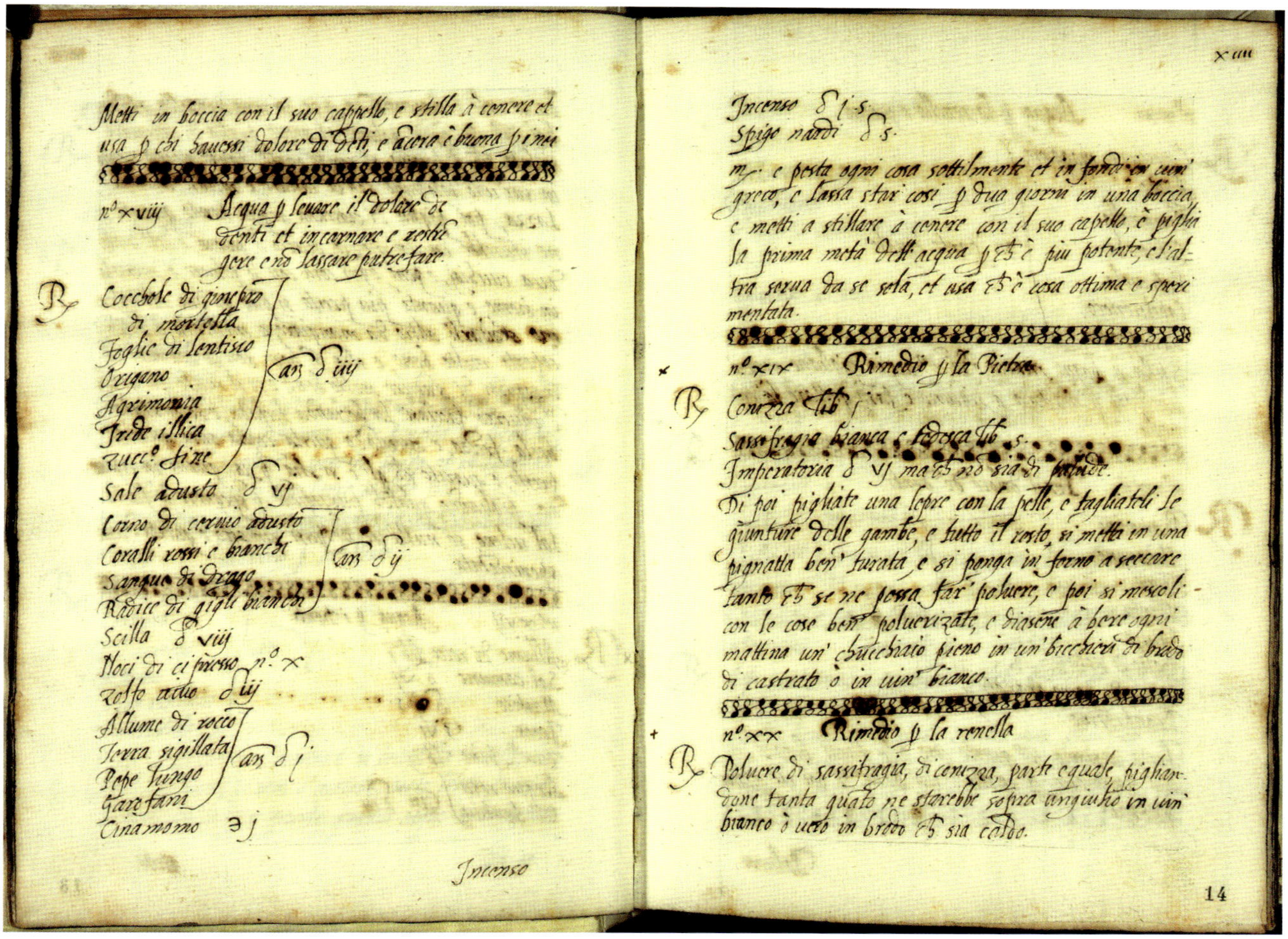

16. This mouthwash is part of a compendium (dated 1576) comprising diverse medicinal and cosmetic formulas, including numerous *acque* intended for various therapeutic uses. Among the ingredients listed in this recipe are substances renowned for their anti-inflammatory, analgesic, and antiseptic properties.

eye salves, 'acqua daocchi fina' and 'acqua daocchi chomune fine', copied one after the other and containing very similar ingredients. On folios 142ʳ–143ᵛ, we find a series of eyewashes ('acqua da occhi') in close succession, many of which share basic ingredients and similar preparation methods.[49]

This tendency to group together similar recipes could develop into whole collections dedicated to a specific ailment or cures for a certain organ or body part. A case in point is a section of the codex Palatino 1023 (fols 49ʳ–55ᵛ), written by a sixteenth-century hand, containing a collection of recipes—mostly *acque*—for the treatment of eye diseases, with detailed descriptions of ingredients, modes of preparation and usage (fig 15).[50] Similarly, the accretion of recipes devoted to a specific organ or disease chiefly proceeded by tweaking the same basic simples with others to produce new medicines.[51] In the collection of the Palatino 1023, for example, the compiler records dozens of remedies for the eyes by recombining a standard number of active ingredients and vehicles (used as solvents or diluents) into different preparations. In the case of the eyewashes here, the active ingredients that reappear in various waters are *tutia* (zinc oxide powder), *canfora* (camphor) and aloe, while the standard solvents are *acqua*

49. BNCF, Magliabechiano MS XV 92, fols 143ʳ⁻ᵛ.

50. BNCF, Palatino MS 1023: 'Experimenti et ricette apiu varie infirmita docchi', fol. 49ʳ.

51. Pugliano, 'Pharmacy, Testing', pp. 237–50.

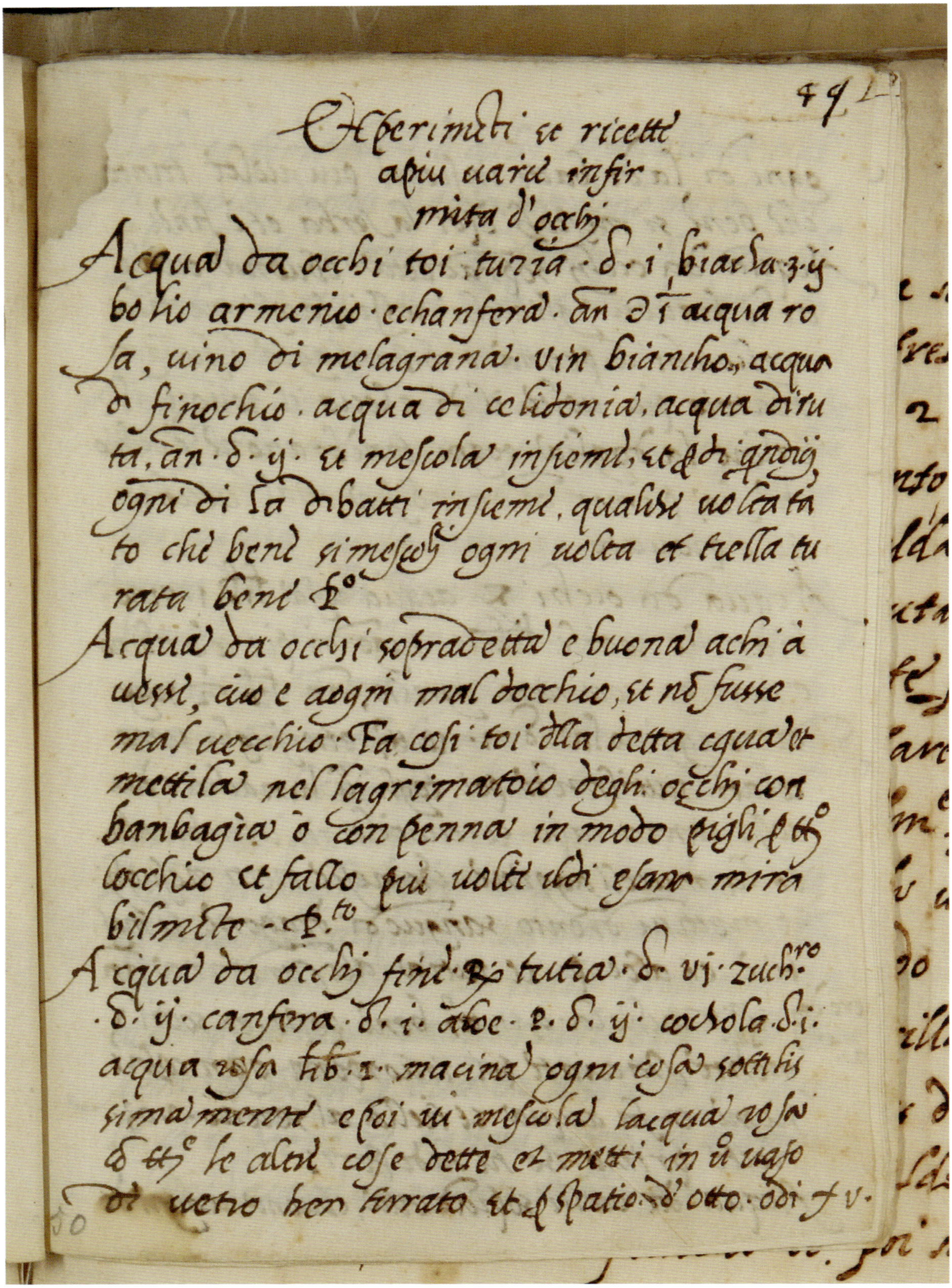

49

Esperimenti et ricette
a più varie infir
mità d'occhi

Acqua da occhi toi tuzia . d. i biacca z. ij
bolo armenio . e chanfora . an. d. i acqua ro
sa, uino di melagrana . vin biancho, acqua
di finochio . acqua di celidonia, acqua di ru
ta, an. d. ij . et mescola insieme, et per giorni
ogni di la dibatti insieme, qualche uolta tan
to che bene si mescoli ogni uolta et tiella tu
rata bene P.o

Acqua da occhi sopradetta e buona a chi à
uessi, cio e a ogni mal docchio, et nō fusse
mal uecchio . Fa cosi toi della detta acqua et
mettila nel lagrimatoio degli occhi con
banbagia o con penna in modo [illegible]
locchio et fallo piu uolte il di e sono mira
bilmente . P.to

Acqua da occhi fine R. tutia . d. vi . zuch.ro
. d. ij . canfora . d. i . aloe . P. d. ij . cocciola d. i .
acqua rosa lib. i . macina ogni cosa sottilis
simamente e poi ui mescola lacqua rosa
[illegible] le altre cose dette et metti in u. uaso
di uetro ben serrato et per spatio d'otto . di [illegible]

17. The image shows the introductory page of a compilation of collyria and eye-salves written by a sixteenth-century hand and preserved within a miscellaneous volume of medical secrets. The collection furnishes instructions on the preparation and application of different eye remedies.

rosa (rose water) and *vino biancho* (white wine).[52] These simples are, in turn, recombined with other ingredients, like coral, incense, cloves, fennel, rosemary, verbena, and celandine, to create new prescriptions. This tweaking approach to recipe compilation is corroborated both internally (within the same manuscript) and externally (recipes copied from other sources and reworked into a new collection).

The general indexing of waters in the manuscript recipe-books also differs from the criteria used in printed pharmacopeias. Instead of classifying preparations by type of remedy, which is the criterion used by the civic pharmacopeias, recipes are often listed using the instructional formula *a fare/a far* ('to make') followed by the specific purpose of the recipe.[53] Alternatively, they may be categorized by the kind of organ that the waters are expected to act upon,[54] the ailment or disease intended to be cured,[55] or more generally by the effect or cure they are expected to provide. Classification and indexation criteria are often eclectic and vary considerably from one collection to the next, but manuscript recipe-books generally avoid or variously supplement the remedy-type arrangement of the printed civic formularies (fig. 18, 19, 20, 21).

Another remarkable difference with the *Ricettario fiorentino* or the early print Italian pharmacopeias is that manuscript recipe-books provide assorted types of instructions for individual preparations, ranging from synoptic indications like those found in the civic pharmacopeia, to highly detailed and customized instructions containing useful recommendations and caveats. For example, the collection of face-washes ('Acque per far bella la facia') in the MS Wellcome 485, attributed to Antonio de Medici (dated 1598), provides detailed information regarding the use of the beauty products and the potential users.[56] The author, for instance, makes fine cosmetic distinctions between the type of lotion (e.g., day / night), and the type of skin (soft or rough complexion), and gives user-friendly advice as to which ingredients to avoid or include depending on the desired effect and the characteristics of the individual user.[57] The codex Palatino 1023 mentioned above also provides detailed information on how to administer specific eyewashes. For example, after the procedures for preparing eye drops the author includes the following instruction:

> Do as follows. Take some of the said water and put it in the tear trough of the eyes with cotton or with a quill so that it covers the whole eye and do this several times and it heals miraculously' (fig. 17).[58]

More elaborate and personalized instructions are to be found, for example, in another volume, the MS Magliabechiano XV 136, a compilation of cosmetic, medical, and technical recipes, along with several *experimenta* and charms, dated 1531. This book offers particularly detailed instructions on how to prepare the various recipes, most of which involve relatively simple chemical procedures, and gives additional first-person recommendations or more meticulous advice on how to use them. Interestingly, the collection opens with a formula for an 'acqua celestiale' (fols 1^{r}–3^{v}), which requires three successive phases of distillation in a still. The final product, according to the author, is a blood-red fluid ('acqua') which must be stored in a flask like a precious stone ('a gemma'). In the long discussion that follows, the author goes on to list the many virtues ('virtù') of this marvelous water. He thus indicates that the resulting waters can be used both externally (as a lotion, eye drops, or bath) and internally to cure wounds and illnesses of all

52. BNCF, Palatino MS 1023: 'Acqua da occhi, fol. 49^{r}; 'Acqua da occhi fine', fol. 49^{r}; 'Acqua da occhi, fol. 49^{v}; 'Acqua da occhi fine', fol. 50^{r}; 'Acqua da occhi', fol. 50^{r}; 'Acqua comune da occhi fine', fol. 52^{v}; 'Acqua da occhi fine di colore azurro', fol. 54^{r}; 'Acqua da occhi che susa infirenze', fol. 54^{v}; 'Acqua da rossori et pizicori d'occhi' and 'Acqua da occhi da ralegrare et allargar il vedere et mandar via le lacrime', fol. 55^{r}.
53. e.g., BNCF, Magliabechiano MS XV 136 (as recorded in the index): 'Affare acqua di buocca', fol. 31; 'Affar dua acque da viso', fol. 3; 'Affare una acqua degnissima', fol. 32; 'Affare acqua grana di verzino', fol. 3; BR, Riccardiano MS 3068: 'Affare aqua da viso dignissima', fols 30^{r-v}; 'A fare agua da viso degna', fols 31^{r-v}; BR, Riccardiano MS 3068: 'A fare biondo licapelli', fol. 6^{r}.
54. BNCF, Magliabechiano MS XV 92: 'Acqua da occhi fine', fol. 56^{r}, 'Acqua de denti', fols 142^{r-v}, 'Acqua da verga', fol. 142^{r}; BR, Riccardiano MS 3057: 'Acqua da verga provata', fol. 46^{v}; BNCF, Magliabechiano MS XV 140: 'Acqua da renella', fol. 13^{v}.
55. BNCF, Magliabechiano MS XV 140: 'Acqua da Cancheri et Fistole', fol. 6^{v}, 'Acque per la memoria e mal caduco', fols 10^{v}–11^{v}; BR, Riccardiano MS 2376: 'Aqua ad scabiem optima', fols 57^{r-v}, 'Acqua magistrale per la rogna approvata', fols 61^{v}–62^{r}; BNCF, Magliabechiano MS XV 92: 'Acqua damale di pietra e fiancho', fol. 144^{r}.
56. Wellcome Library, MS 485, fols 50^{v}–75^{v}.
57. Wellcome Library, MS 485, fols 61^{v} and 67^{v}.
58. 'Fa cosi. toi della detta aqua et mettila nel lagrimatoio degli occhi con banbagia o con penna in modo pigli per tutto locchio et fallo piu volte adi esana mirabilmente'. BNCF, Palatino MS 1023, fol. 49^{r}.

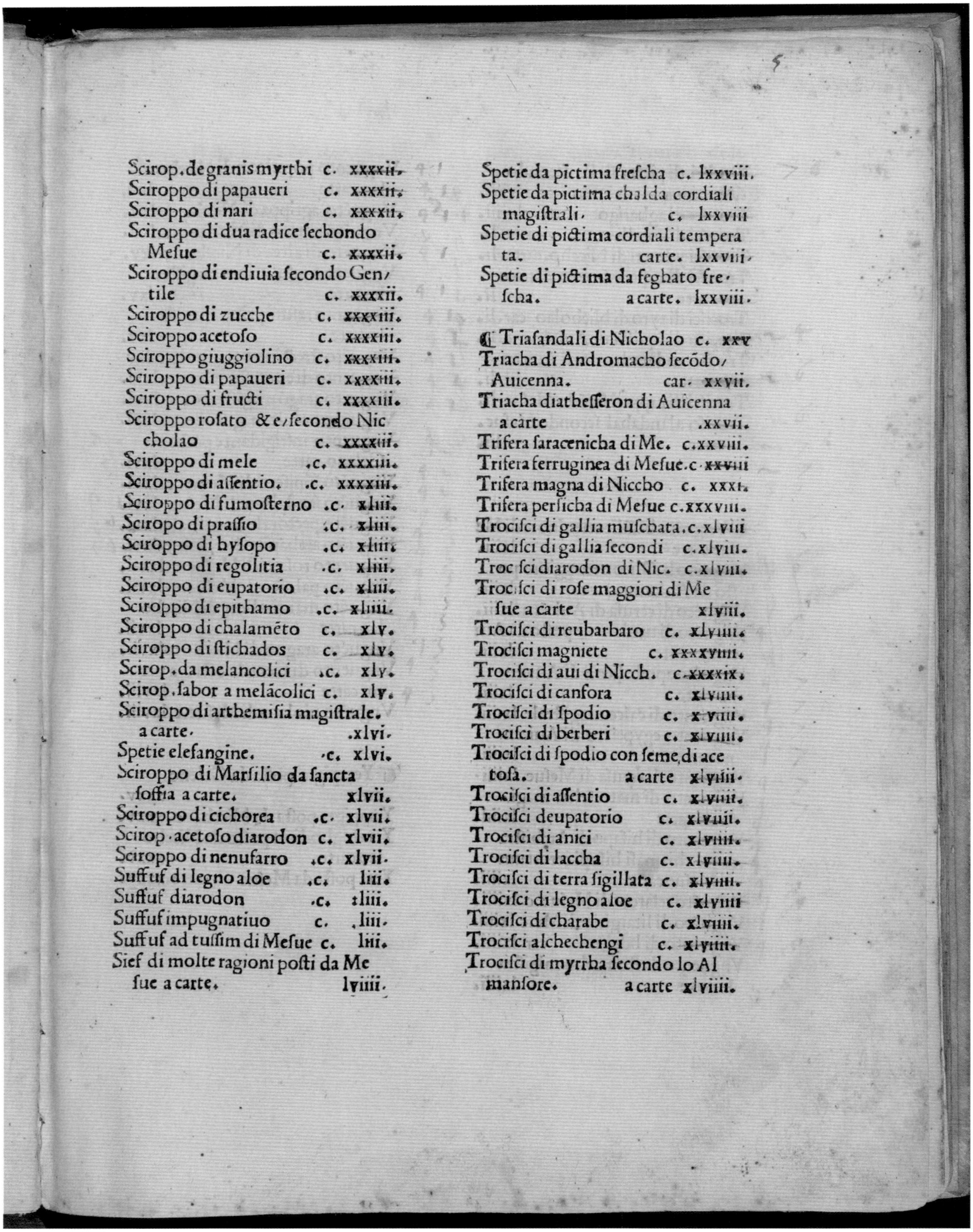

Scirop.de granis myrthi c. xxxxii.
Sciroppo di papaueri c. xxxxii.
Sciroppo di nari c. xxxxii.
Sciroppo di dua radice ſechondo Meſue c. xxxxii.
Sciroppo di endiuia ſecondo Gen/tile c. xxxxii.
Sciroppo di zucche c. xxxxiii.
Sciroppo acetoſo c. xxxxiii.
Sciroppo giuggiolino c. xxxxiii.
Sciroppo di papaueri c. xxxxiii.
Sciroppo di fructi c. xxxxiii.
Sciroppo roſato &c/ſecondo Nicholao c. xxxxiii.
Sciroppo di mele .c. xxxxiii.
Sciroppo di aſſentio. .c. xxxxiii.
Sciroppo di fumoſterno .c. xliii.
Sciropo di praſſio .c. xliii.
Sciroppo di hyſopo .c. xliii.
Sciroppo di regolitia .c. xliii.
Sciroppo di eupatorio .c. xliii.
Sciroppo di epithamo .c. xliii.
Sciroppo di chalaměto c. xlv.
Sciroppo di ſtichados c. xlv.
Scirop.da melancolici .c. xlv.
Scirop.ſabor a melăcolici c. xlv.
Sciroppo di artbemiſia magiſtrale. a carte. .xlvi.
Spetie eleſangine. .c. xlvi.
Sciroppo di Marſilio da ſancta ſoffia a carte. xlvii.
Sciroppo di cichorea .c. xlvii.
Scirop.acetoſo diarodon c. xlvii.
Sciroppo di nenufarro .c. xlvii.
Suffuf di legno aloe .c. liii.
Suffuf diarodon .c. liii.
Suffuf impugnatiuo c. liii.
Suffuf ad tuſſim di Meſue c. liii.
Sief di molte ragioni poſti da Meſue a carte. lviiii.

Spetie da pictima freſcha c. lxxviii.
Spetie da pictima chalda cordiali magiſtrali. c. lxxviii
Spetie di pictima cordiali temperata. carte. lxxviii.
Spetie di pictima da feghato freſcha. a carte. lxxviii.

¶ Triaſandali di Nicholao c. xxv
Triacha di Andromacho ſecŏdo Auicenna. car. xxvii.
Triacha diatheſſeron di Auicenna a carte .xxvii.
Trifera ſaracenicha di Me. c.xxviii.
Trifera ferruginea di Meſue.c. xxviii
Trifera magna di Niccho c. xxxi.
Trifera perſicha di Meſue c.xxxviii.
Trociſci di gallia muſchata.c.xlviii
Trociſci di gallia ſecondi c.xlviii.
Trociſci diarodon di Nic. c.xlviii.
Trociſci di roſe maggiori di Meſue a carte xlviii.
Trociſci di reubarbaro c. xlviii.
Trociſci magniete c. xxxxviiii.
Trociſci di aui di Nicch. c.xxxxix.
Trociſci di canfora c. xlviii.
Trociſci di ſpodio c. xlviii.
Trociſci di berberi c. xlviii.
Trociſci di ſpodio con ſeme di acetoſa. a carte xlviii.
Trociſci di aſſentio c. xlviii.
Trociſci deupatorio c. xlviii.
Trociſci di anici c. xlviii.
Trociſci di laccha c. xlviii.
Trociſci di terra ſigillata c. xlviii.
Trociſci di legno aloe c. xlviii
Trociſci di charabe c. xlviii.
Trociſci alchechengi c. xlviii.
Trociſci di myrrha ſecondo lo Almanſore. a carte xlviii.

18. The table displays preparations categorized by remedy-type under a section of letter S, notably *sciroppo*, *sulfuf*, *sief*, and *spetie*.

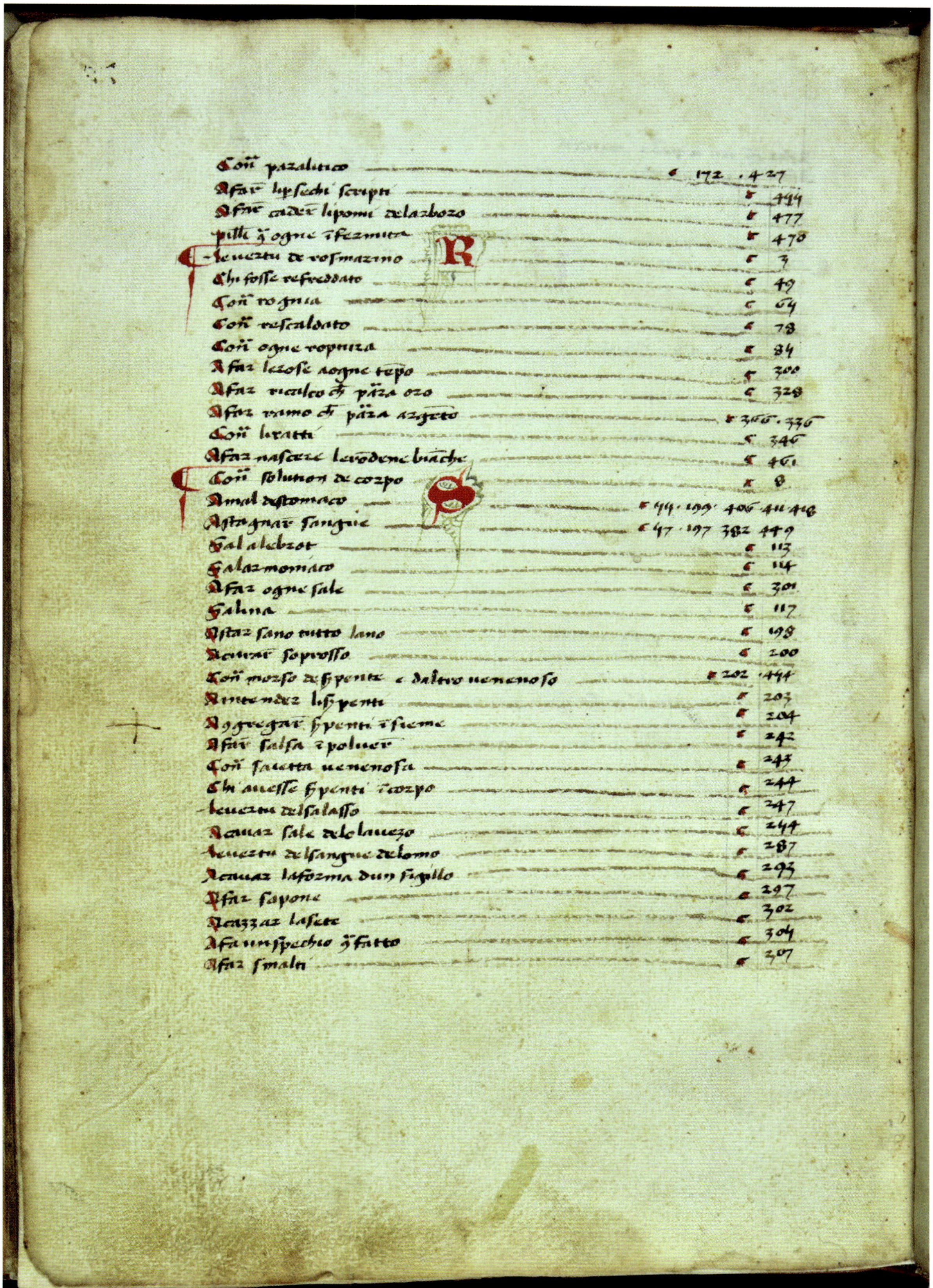

19. The image shows a segment of the alphabetical index under letter S, structured by various miscellaneous keywords such as *stomaco, sangue, sal, sano, serpente, sapone, sigillo, sete, spechio, smalti*, etc.

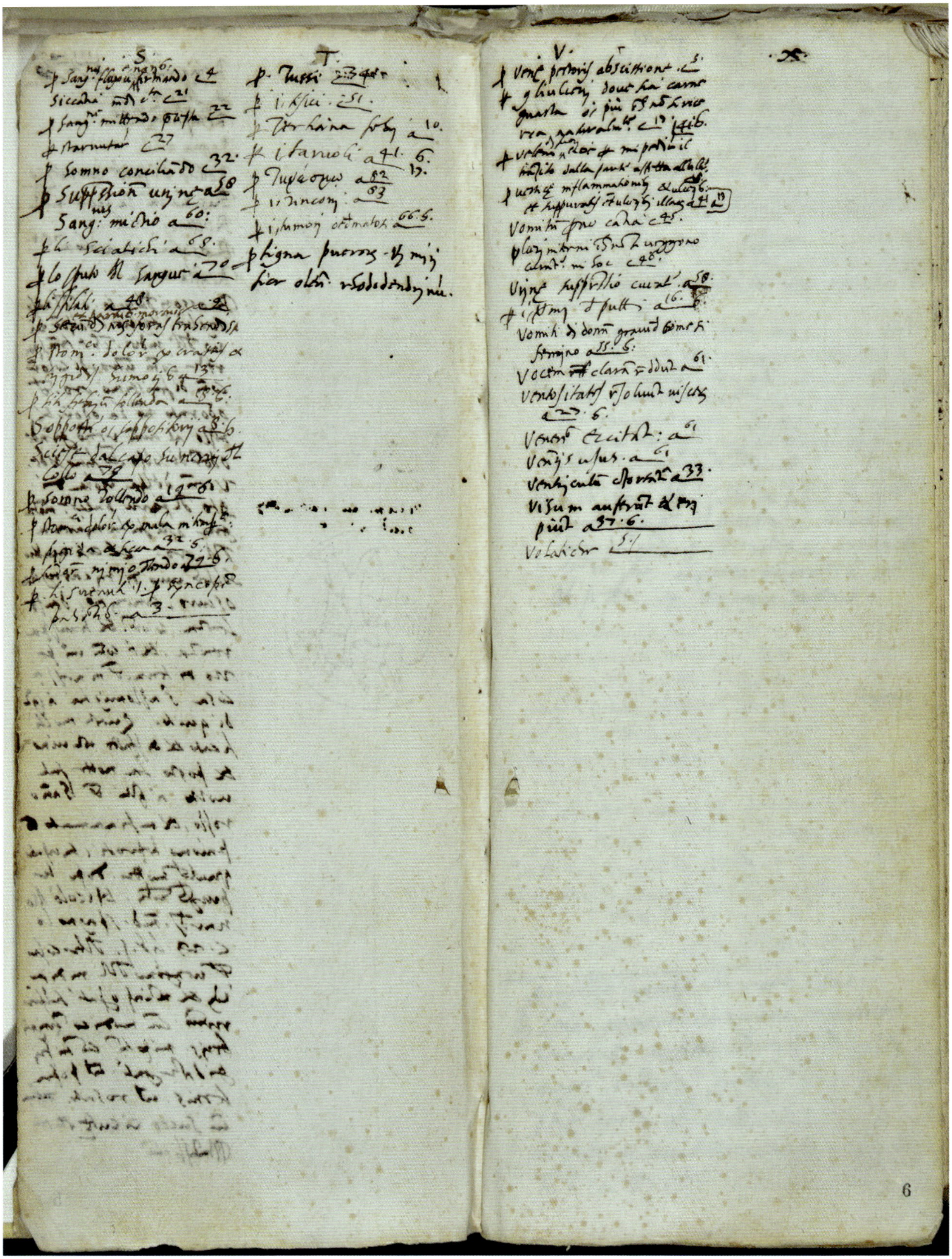

20. A hybrid sixteenth century notebook indexing recipes in both Latin and Italian under the letter S, including assorted entries like: *sanguinis fluxu, siccantia, somno conciliando, sciatichi, sputo del sangue, somno tollendo*, etc.

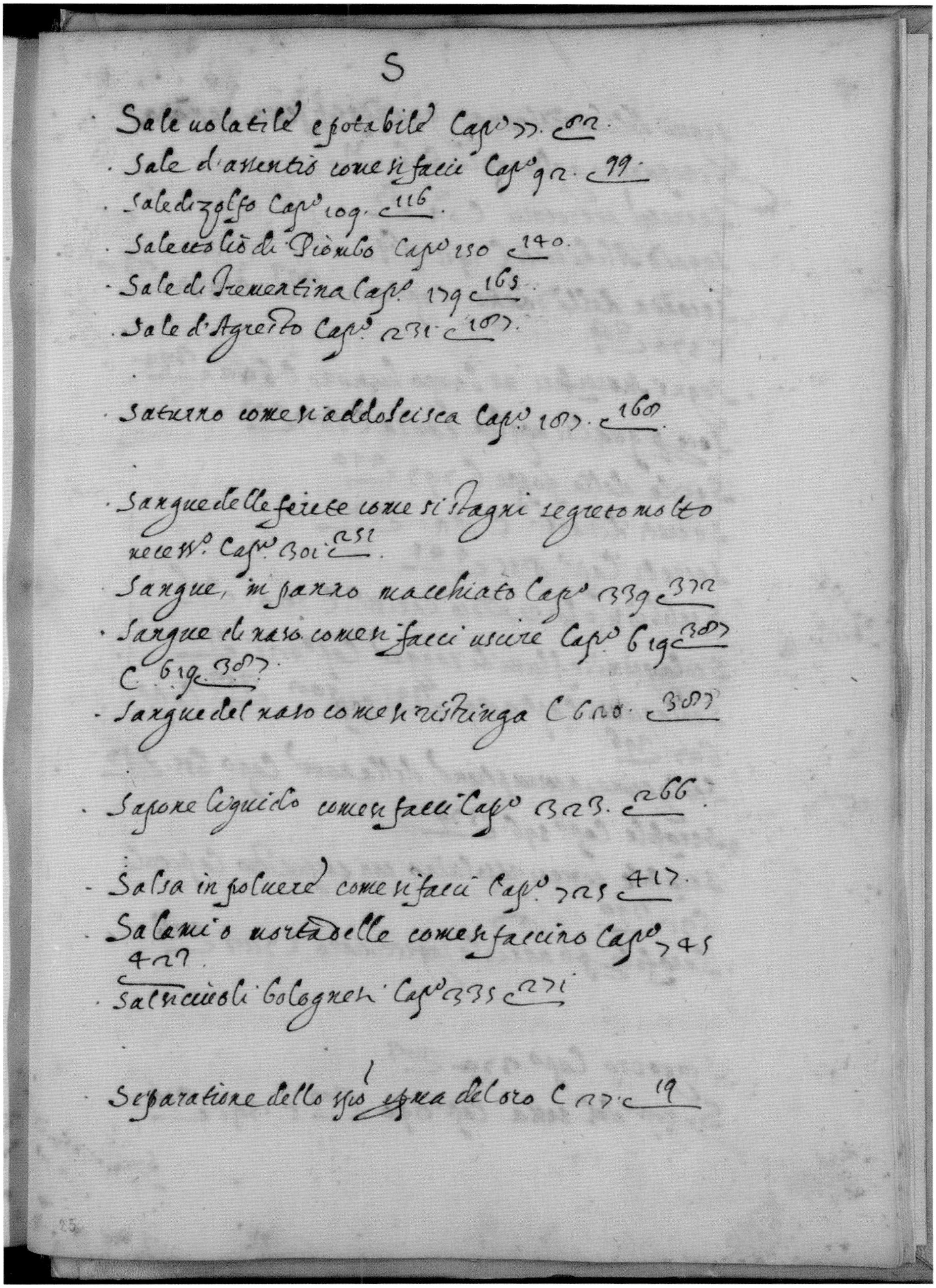

S

Sale uolatile e potabile Cap.° 77. c 82.
Sale d'argento come si facci Cap.° 92. c 99.
Sale di zolfo Cap.° 109. c 116.
Sale e olio di Piombo Cap.° 130 c 140.
Sale di Trementina Cap.° 179 c 165.
Sale d'Agresto Cap.° 231. c 187.

Saturno come si addolcisca Cap.° 187. c 160.

Sangue delle ferite come si stagni segreto molto necess.° Cap.° 301. c 251.
Sangue, in panno macchiato Cap.° 339 c 372
Sangue di naso come si facci uscire Cap.° 619 c 387
C 619. 387.
Sangue del naso come si ristringa C 620. c 387

Sapone liquido come si facci Cap.° 323. c 266.

Salsa in poluere come si facci Cap.° 725 c 417.
Salami o mortadelle come si faccino Cap.° 745 c 427.
Salsiccioli Bolognesi Cap.° 335 c 271

Separatione dello sp.° acqua del oro C 27. c 19

21. Alphabetical index under Letter S from the 'Apparato della Fonderia dell'Illustrissimo et eccellentiss. Sig. D. Antonio Medici,' 1604. Recipes in the collection are indexed following assorted classification criteria: by remedy-type (e.g., *syropo*), body part (e.g., *stomaco*), effect (e.g., *sonnifero*), substance (e.g., *sale*), ailment (e.g., *scrofole*), and other miscellaneous categories (e.g., *secreti*).

kinds, but also as an eyewash, for menstrual pains, and for other more miraculous effects.

While some recipe-books reproduce the impersonal language of the printed pharmacopeias, other manuscripts advertise the effects of certain waters through an extravagant language that promises miraculous cures. In some cases, authors provide first-hand evidence of such effects. The connection between waters and miracles is certainly not new. Indeed, medieval manuscripts devoted to marvelous waters, often anonymous or spuriously attributed to famous men like Aristotle, Peter of Spain, Albert the Great or Arnald of Villanova, were part of a pseudo-scientific literature that predated the early modern fascination with water therapies.[59] In line with this tradition, the titles recorded in the early modern *ricettari* often highlight the marvelous effects of certain waters through the use of eye-catching qualifiers like admirable (*mirabile*) and miraculous (*miracoloso*). Examples include: 'Acqua di Aldobrandino da ferite et sana in pochi giorni cosa miracolosa';[60] 'Acqua mirabile et perfectissima a sanare tutte le piaghe';[61] 'Acqua con sollimato mirabile da far bianche et morbide le carni';[62] and 'Aqua mirabile da ochi'.[63] In other cases, the authors spell out the miraculous effect more eloquently, or provide evidence thereof. Following the long instructions to produce the *acqua celestiale* mentioned above, the author concludes that the water in question has indeed additional miraculous effects, such as 'rejuvenating the elderly' ('di vechio fa giovane') or bringing back doctors who have abandoned their patients.[64] In other sections of the manuscript, he corroborates in the first person the curative properties of certain waters. He recounts, for example, the case of a girl whose arm had begun to decay and risked amputation, but who finally managed to spare her limb by aspersion with the 'acqua da fra Giovanni da rimino degnia' (fols 3^{v}–4^{r}). Elsewhere, confirmation of the wondrous effects may call for the authority of third parties. Thus, the anonymous author of the fifteenth-century Palatino 857 describes a balsam that cleanly pierces a person's hand without causing an injury, an opinion also confirmed by a clergyman and a cardinal.[65]

Miraculous waters are advertised profusely in another popular genre of medical and technical literature, the so-called *libri di secreti* (books of secrets), which became a runaway editorial success in the mid-sixteenth century.[66] For example, the immensely popular *De' secreti del reverendo donno Alessio Piemontese* (The Secrets of the Reverend Master Alexis of Piedmont, 1555) features dozens of cosmetic and medicinal waters,[67] some of which promise to have 'miraculous effects' ('effetto miracoloso').[68] Another popular book of secrets attributed to Gabrielle Falloppio (but probably authored by Leonardo Fioravanti), the *Secreti diversi et miracolosi ne' quali si mostra la via facile di risanare le infirmità del corpo humano* (Various Miraculous Secrets that Reveal the Easy Way to Heal the Infirmities of the Human Body, 1563),[69] also indexes dozens of recipes as *acque* with medicinal and cosmetic properties, displaying a particularly attention-grabbing diction that highlights their extraordinary effects.[70] Cosmetic and scented waters, often advertised through hyperbolic language, were not only an integral part of the secrets literature, both manuscript and printed, but also thrived in mid-sixteenth-century publications supposedly composed by or specifically addressed to women. Thus, the book *I secreti della signora Isabella Cortese* (The Secrets of Signora Isabella

59. See Forbes, *History of Distillation*, pp. 69–70.
60. BR, Riccardiano MS 3057, fols 89^{v}–90^{v}.
61. BR, Riccardiano MS 3057, fols 140^{v}–141^{r}.
62. BNCF, Palatino MS 1026, fol. 11^{r}.
63. BR, Riccardiano MS 3056, fol. 76^{r}.
64. BNCF, Magliabechiano MS XV 136, fols 1^{r}–3^{v}.
65. BNCF, Palatino MS 857, fol. 22^{r}. See Gentile, *I codici Palatini*, 2, p. 367.
66. On secrets and books of secrets, see Leong and Rankin, *Secrets and Knowledge*, pp. 7–20.
67. cf. Piemontese, *De' secreti*: 'acqua pettorale', pp. 77–79; 'acqua da sanare in cinque giorni[...]', pp. 87–88; 'acqua odorifera e molto buona', pp. 155–58 (ten recipes); 'a far acqua che fa le carni colorite, a chi l'ha palide', p. 214 and other recipes (pp. 215–17); 'a far acqua di melloni bianchi per far bella carnatura', pp. 219–20; 'acqua perfetta di xucche o cocozze domestiche da mangiare o delle salvatiche', p. 220; 'acqua di talco perfettissima', p. 223; 'a fare acqua che imbianchisce il volto', p. 229; 'a fare un'acqua che manda via ogni tintura, e macchia delle mani', pp. 231–33, 260, 265, etc.
68. Piemontese, *De' secreti*, p. 52.
69. On the attribution of Fallopio's book to Fioravanti, see Eamon, *Science and the Secrets of Nature*, pp. 166–68.
70. Fallopio, *Secreti divesi:* 'Acqua divina per sanar l'infirmita degli occhi', p. 168; 'a far un acqua odorifera [...]', p.169; dozens of recipes indexed as waters for various purposes, medicinal, cosmetic, chemical, etc., pp. 170–208; 'acqua miracolosa', p.181; 'acqua per ogni piaga et ferita miracolosa', p. 185; 'un'acqua con molte et diverse proprieta naturali et miracolose', p. 200, etc.

Cortese, 1565), attributed to an unidentified female writer,[71] includes recipes for the preparation of various such cosmetic, medicinal, and perfumed waters.[72] Another contemporary work, *Gli ornamenti delle donne* (Women's Adornments), written by Giovanni Marinello (1562), includes over fifty recipes indexed as waters. A veritable handbook of feminine cosmetics, Marinello's work includes waters to soften and whiten the skin and remove all kinds of blemishes and imperfections (pp. 238, 246, 248, 252, etc.), hair-dyes, hair-moisturizers, and shampoos (pp. 40, 51, 56, 58, 61, 63, 70, 78, etc.), mouth-washes, teeth-whitening waters (pp. 176, 173), eye drops and eyewashes (pp. 104, 147), perfumed waters and colognes (pp. 5, 12, 13) along with other assorted medicinal waters. The adjective 'miraculous' and other cognates are used over forty times in the treatise, especially to publicize the marvelous effects of a certain remedy. For example, in a section on 'Scented waters and liquors' ('Acque et liquori odoriferi'), Marinello informs the readers that he would reveal 'a miraculous secret' ('un miracoloso secreto') for preparing a specific kind of water, as well as other sweet-scented perfumes.[73] In sum, the publishing success of books of secrets confirms the spread and popularity of medicinal and cosmetic waters in the early modern period. However, it should be noted that the printed secrets were only the most visible and external expression of a long-established tradition of experimentation with waters and other substances that had previously circulated (and continued to circulate) in manuscript form as collections of *experimenta* and *secreta*.

In the surveyed manuscripts, medicinal waters are obtained both through the traditional method of decoction, but most notably through distillation. Contrary to what the editors of the 1499 *Ricettario fiorentino* recorded, remedies obtained by distillation were fundamental to medieval and early modern pharmacology. In fact, lists of simple distilled waters are not uncommon in manuscript recipe-books. Thus, for example, a collection of medical recipes similar to the 1499 *Ricettario fiorentino*, and possibly the one used in apothecaries' shops before Grand Duke Cosimo I had it reformed and printed, the MS Magliabechiano XV 118 (c. 1470), includes a list of nearly one hundred waters that can be obtained by distillation.[74] An Italian book containing a number of receipts, description of diseases and cures, with sparse marginal illustrations, the MS Wellcome 174, written in 1529, also gives the description and therapeutic uses of simple waters obtained by distillation and decoction in several folios, classing them according to the four properties in the Galenic pharmacological theory (cold, hot, wet, and dry). According to the author of this book, a barber by the name of Gasparo di Cagali, much of the information in this section is drawn from a certain Maximo da Milan. Inside the lower cover, the volume includes two fine drawings of distilling apparatuses.

Recipes for waters including distillation are frequent in fifteenth-century manuscripts, although they will become far more widespread in the following century. For example, the author of the MS Palatino 857, a fifteenth-century book of medical, alchemical, and industrial secrets written in a hybrid Latin and Italian dialect,[75] employs a three-stage distillation process for the preparation of a medicinal water ('Aqua che si chiama matre balsami', fols. 19ʳ–23ʳ). The author explains that 'the first water that is distilled is called balsam water // the second balsam oil // the third artificial balsam //and the first is good // the second better // the third optimal'.[76] But distillation is also used for other remedies in the collection, like a collyrium and a wound-healing powder.[77] Similarly, the MS Magliabechiano XV 76, written in 1468, contains a miscellany of alchemical, medicinal and cosmetic recipes, some of which include distillation processes. For example, on folio 18ᵛ, the author indexes a certain 'water to break any metal' ('acqua da rodere ogni metallo') which has also multiple other marvelous uses as a hair dye and as a writing ink, when combined with tin and copper filings. According to the

71. On Cortese, see the introduction to Leong and Rankin, *Secrets and Knowledge in Medicine and Science*, pp. 16–17, and Eamon, 'How to Read a Book of Secrets', pp. 28–34.
72. Cortese, *I secreti*: 'A fare acqua azurra', p.67; perfumed waters, pp. 121–23; mouthwash, p. 124; facewashes ('acqua da viso'), pp. 135–36, 142–44, 160; as well as other perfumed and cosmetic waters, pp. 190–98.
73. Marinello, *Gli ornamenti*, p. 5.
74. BNCF, MS Magliabechiano XV 118, fols 10ᵛ–11ᵛ. The list is preceded by the following legend: 'Tutte queste sono laqque medicinali che semprecemente sistillano'.
75. See Gentile, *I codici Palatini della Biblioteca Nazionale*, II, p. 367.
76. 'E Sapi che la prima aqua che distilla si chiama aqua balsami//la seconda ollio di balsamo //la terza balsamo artificiale // e la prima bona //la seconda mejo // la terza otima', fol. 20ʳ.
77. BNCF, MS Palatino 857, fol. 39ᵛ, and fols 36 ʳ⁻ᵛ.

author, this water is obtained through distillation in a still and requires that the person in charge carefully observe changes in color as the process unfolds.[78]

The number of water recipes using distillation increases dramatically toward the second half of the sixteenth century. In various manuscripts, distillation processes in the preparation of remedies, including but not limited to waters, are often explained in great detail. For example, a neatly copied collection of secrets attributed to Prince D. Antonio de Medici, the MS Magliabechiano XV 140, provides detailed instructions for the preparation of ten different *acque*, all of which involve one or more stages of distillation[79] (fig. 20). A standard procedure reads as follows:

> Crush the things to be pounded and put them in the acqua vita (water of life), in a vessel, sealing it very well, and let it stand for three days, and thus sealed you will put it in a bain-marie with a little fire for another three days, and then you will put the stopper with its container, and you will put it on the fire for another three days, or for as long as it distils, and what will come out of it will be the Matrebalsam water, which you will keep well sealed. From the residue that remains, make oil in this way [...][80]

Overall, preparing the various waters listed in this manuscript requires a series of standardized steps or phases, such as grinding and sieving the ingredients, distilling in a bain-marie, adding more ingredients if necessary (further infusion), distilling again, increasing or decreasing the fire as required, and finally collecting the distilled water (and also essential oils) and storing it in a tightly closed flask. In sum, distillates were part and parcel of the early modern pharmacopeia. The manuscript recipe books provide evidence of the widespread use and increasing popularity of distillation methods, thus rectifying the distorted view offered by the official pharmacopeias.

In the manuscript tradition, recipes are part of a genre of craft practice that primarily involves experimentation with substances and materials. Thus, recipe-books often amalgamate *materia medica*, pharmacology, cosmetics, secrets, alchemy, and craftsmanship of various kinds without making clear-cut distinctions between fields of expertise.[81] The underlying criterion seems to be the gathering of vernacular lore pertaining to the try-and-test approach to nature. This overlap and cross-pollination of knowledge domains is precluded by the regulatory civic approach to public health displayed in the printed pharmacopeias. In the 16th century, however, an apparently contrary phenomenon emerges, namely the compilation of recipes belonging to more distinct domains of artisanal experimentation. Cosmetics, for example, which gradually emerged as a branch of experimental medicine and chemistry, was one of the areas that flourished in the sixteenth century and produced more tightly organized collection of recipes.

Several manuscripts attest to this increasing specialization and categorization into individual craft domains. The MS Palatino 941, for example, is a remarkable sixteenth-century handbook containing myriad secrets and recipes both for medicinal, cosmetic, and industrial purposes. Written in calligraphic cursive hand, and featuring neatly defined red-ink rubrics, the book contains a rare and highly detailed, user-friendly index which follows specific classification criteria. Waters, for example, are divided here into two broad categories: 'waters for women' ('acque per donne') and 'scented waters' ('acque odorifere'). The former category comprises over sixty recipes, mainly skin lotions, while the latter indexes over forty different perfumes and colognes. This twofold

78. BNCF, MS Palatino 857, fol. 18^{v}.

79. BNCF, MS Magliabechiano XV 140, 'Segreti Sperimentati dall'Illumo et Eccmo Sigr. Principe D. Antonio de Medici Nella sua Fonderia del Casino': 'Acqua e Olio Matrebalsamo', fol. 3^{r}; 'Alli occhi Acqua conservativa della Sanità', fols 5^{v}–6^{r}; ' Acqua da Cancheri et Fistole', fol. 6^{v}; 'Acque per la memoria e mal caduco', fols 10^{v}–11^{v}; 'Acqua da Petecchie', fols 11^{v}–12^{r}; 'Acqua per li nervi che hanno patito per causa di catarro o gocciola', fol. $12^{r\text{-}v}$; 'Acqua per incarnare li denti et mantenerli bianco', fol. 13^{r}; 'Acqua da Renella', fol. 13^{v}; 'Acqua perfetta a dolor di fianco et catarri et altri mali causati da ventosita', fols 13^{v}–14^{v}; 'Acqua et Olio Matrebalsamo', fols $20^{r\text{-}v}$.

80. 'Pesta le cose da pestare, et infondi nell'acqua vite, in boccia, turandola molto bene, et lascia stare per tre giorni, et cosi turata la porrai a bagno maria con poco fuoco per tre altri di, et poi gli metterai il cappello con in suo recipiente, et tutto ben turato, et li darai fuoco per tre altri di, o vero tanto quanto stillerà, e quello, che n'uscira e l'acqua Matrebalsamo, la quale conserverai benissimo turata. Delle feccie che resteranno, si trahe l'Olio in questo modo [...]', fol. 3^{r}.

81. Examples of miscellaneous manuscripts, including medical, cosmetic, industrial and alchemical recipes, are: BNCF MS Magliabechiano XV 136 (dated 1531); MS Magliabechiano XV 92 (1515), MS Palatino 851 (S. XV), fols 1^{r}–29^{v}; MS Palatino 885 (S. XVI), fols 35^{r}–50^{v}, 88^{r}–94^{v}; MS Palatino 891 (1538-1553), fols 126^{v}–161^{v}; MS Palatino 916 (S. XV. metà), fols 1^{r}–154^{v}; MS Palatino 1026 (Zibaldone strozziano, S. XV-XVI).

classification shows that waters are interpreted here primarily as beauty or cosmetic products rather than as an all-encompassing category, as is mostly the case in the rest of the surveyed manuscripts. Other volumes are entirely devoted to cosmetics and offer clearly distinct sections for specific kinds of preparations. Such is the case of the elegant MS Riccardiano 3058, a sixteenth-century cosmetics handbook, which organizes recipes into seven different sections according to the type of cosmetic product: *acque da viso et liscie et acque odorifere* (fols 1^{r}–33^{v}), *composizioni d'olii, come si fanno* (fols 37^{r}–41^{r}), *composizioni delle pomate et saponi di diverse ragioni* (fols 44^{r}–51^{v}), *poveri odorifere di piu ragioni* (fols 55^{v}–62^{r}), *profumi di diverse ragioni* (fols 65^{r}–70^{r}), *ricette medicinali* (fols 71^{r}–80^{r}) and *saponi, torte e altre cose* (fols 82^{v}–84^{v}) It is interesting to see in this example how medicinal products (*ricette medicinali*) actually become a subcategory of cosmetic products more largely. Overall, while the most prevalent manifestation was that of miscellaneous collections of artisanal experiments including medical, alchemical, and industrial products, the opposite phenomenon of growing specialization and focused compilations can also be observed.

CONCLUSION

By the late sixteenth century, water, and waters (in the plural) had become an integral part of medicine, cosmetics, diet, self-care, and preventive therapies in Renaissance Florence. In this context, manufactured waters enjoyed tremendous success. The expansion of this loose category of medicinal-cosmetic remedies designated as *acque* was coextensive with the diversification of other traditional pharmaceutical products during the sixteenth century. But unlike other types of medicines, such as oils, ointments, electuaries and pills, waters grew into a *sui generis*, all-encompassing category of remedies that served a variety of purposes, most of which were not recorded in the civic formularies. The proliferation of aqueous products of all kinds, such as baths, simple and complex distilled waters, eye-salves, lotions, colognes and tonics, may also be interpreted as a corollary of a culture that exploited and cultivated the therapeutic properties of water more generally, as evidenced by the growing interest in balneology, regimes of health, and water cures.

The wide assortment of preparations designated as waters in the manuscript sources, compared to the limited records in the civic formularies, indicates a divide between two discursive domains: that of medical theory, which fostered a conservative and prescriptive approach to public health, and relied on time-tested recipes recorded in medieval formularies, and that of medical practice, which incorporated a much wider variety of individuals across the social spectrum, and adopted eclectic and increasingly innovative medical therapies and treatments. However, this gap between theory and practice partially began to narrow over the course of the sixteenth century. Thus the 1574 edition of the civic *ricettario* offered a more extensive treatment of distillation methods and equipment, probably reflecting the popularity of vernacular distillation manuals and the impulse given by the Medici family to alchemical experimentation more generally, along with the diffusion of Paracelsian chemical medicine in Northern Italy. Notwithstanding, the civic pharmacopeias barely reflected the diversity of waters available. This fact therefore points to the importance of considering vernacular knowledge to properly gauge the scientific developments in the early modern period.

The case of medicinal waters also offers insight into the vernacular modes of recording and transmitting medical knowledge more largely. As shown in the sources, recipes were not normally indexed by remedy-type, as in the civic formularies, but by the kind of effect or cure they were expected to provide, thus revealing an organization that was centered on the patient rather than the medical specialist. As amply illustrated by the proliferation of waters, the accrual of recipes within or across recipe-books was often the result of simple repetitions of the same title and preparation, the tweaking of headings, or the intermingling of basic ingredients. The procedural section of the individual recipes offered the greatest margin for innovation. Indeed, the length, degree of detail, register and mode of enunciation of the procedures and recommendations for use varied considerably from one manuscript to the next. The case of waters thus reveals that the recipe-book format is highly malleable and context-sensitive, and sheds light on the way different communities of learning and practice adapt medical knowledge to specific ends.

Finally, the evidence in the manuscript recipe-books illustrates the empirical base of pharmaceutical innovation in the sixteenth century. Indeed, these developments resulted from the overlap of various knowledge domains (*materia medica*, pharmacology, cosmetics, secrets, alchemy, and craftsmanship of various kinds), often without precise distinction between areas of expertise, and the interaction of a range of health-related individuals, from learned physicians to empirics and laypeople more generally. This experimental approach to water therapies—and pharmaceutical knowledge more generally—contrasted with the conservative and prescriptive approach to public health as featured in the civic pharmacopeias issued by the Collegio dei Medici. Further research may help us understand how these waters were produced, marketed, and consumed by individual social actors in Renaissance Florence and beyond.

WORKS CITED

Printed Primary Sources

Augustis, Quiricus de, *Lumen apothecariorum* (Turin: Nicolaus de Benedectis, 1492).

Biringuccio, Vannuccio, *Pirotechnia... Nuovamente corretta, et ristampata* (Venice: Gironimo Giglio, 1559).

Brunschwig, Hieronymus, *The Vertuose Boke of Distyllacyon of the Waters of All Maner of Herbes* (London: Laurens Andrewe, 1527).

Cardano, Girolamo. 'De subtilitate', in *Opera Omnia*, 10 vols (Lyon: Jean Antoine Huguetan/ Marc Antione Ravaud, 1663).

Fallopio, Gabrielle, *Secreti diversi e miracolosi* (Venice: Marc'Antonio Bonibelli, 1597).

Fioravanti, Leonardo, *Dello specchio di scientia universale...Libri Tre* (Venice: Vincenzo Valgrisi, 1564).

Gessner, Conrad, *Thesaurus Euonymi Philiatri de remediis secretis* (Zürich: Andrea Gessner, 1552).

Manardo, Giovanni, *Ioannis Manardi...Epistolarum medicinalium lib. XX* (Venice: Petrus Schoeffer, 1542).

Manlio del Bosco, Giovanni Giacomo, *Luminare maius* (Venice: Ioan. Gryphium, 1551).

Marinello, Giovanni, *Gli ornamenti delle donne* (Venice: Giovanni Valgrisio, 1574).

Mattioli, Pietro Andrea, *Commentarii in Sex libros Pedacii Dioscoridis Anazarbei De medica materia* (Venice: Vincenzo Valgrisi, 1565).

Saladinus di Asculo, *Compendium aromatariorum* (Bologna: Benedictus Hectoris, 1488).

Suardo, Paolo, *Thesaurus aromatariorum* (Milan: Leonardus Pachel, 1496).

Secondary Sources

Abraham, Lyndy, *A Dictionary of Alchemical Imagery* (Cambridge: Cambridge University Press, 1998).

Barker, Sheila, 'Cosimo I de' Medici and the Renaissance Sciences: "To Measure and to See"', in *A Companion to Cosimo I de' Medici*, ed. by Alessio Assonitis and Henk Th. van Veen (Leiden: Brill, 2021), pp. 520–80.

Beck, Emily, 'The Ricettario Fiorentino and Manuscript Recipe Culture in Sixteenth- Century Florence', in *Drugs on the Page. Pharmacopoeias and Healing Knowledge in the Early Modern Atlantic World*, ed. by Matthew James Crawford and Joseph Gabriel (Pittsburgh: University of Pittsburgh Press, 2019).

Bellorini, Cristina, *The World of Plants in Renaissance Tuscany* (Farnham: Ashgate, 2016).

Bénézet, Jean Pierre, *Pharmacie et médicament en Méditerranée Occidentale, XIIIe-XVIe siècles* (Paris: Champion, 1999).

Camporesi, Piero, *Camminare il mondo. Vita e avventure di Leonardo Fioravanti medico del Cinquecento* (Milan: Garzanti, 2007).

Cavallo, Sandra, 'Health, Beauty and Hygiene', in *At Home in Renaissance Italy*, ed. by Marta Ajmar-Wollheim and Flora Dennis (London: Victoria and Albert Museum, 2006), pp. 174–87.

Cavallo, Sandra and Tessa Storey, *Healthy Living in Late Renaissance Italy* (Oxford: Oxford University Press, 2014).

Cifuentes, Lluís, 'El receptari mèdic baixmedieval i renaixentista: un gènere vernacle', in *Els manuscrits, el saber i les lletres a la corona d'Aragó, 1250-1500*, ed. by Lluís Cifuentes and others (Barcelona: Publicacions de l'Abadia de Montserrat, 2016), pp. 103–60.

Cingolani, Enrico and Leonardo Colapinto, *Dagli antidotari alle moderne farmacopee*, (Rome: Renzi editore, 2000).

Cipriani, Giovanni, *Il trionfo della ragione. Salute e malattia nella Toscana dell'Età Moderna* (Florence: Nicomp Laboratorio Editoriale, 2005).

Clericuzio, Antonio, 'Chemical Medicine and Paracelsianism in Italy, 1550–1650', in *The Practice of Reform in Health, Medicine, and Science, 1500–2000: Essays for Charles Webster*, ed. by Margaret Pelling and Scott Mandelbrote (Aldershot: Ashgate, 2005), pp. 61–70.

Conticelli, Valentina, *"Guardaroba di cose rare et preziose": lo studiolo di Francesco I de' Medici* (Lugano: Agorà, 2007).

Corradi, Alfonso, *Le prime farmacopee italiane, ed in particolare Dei Ricettari Fiorentini. Memoria* (Milan: Fratelli Rechiedei Editori, 1887).

Cortese, Isabella, *I secreti de la Signora Isabella Cortese* (Venice: Giovanni Bariletto, 1565).

Crisciani, Chiara, 'Ricette e medicina: tre zibaldoni nel Quattrocento', Doctor *Virtualis* 13 (2015), 11–37.

Debus, Allen, *The Chemical Philosophy: Paracelsian Science and Medicine in the Sixteenth and Seventeenth Centuries,* 2 vols (Mineola, NY: Courier Dover Publications, 2002).

Eamon, William, *Science and the Secrets of Nature: Books of Secrets in Medieval and Early Modern Culture* (Princeton: Princeton University Press, 1994), pp. 164–93.

Eamon, William, 'How to Read a Book of Secrets', in *Secrets and Knowledge in Medicine and Science, 1500–1800*, ed. by Elaine Leong and Alisha Rankin (Farnham: Ashgate, 2011), pp. 23–46.

Forbes, Robert, A *Short History of the Art of Distillation: from the Beginnings up to the Death of Cellier* (Leiden: Brill, 1970).

Gentilcore, David, *Medical Charlatanism in Early Modern Italy* (Oxford: Oxford University Press, 2006).

Gentilcore, David, 'From "Vilest Beverage" to "Universal Medicine": Drinking Water in Printed Regimens and Health Guides, 1450–1750', *Social History of Medicine*, 33.3 (2020), pp. 683–703.

Gentile, Luigi, *I codici Palatini della Biblioteca Nazionale Centrale di Firenze*, II (Rome: Ministero della Pubblica Istruzione, 1885).

Hedesan, Georgiana, 'Alchemy and Paracelsianism in the Casino di San Marco in Florence', *Nuncius* 37 (2022), 119–43.

Henderson, John, *The Renaissance Hospital: Healing the Body and Healing the Soul* (New Haven: Yale University Press, 2006).

Hirsch, Rudolph, 'The Invention of Printing and the Diffusion of Alchemical and Chemical Knowledge', *Chymia*, 3 (1950), 115–41.

Klein, Ursula and Emma C. Spary, *Materials and Expertise in Early Modern Europe: Between Market and Laboratory* (Chicago: University of Chicago Press, 2010).

Leong, Elaine and Alisha Rankin, 'Introduction: Secrets and Knowledge' in *Secrets and Knowledge in Medicine and Science*, ed. by Elaine Leong and Alisha Rankin (Farnham: Ashgate, 2011), pp. 1–22.

Long, Pamela, *Openness, Secrecy, Authorship: Technical Arts and the Culture of Knowledge from Antiquity to the Renaissance* (Baltimore, MD: Johns Hopkins University Press, 2001).

Mahmoud Salem, Elsheikh, *Medicina e farmacologia nei manoscritti della Biblioteca Riccardiana di Firenze* (Rome: Vecchiarelli, 1990).

Mocarelli, Luca, 'Attitudes to Work and Commerce in the Late Italian Renaissance: A Comparison between Tomaso Garzoni's *La Piazza Universale* and Leonardo Fioravanti's *Dello Specchio Di Scientia Universale*', *International Review of Social History, 56* (S19) (2011), 89–106.

Moran, Bruce, *Distilling Knowledge: Alchemy, Chemistry, and the Scientific Revolution*, (Cambridge, MA and London: Harvard University Press, 2005).

Palmer, Richard, 'Pharmacy in the Republic of Venice', in *The Medical Renaissance of the Sixteenth Century*, ed. by Andrew Wear, Roger K. French, and Iain M. Lonie (Cambridge: Cambridge University Press, 1985), pp. 100–17.

Perifano, Alfredo, *L'alchimie à la Cour de Côme Ier de Médicis: savoirs, culture et politique* (Paris: Honoré Champion, 1997).

Piccardi, Giovanni, *La farmacia granducale* (Florence: Olschki, 2018).

Piemontese, Alessio, *De' secreti del reverendo donno Alessio Piemontese: prima parte, divisa in sei libri: opera utilissima* (Lyon: Theobaldo Pagano, 1558).

Pugliano, Valentina, 'Pharmacy, Testing, and the Language of Truth in Renaissance Italy', *Bulletin of the History of Medicine* 91.2 (2017), 233–73.

Ruland, Martin, *Lexicon Alchemiae* (Hildesheim, Zürich, New York: Georg Olms Verlag, 1987).

Smith, Pamela, *The Body of the Artisan: Art and Experience in the Scientific Revolution* (Chicago: University of Chicago Press, 2004).

Smith, Pamela, 'Science on the Move: Recent Trends in the History of Early Modern Science', *Renaissance Quarterly*, 62.2 (2008), 345–75.

Smith, Pamela, 'What is a Secret? Secrets and Craft Knowledge in Early Modern Europe' in *Secrets and Knowledge in Medicine and Science, 1500–1800*, ed. by Elaine Leong and Anisha Rankin (Farnham: Ashgate, 2011), pp. 47–68.

Spicer, Jacqueline Nicole, 'A Fare Bella: The Visual and Material Culture of Cosmetics in Renaissance Italy (1450-1540)' (doctoral dissertation, University of Edinburgh, 2015).

Stannard, Jerry, 'Medieval Herbalism and Post-Medieval Folk Medicine', *Pharmacy in History*, 55.2/3 (2013), 47–54.

Stolberg, Michael, *Learned Physicians and Everyday Medical Practice in the Renaissance* (Berlin: De Gruyter, 2022).

Storey, Tessa, 'Face Waters, Oils, Love Magic and Poison: Making and Selling Secrets in Early Modern Rome', in *Secrets and Knowledge in Medicine and Science, 1500-1800*, ed. by Elaine Leong and Alisha Rankin (Farnham: Ashgate, 2011), pp. 143–166.

Taape, Tillmann, 'Distilling Reliable Remedies: Hieronymus Brunschwig's *Liber de arte distillandi* (1500) Between Alchemical Learning and Craft Practice', *Ambix* 61(3) (2014), pp. 236–56.

Targioni Tozzetti, Giovanni, *Catalogo generale dei manoscritti Magliabechiani, vol 5 (Classi XIII-XVI)* (Firenze, Biblioteca Nazionale Centrale, Sala maonscritti e rari, Cataloghi, 45).

8

Circulating and Consuming Drugs in Late Seventeenth-Century Venice:

Between Theory and Practice

Sabrina Minuzzi

This chapter adopts a distinctive interpretation of theory: theory not as the elucidation of medical-philosophical principles, but as the set of regulations governing medical practice established by the health and political authorities responsible for its formulation. Thus, it explores the deviation of commonly accepted practice from those normatively established principles. However, as we shall see, even regulations are influenced by the cultural climate of the scientific context in which they originated, albeit indirectly and filtered through politically sensitive orientations. The framework outlined below emerges from the comparison between documents related to the provisions that regulated the secular and religious pharmacopeias and other sources shedding light on the actual local circulation of drugs, sometimes even in contravention of the former. Although geographically centered on the Venetian area, the resulting framework could be extended to various urban realities in early modern Western Europe and can certainly serve as a point of comparison for other regions.

Typically, a gap persists between theory and practice, varying in degree across different contexts. Acknowledging this disconnection is crucial, although documentation of such discrepancies is often partial and fragmentary.

Two printed sources outlined the normative principles that governed the manipulation and trade of medicines in the early modern period: official pharmacopeias and medicinal tariffs. 'Official' or 'public' pharmacopeias were typically drafted by a collegiate physician on behalf of the local health authority. They were distinct from so-called 'private' pharmacopeias, which were authored by individuals—rarely pharmacists, more often physicians—who had not received any official appointment and pursued this task out of personal interest, often coupled with the social and professional prestige associated with such an undertaking. The official pharmacopeia, however, had a far broader and more pervasive application compared to any private pharmacopeia, at least in the intentions of the endorsing authorities.[1] These were essentially pharmaceutical codes that apothecaries had to follow when making drugs. They listed the natural substances (generally called 'simples'[2]) that apothecary shops were required to stock in optimal condition, under penalty of fines that could be issued during periodic inspections. Additionally, they listed the compound remedies that apothecaries could prepare and illustrated this process by specifying the ingredients, correct quantities, and best modes of making them for commercial sale.

Arising from the need to standardize (and thus control) diverse territorial pharmaceutical practices across territories, official pharmacopeias serve as crucial tools to reconstruct what was intended to be pharmaceutical orthodoxy in various locales. They all embodied, even inadvertently, the scientific inclinations of local medical Colleges and of the political-territorial entities under whose auspices they were established. This attitude is especially evident in the degree of openness towards

1. The significant distinction between these two types of pharmacopeias was clearly delineated long ago by Corradi, *Le prime farmacopee italiane*. There is no comprehensive study on official European pharmacopeias, which are sometimes confused with private ones and whose first editions are often quoted erroneously. A still useful summary is in Urdang, 'Pharmacopeias as Witnesses of World History'.
2. The ancient pharmacopeia referred to 'simples' as the plant, animal, and mineral substances constituting the *materia medica*. When combined, these simples formed compound remedies.

chemical processes (distillation, sublimation, calcination, etc.), as opposed to the more traditional Galenic approaches (decoctions) to medicinal preparation.[3]

Italy was the earliest region in Europe to develop an official pharmaceutical code, which was published in Florence in January 1499 (1498 *ab Incarnatione*), inaugurating a phenomenon that soon became established in Italy and across Europe with the advent of printing press.[4] During the sixteenth and seventeenth centuries, many Italian states—much like many European countries—developed their own antidotaries or official pharmacopeias, which listed the medicinal remedies in current local use. These official Italian pharmacopeias functioned as barriers to the spread of some of the most important contributions of the Paracelsian revolution: the use of mineral substances and the chemical manipulation of ingredients.[5]

Conversely, the German countries, represented the cradle of alchemical and later chemical studies, and this was also prominently reflected in their official pharmacopeias.[6] In France, a polarity emerged between the medical faculty in Paris—a stronghold of Galenism—and the advocates of chemical innovation in Montpellier, who produced abundant chemical pharmacopeias.[7] Much of the drafting of the London pharmacopeia was the work of a Genevan doctor, Théodore Turquet de Mayerne, a Huguenot expelled from France who had studied medicine in Paris and Heidelberg, and then iatrochemistry in Montpellier. In 1611, Mayerne, who believed in reconciling iatrochemistry with Galenic medicine, had become personal physician to James I. By 1616, he became a member of the Royal College of Physicians in London, simultaneously taking on the responsibility and honor of completing the demanding project of the *Pharmacopoea Londinensis*. This endeavor provided him with the opportunity to incorporate all his knowledge of Paracelsian medicine and chemical remedies.[8]

Across much of Northern Europe, public pharmacopeias flourished—either directly or following lively debates—bearing a strong spagyric and chemical imprint. These publications provided instructions on techniques like distillation, sublimation, calcination, etc., for producing waters, oils, extracts, salts, and tinctures. They heavily advocated the use of mineral substances. In stark contrast, the official Italian pharmacopeias reflected a disquieting backwardness. Primarily entrenched in prescribing ancient Galenic decoctions, they remained limited to ingredients predominantly of plant and animal origin. Except for the Bolognese antidotary, which from 1641 provided a twenty-page *Appendix of Chemical Remedies* (out of a total of more than 500 pages), and the openness to chemistry shown by the doctors of the Studio Felsineo, Italian health authorities generally shunned chemical remedies.[9] Chemistry thus filtered into official pharmaceutical codes in only small amounts. It struggled to enter even into the later editions of the Florentine pharmacopeia, notwithstanding the interest in chemical and alchemical experimentation shown by various members of the Medici family, in line with trends at other European courts, at the end of the sixteenth century.[10] In

3. For official pharmacopeias from Atlantic contexts over the centuries, see the contributions in Crawford and Gabriel, *Pharmacopeias and Healing Knowledge*.
4. *Nuovo receptario*.
5. A framework of official Italian pharmacopeias that takes these aspects into consideration, with reference to foreign examples, is in Minuzzi, *Sul filo dei segreti*, pp. 45–56.
6. The Nuremberg code, authored by the physician, chemist, and botanist Valerius Cordus, stood among the early documents that embraced the principles of chemistry; it was soon translated into French, Italian, and other European languages. The *Pharmacopeia Londonensis*, which was first published relatively late (1618), was so successful that it was adopted not only by neighboring areas, but on a national level, with over sixty editions by the end of the eighteenth century. See Jepson, 'From Secret Remedies'.
7. The first among these was Joseph Du Chesne's 1607 *Pharmacopoea*, which met with extraordinary success. Meanwhile, Jean de Renou, a professor of medicine in Paris, published the *Institutionum pharmaceuticarum libri* (1608), with a Galenic approach. The hostility of the Parisian Galenists, who had spoken out against the use of chemical medicines in 1615, was effectively nullified by the support shown by the royal court to Paracelsian medical practitioners and chemical experimentation, to the point that in 1640 a royally designated Chair of Chemistry was designated at the Parisian Jardin des Plantes. See Debus, 'La medicina chimica', ibid., *Chemistry, Alchemy and the New Philosophy*.
8. Debus, 'La medicina chimica'; Jepson, 'From Secret Remedies'. England opened its doors to chemistry in a less dramatic way than in France, and in 1671, a central chemistry laboratory was opened in London to supply all members of the Society of Apothecaries with both basic and more elaborate chemical preparations at wholesale prices to guarantee quality and uniformity.
9. Aldrovandi (1522-1604), *Antidotarium Bononiense*.
10. The protection offered by royal courts often made them centers of study and the dissemination of the newest scientific trends. Moran, *Patronage and Institutions*. For Paracelsian medicine in specific, see Moran, 'Courts and Academies'. For the Tuscan case under the Medici, see Galluzzi, 'Motivi paracelsiani nella Toscana di Cosimo II e di don Antonio dei Medici'.

the State of Milan, chemical remedies were banned entirely and the health authorities adopted the *Roman Antidotary* and its strict Galenic approach (with recipes that were prevalently vegetal and made through mechanical processes). This was replaced in 1668 by their own Milanese Antidotary, with similar characteristics.[11]

As for Venice, its apothecaries had established a College as early as 1258 with the 'Capitulare de specialibus' (*Capitular of the apothecaries*), the oldest surviving document of its kind. Drawn up almost simultaneously with that of the Medical College, with which it shares many similarities, it began with one of the longest oath sworn on the Gospel and was strongly grounded in ethical principles.[12] More regulatory and concerned with the practical aspects of the profession was the *Capitular* of the apothecaries, approved in November of 1565: it laid down a series of obligations and guarantees for the members of the College (figs. 22a-b).[13] Chapter XXVIII of the 1565 *Capitular* mandated that apothecaries must use a recipe book to ensure universally consistent doses and packaging standards for the compounds prescribed by medical practitioners. The College of Physicians was to be responsible for drafting the book, while the College of Apothecaries would handle its publication and distribution to the shops.[14]

A second important source of information on the circulation of medicines in early modern European society is provided by tariffs. If pharmacopeias as sources in themselves have received limited attention from historians, tariffs have been virtually ignored, partly because very few have survived. They were ephemeral materials for everyday use, and only rare examples can be found in the catalogs of a few libraries.[15] Chapter XLI of the 1565 *Capitular* introduced the use of tariffs in Venice, which were also called 'limitations' (*Limitationi*) or 'medicinal taxes' (*Taxa medicinalium)*:

'Chapter XLI. The prices of the compositions are established every year.

[...] every year on the first of March [...] this College [of Apothecaries] shall be obliged to print these Limitations, so that every medical apothecary has one at no cost; & any who fails to go to or send [someone] to fetch it from the College prior in eight days' time, will be subject to the penalty of paying one ducat, which goes to the College.'[16]

Printed on a few pages, it was obligatory to keep and use the tariff in apothecary shops for one year, after which it would be replaced by a new tariff with updated prices. In the Venetian *Mariegola* (or *Matricula*, a list of collegiate members), the Capitulare was followed by a price list that was republished annually, with blank spaces for prices that were updated over the years: the *Limitations of the Prices of All the Compositions and Medical Stuffs Made by the Prior and Counselors of the College of Apothecaries of the Illustrious City of Venice* [...] *MDLXVI.*[17]

Thanks to the valuable work of Richard Palmer, we can explore one notable group of Venetian tariffs found among the papers of the Fraterna dei Battuti di Udine, a devotional confraternity that, in the early fourteenth century, had been transformed into a charitable institution with the foundation and administration of the hospital of Santa Maria della Misericordia.[18] Published between 1636 and 1713, the forty or so surviving medicinal tariffs

---

11. After 1680, only two apothecaries were authorized to prepare and sell chemical medications in Milan, and only one century later (1780), their production and sale was permitted in private pharmacies in the territory. See Brambilla, 'Dagli antidoti contro la peste', pp. 316–17. For the Roman context, see Ait, *Tra scienza e mercato*; Kolega, 'Speziali, spagirici'.
12. A modern edition of the Venetian *Capitular* is available in Marangoni, *Le associazioni di mestiere*, pp. 179–82, but the classic (and still useful) critical edition is that of Monticolo, *I capitolari delle arti veneziane*. Chapters I-XVIII are followed by the additions of Chapters XIX-XXVIII, which are adequately annotated.
13. The statute, printed on parchment and decorated with an illuminated frontispiece and initial capitals, occupies pages 11–27 of the '*mariegola*' (or *Matricula*, a list of the members) and is conserved in BNMVe, MS. It. VII 1971 (=9042), *Capitolare dell'arte degli speziali*.
14. Ibid., pp. 21–22.
15. A quick summary tracing the history of Italian tariffs available in the OPAC and MetaOPAC currently leads to the identification of very few titles, almost always surviving as a single copy: the Florentine *Tariffa et prezzi del medicinale* of 1593 (https://edit16.iccu.sbn.it/titolo/CNCE062128), the Luccan *Tariffa* of 1594 (https://edit16.iccu.sbn.it/titolo/CNCE055871) and *Tariffa* of 1640 (http://id.sbn.it/bid/LUAE007074), and the Venetian *Taxa* of 1690 (http://id.sbn.it/bid/UBOE045278) and 1694 (OCLC 257471260).
16. BNMVe, MS. It. VII 1971 (=9042), p. 27: 'Cap. XLI *Li pretii delle compositioni siano ogni anno limitati* | [...] ogni anno per il primo di marzo [...] sia obligato esso Collegio [degli speziali] far stampare essa Limitatione, acciocché ogni spetiale medicinale ne habbia una senza spesa; & cadauno che mancarà di andare o [di] mandare a tuorla dal Priore in tempo di giorni otto, cada nella pena di pagare duc. uno, il qual vada al Collegio'.
17. Ibid., pp. 31–42.
18. Palmer, 'Pharmacy in the Republic of Venice', endnote 46. For the activities of the fraternity and hospital, see the introductions to Cargnelutti, *Inventario*, and Villotta, *L'archivio storico*. In 1344, documents first speak of a 'hospital' in the sense of a shelter for the poor, but it wasn't until the

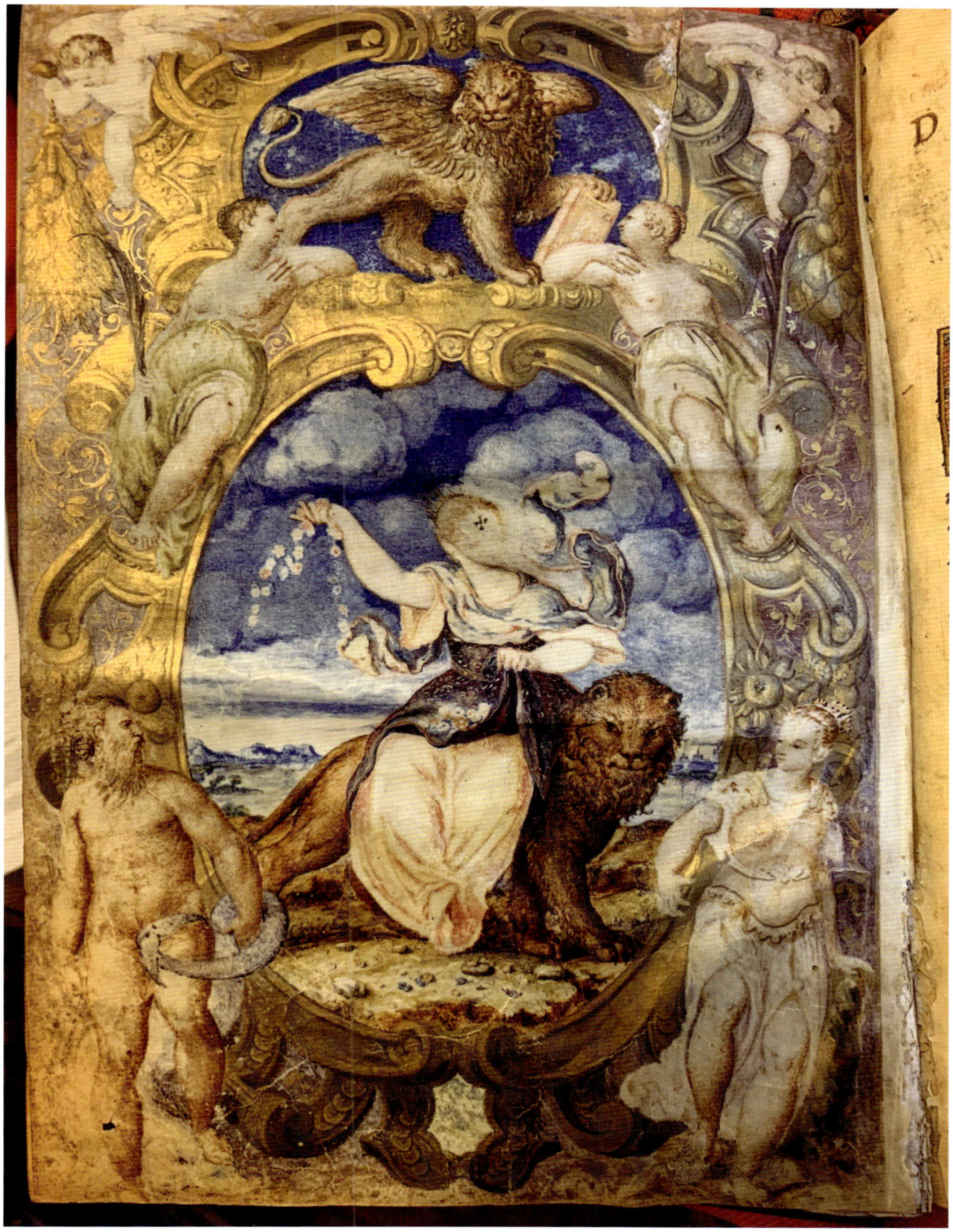

22a. Illuminated frontispiece of the *Capitular on the Art of Apothecaries* of 1565.

exhibited specific characteristics linked to their intended use. They were written in the vernacular but more frequently in Latin, as pharmacists were well-versed in Latin due to their education and the necessity of consulting official antidotaries, which were often in that language. Typically in folio format, these tariffs were about twenty pages long, printed on durable paper, and displayed a growing emphasis on elegance in their presentation over

sixteenth century that the structure managed by the Battuti took on the meaning of a hospital in the modern sense, combining therapeutic activity with support for the needy, orphans, and foundlings.

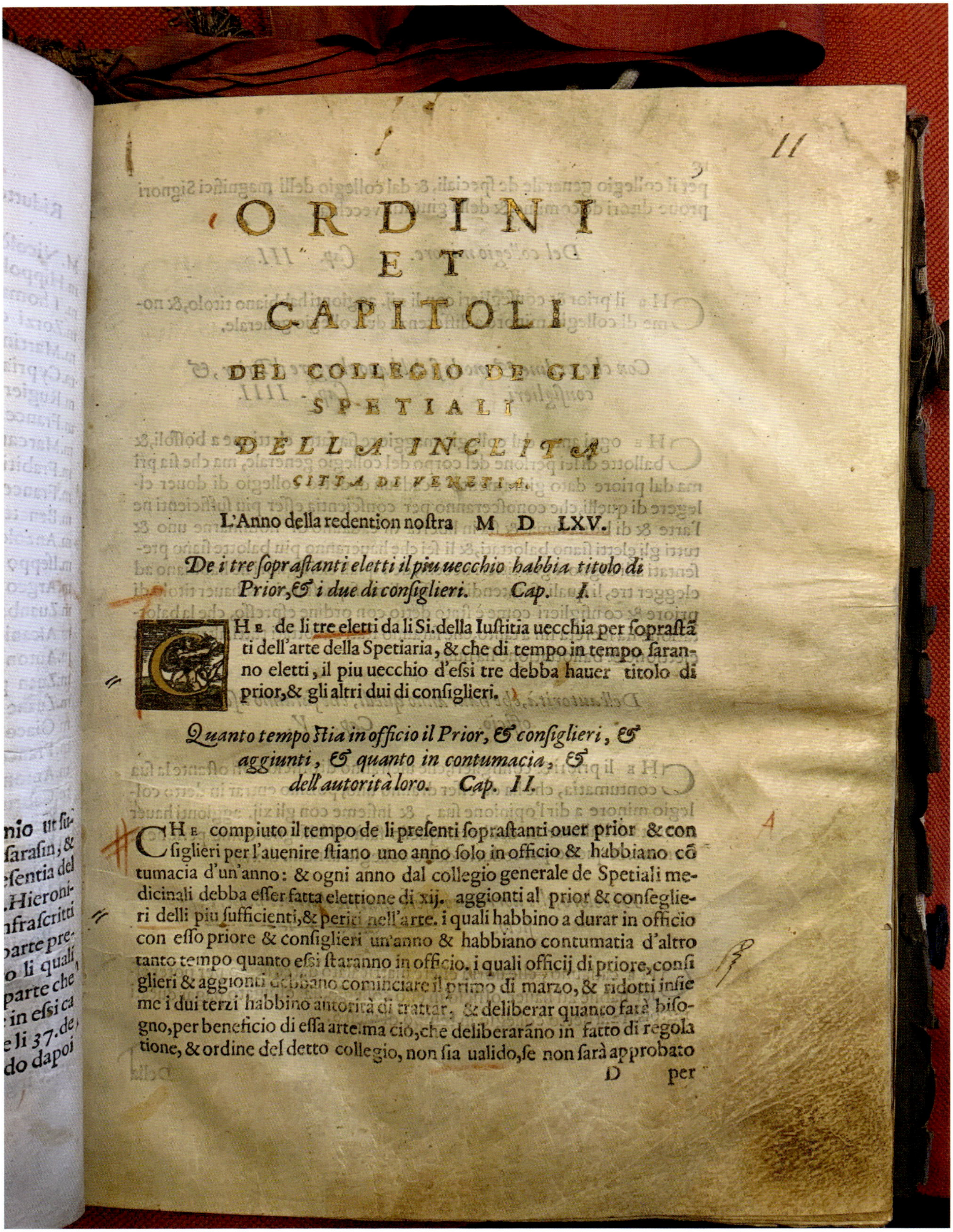
ORDINI
ET
CAPITOLI
DEL COLLEGIO DE GLI
SPETIALI
DELLA INCLITA
CITTA DI VENETIA.
L'Anno della redention nostra M D LXV.

De i tre soprastanti eletti il piu uecchio habbia titolo di Prior, & i due di consiglieri. Cap. I.

CHE de li tre eletti da li Si. della Iustitia uecchia per soprastanti dell'arte della Spetiaria, & che di tempo in tempo saranno eletti, il piu uecchio d'essi tre debba hauer titolo di prior, & gli altri dui di consiglieri.

Quanto tempo stia in officio il Prior, & consiglieri, & aggiunti, & quanto in contumacia, & dell'autorità loro. Cap. II.

CHE compiuto il tempo de li presenti soprastanti ouer prior & consiglieri per l'auenire stiano uno anno solo in officio & habbiano cōtumacia d'un'anno: & ogni anno dal collegio generale de Spetiali medicinali debba esser fatta elettione di xij. aggionti al prior & conseglieri delli piu sufficienti, & periti nell'arte. i quali habbino a durar in officio con esso priore & consiglieri un'anno & habbiano contumatia d'altro tanto tempo quanto essi staranno in officio. i quali officij di priore, consiglieri & aggionti debbano cominciare il primo di marzo, & ridotti insieme i dui terzi habbino autorità di trattar, & deliberar quanto sarà bisogno, per beneficio di essa arte. ma cio, che deliberarāno in fatto di regolatione, & ordine del detto collegio, non sia ualido, se non sarà approbato
D per

22b. Page 11 of the *Capitular on the Art of Apothecaries* of 1565. Printed on parchment.

time.[19] In the 1671 tariff, the previous woodcuts were replaced with more refined engravings by Antonio Bosio, a printer, bookseller, and engraver who was entrusted with their printing until 1685, after which other well-known local printers would continue in the same style.[20] Bosio's tariffs are distinguished from their predecessors by their attractive covers, decorated with typographical motifs and woodcut borders, which suggests that these were tools meant to be placed on counters within sight of customers (figs. 23a-d). The list of prices, which was updated annually, was simultaneously a point of reference for apothecary managers and a guarantee for customers, who could verify the tariffs set by local health authorities and compare them with the cost of their purchases, determined by the discounts offered (as we shall see, discounts were almost universally applied).

We have thus outlined the features of the two main regulatory sources that governed pharmaceutical practices in the early modern period. In the following sections of the chapter, we will see how the prescriptions from antidotaries and tariffs were applied in everyday life. Other sources—some well-studied, others almost unknown—suggest that deviation from these norms was common. These deviations of practice from the theorized norm have significant socio-cultural implications and prompt a series of questions: What was the relationship between the medicines actually in circulation and those described in the pharmaceutical codes? What was the pricing policy in the drug market? What were the alternative methods of circulating medicines, other than buying and selling them, and what factors influenced them? And since, as we shall see, secular apothecaries were flanked by monastic ones, did different people make use of religious and secular apothecaries? How much did ordinary people and medical professionals trust religious apothecaries?

As these questions suggest, examining practices in relation to normative sources will also provide an opportunity to compare the management and perception of secular pharmacies with those of religious ones, an issue often overlooked in historical research. There is undoubtedly a wealth of documentation about these subjects awaiting to be studied, as suggested by a recent historical and artistic survey of the gardens and orchards—almost always associated with pharmaceutical activity—of various religious orders in Italy.[21] However, studies dedicated to monastery or hospital apothecaries remain rather limited, despite some enlightening contributions regarding the Florentine territory in the Renaissance.[22] Established to meet the medicinal needs of the religious institution, apothecaries run by internal staff often became independent commercial entities whose services extended beyond the monastery walls.[23] Despite both religious and secular regulations prohibiting it, as we will see, the religious apothecary actually achieved a high degree of integration into the economy and daily life of the city.

BEYOND OFFICIAL PHARMACOPEIAS: PRIVILEGED SECRETS, INVENTORIES, AND BOOKS

The pharmaceuticals in circulation were far more numerous than those anticipated by official pharmacopeias. It is also clear that apothecaries were not the only ones making and selling drugs. In recent decades, there has been a proliferation of historical studies about the many figures who practiced pharmacy, including those authorized, unauthorized, or allowed to deviate from established laws: charlatans and empirics (often, unfortunately, blurred together), men and women, and—more often than one might imagine—entire families.[24] European rulers granted privileges at their own discretion to inventors of miraculous antidotes against both natural and malicious poisoning, and by the end of the sixteenth century, medicines became subject to testing to verify their efficacy and place them within the scope of

19. ACUd, Ospedale di S. Maria della Misericordia, b. 1064. Thirty-eight of the tariffs date back to the seventeenth century, while only one is from the eighteenth (1713).
20. These other printers included Giovanni Francesco and then Giacomo Valvasense. For Bosio's work, see Minuzzi, *Il secolo di carta*, and *Inventario di bottega*.
21. Benocci, *A ciascuno il suo paradiso*.
22. Strocchia, 'The nun apothecaries of Renaissance Florence'; Henderson, *The Renaissance Hospital*, chap. 9.
23. Especially in the case of enterprising nuns from Florentine convents, see *Forgotten Healers*, chap. 3. In Venice, in many cases, the explicit motivation for opening an apothecary was to curb the excessive expenses for medicines of the religious institution (see documentation from the monastery of SS. Giovanni e Paolo).
24. Minuzzi, review of Alisha Rankin, *The Poison Trials*.

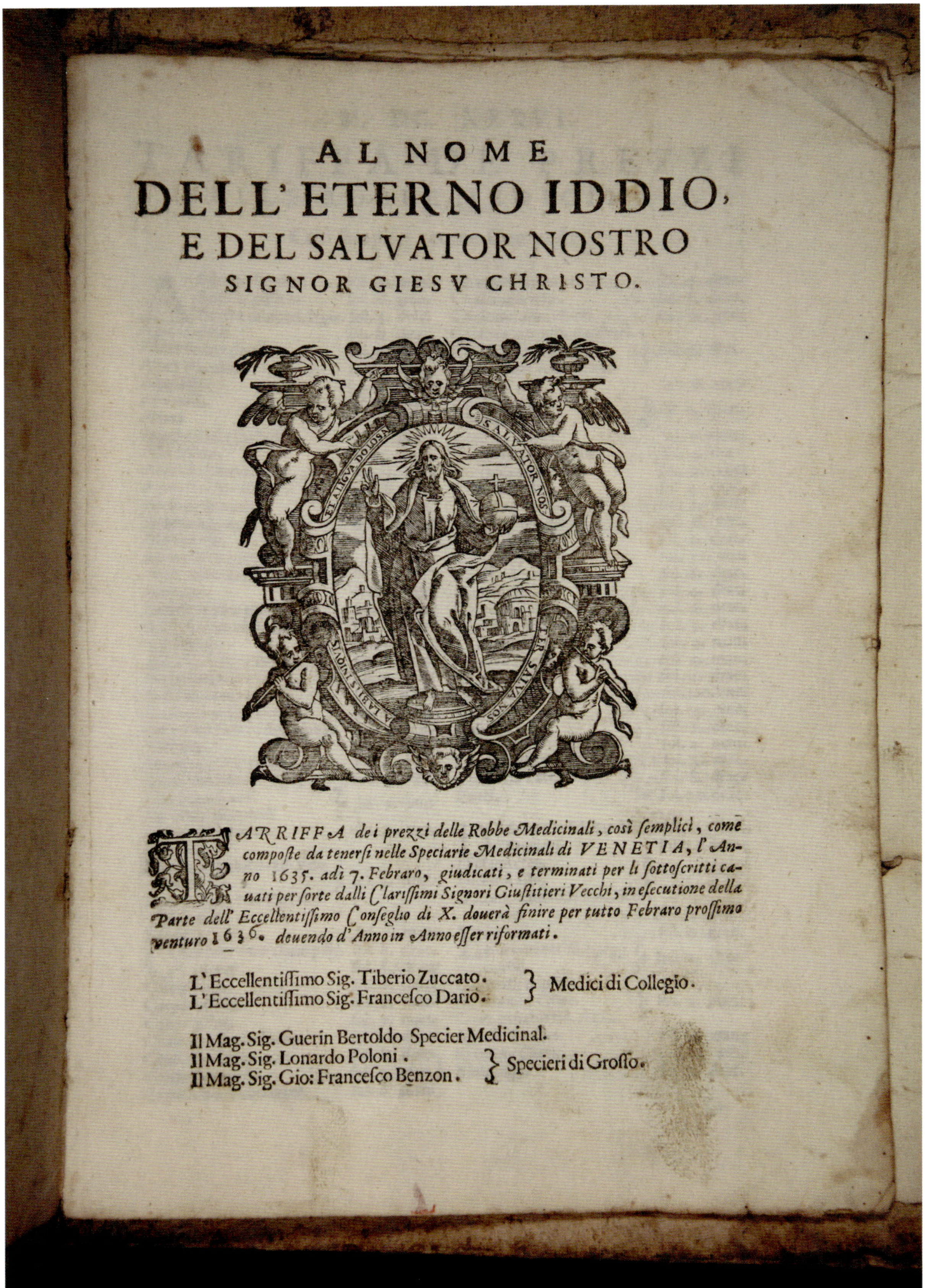

AL NOME
DELL' ETERNO IDDIO,
E DEL SALVATOR NOSTRO
SIGNOR GIESV CHRISTO.

TARRIFFA dei prezzi delle Robbe Medicinali, così semplici, come composte da tenersi nelle Speciarie Medicinali di VENETIA, l'Anno 1635. adì 7. Febraro, giudicati, e terminati per li sottoscritti cauati per sorte dalli Clarissimi Signori Giustitieri Vecchi, in esecutione della Parte dell' Eccellentissimo Conseglio di X. douerà finire per tutto Febraro prossimo venturo 1636. deuendo d'Anno in Anno esser riformati.

L'Eccellentissimo Sig. Tiberio Zuccato.
L'Eccellentissimo Sig. Francesco Dario. } Medici di Collegio.

Il Mag. Sig. Guerin Bertoldo Specier Medicinal.
Il Mag. Sig. Lonardo Poloni.
Il Mag. Sig. Gio: Francesco Benzon. } Specieri di Grosso.

23a. Frontispiece (and first page) of the 1636 Tariff with a woodcut vignette of Christ

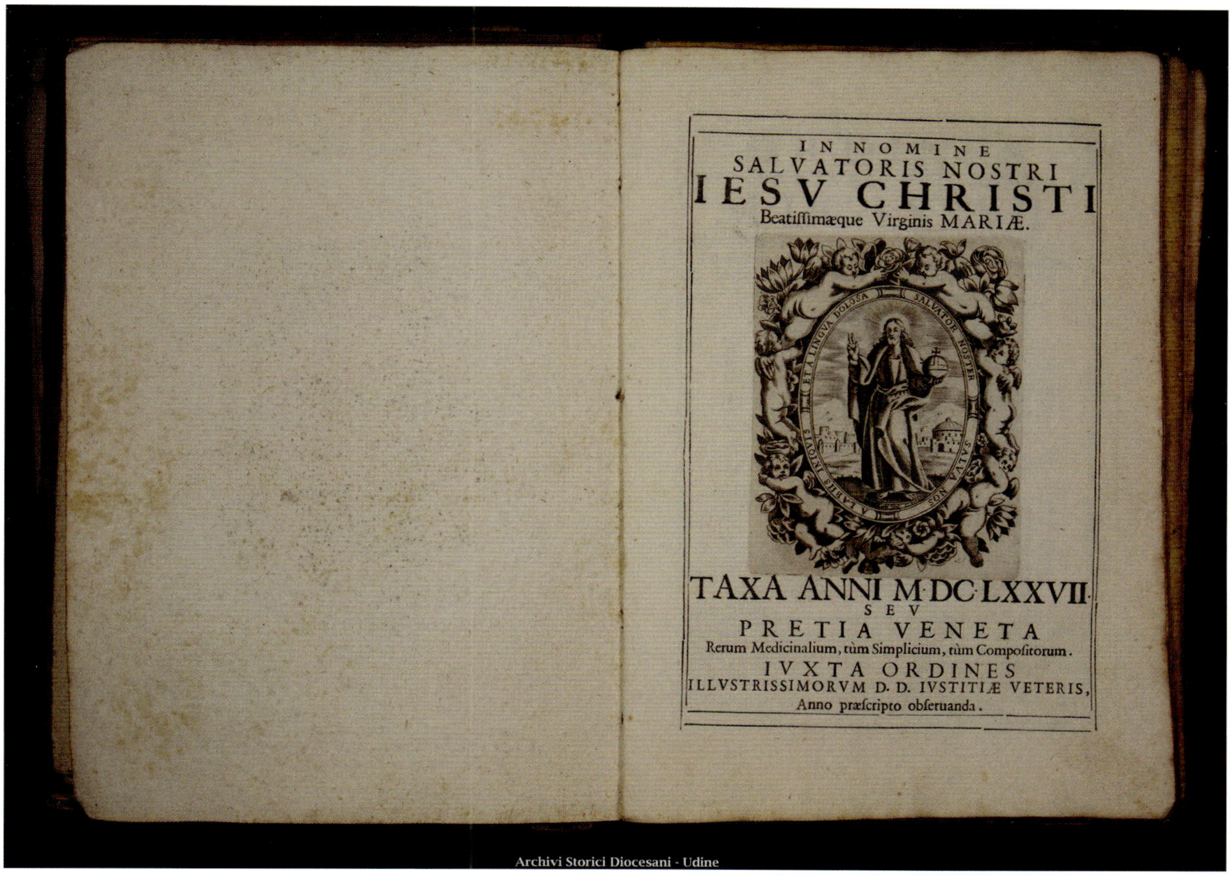

23b. Tariff (Taxa) for 1672 printed by Antonio Bosio, with engraved vignette by the same.

approved pharmaceuticals.[25] Generally, however, the licenses issued by lay authorities and high prelates only occasionally involved local medical Colleges, frequently creating friction between medical professionals.[26]

In different countries, the production of so-called 'secrets,' or even of common medicines that circulated outside apothecary shops, was subject to different levels of control. England, for example, stands out for its lack of systematic control by the authorities: from the mid-1500s, it was common practice for stationers and booksellers—and occasionally typographers and even bookbinders—to sell some pills and syrups, which they advertised themselves on leaflets and in early printed newspapers.[27] A large quantity of English advertising leaflets and booklets survive, listing, at the end of the description of a 'secret"s properties, up to thirty bookshops and similar venues where the medicine was available for sale, even in cities quite distant from each other.[28] The link between medicinal secrets and English booksellers, which had always been tight, was reinforced during the 1730s thanks to the dense distribution network of provincial gazettes and newspapers, which were more widely read than in Italy.[29]

25. Rankin, Rivest, 'Medicine, Monopoly, and the Premodern State'; Rankin, *The Poison Trials*.
26. Physicians in the French royal entourage sometimes enjoyed privileges for new medicines in conflict with the Parisian Faculty of Medicine. In the eighteenth century, some personally profited by investing in pharmaceutical patents, introducing a new level of corruption in the system. See Jones, 'The French King's Physicians'. For the medicines authorized in England and France, see Brockliss, Jones, *The Medical World*, passim; Porter, *Health for Sale*, pp. 9, 28, and passim; Jepson, 'From Secret Remedies', pp. 223–26.
27. Furdell, *Publishing and Medicine in Early Modern England*, p. 131.
28. See the description of seventy-two advertisements for medicinal secrets in Alden, 'Pills and Publishing'. One sheet from 1679 advertised a remedy based on Cochlearia root for sale at twenty-four booksellers. William Stoughton's *elixir magnum stomachium* was sold at thirty locations, though the average distribution for medications was at two to three booksellers.
29. In 1786, the editor of the *Bristol Gazette* listed fifty-three medicinal secrets for sale in his bookshop. See Isaac, 'Pills and Print', p. 35. Isaac makes a brief but clear review of the so-called 'proprietary medicines', which were remedies sold directly by their creator, often a figure in the world of

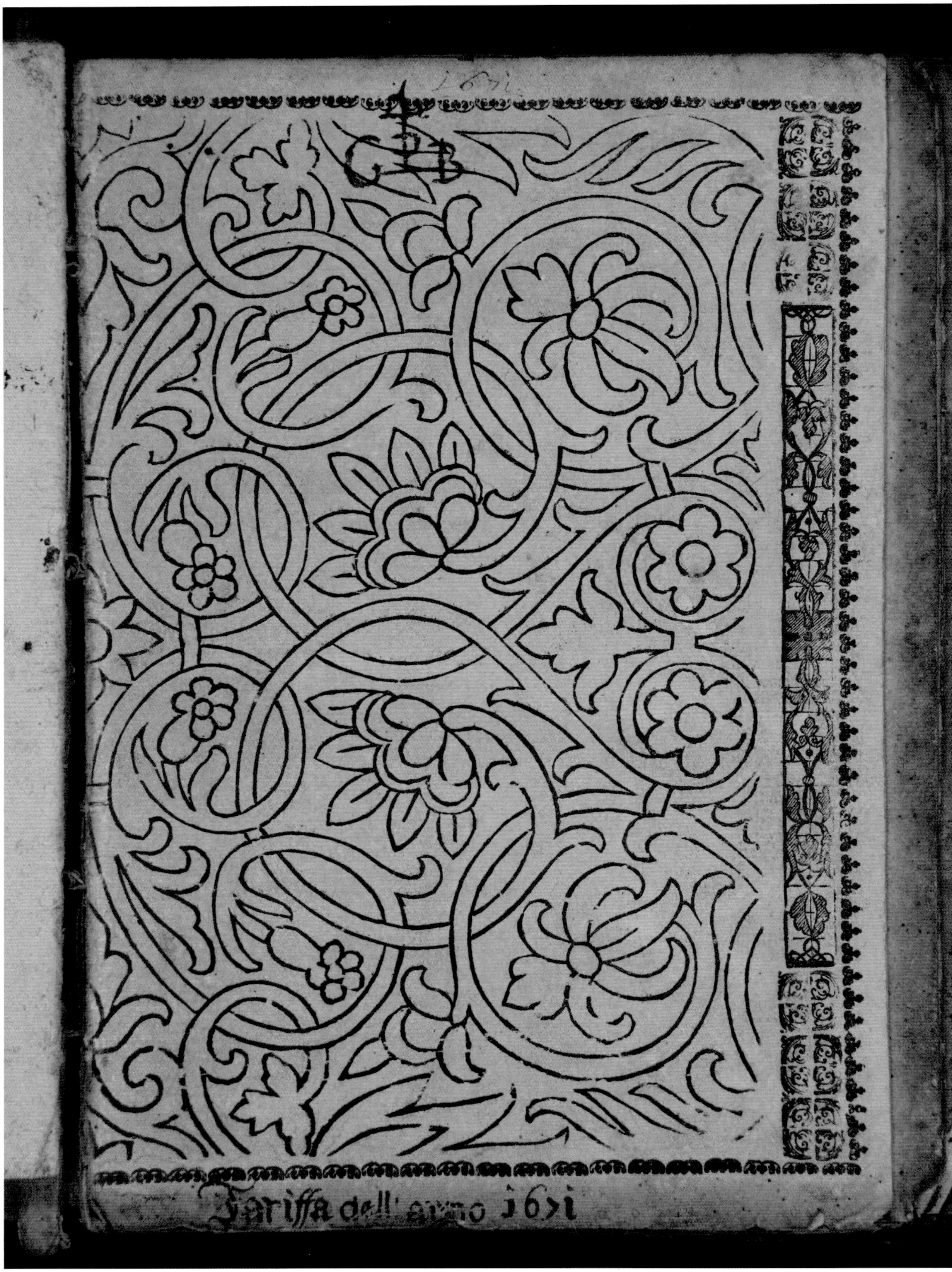

23c and d. Covers of the 1671 and 1685 Tariffs.

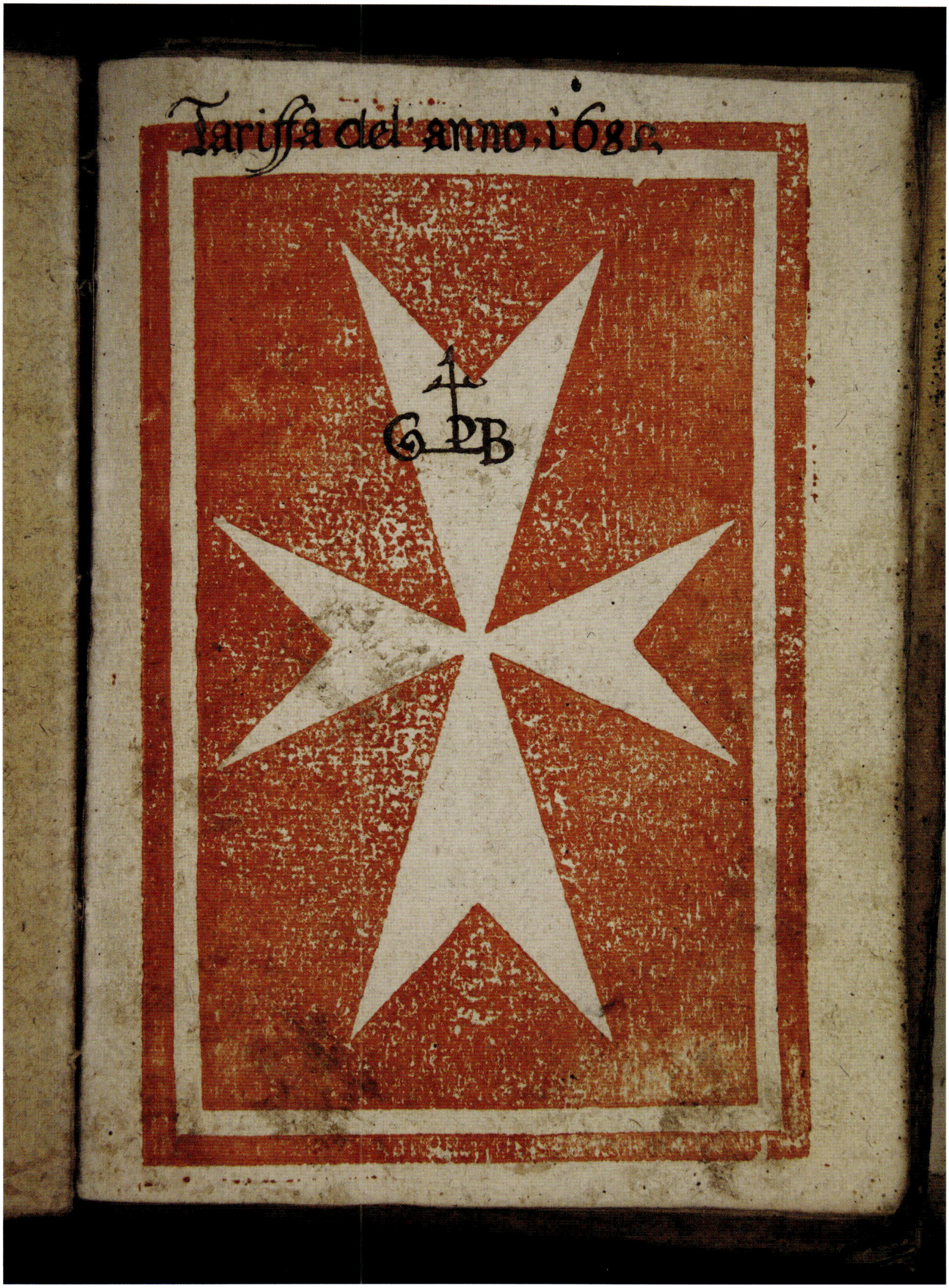
Tariffa del' anno, 1685,
G PB

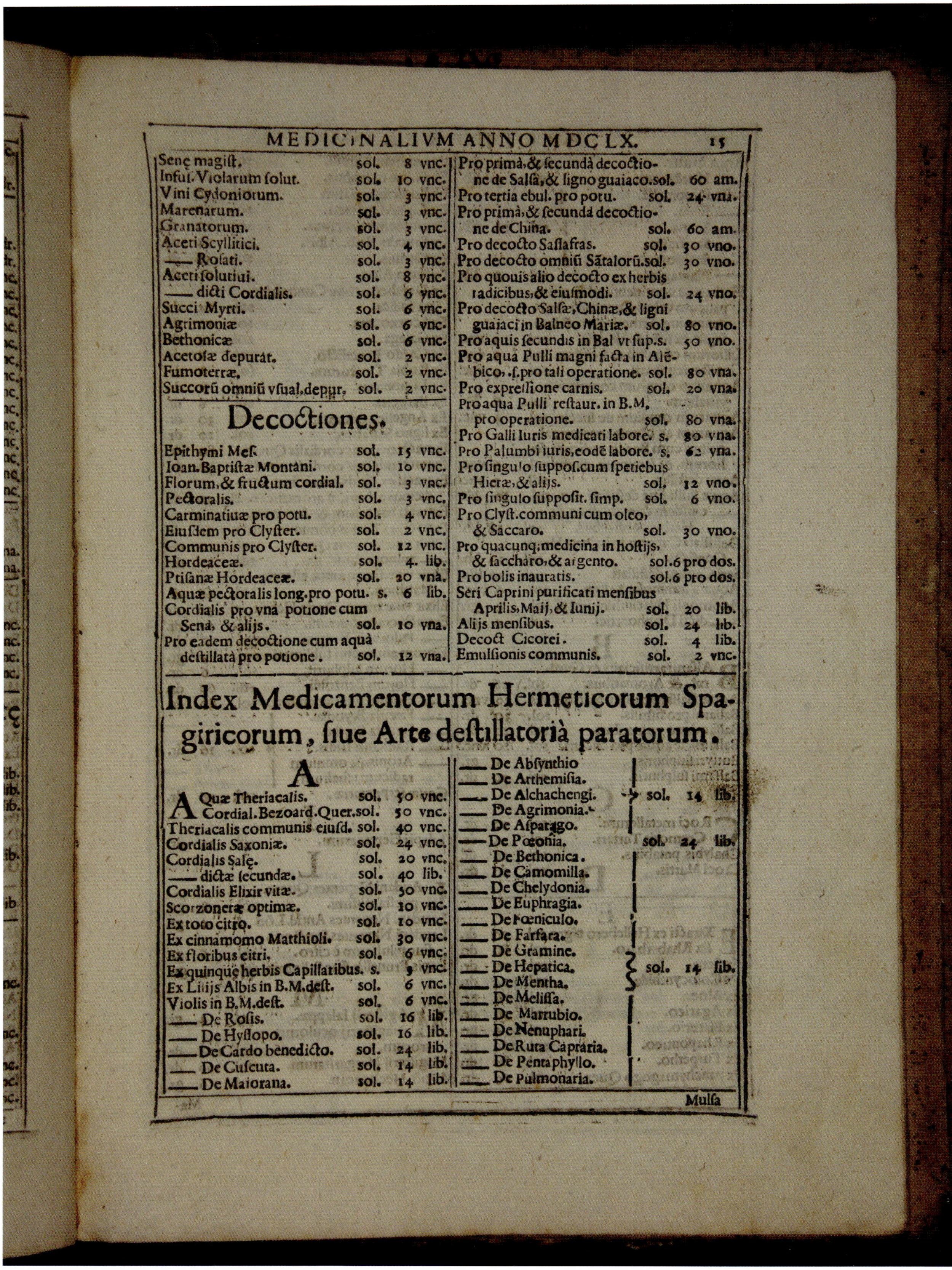
MEDICINALIVM ANNO MDCLX. 15

Senę magiſt. sol. 8 vnc.
Infuſ. Violarum ſolut. sol. 10 vnc.
Vini Cydoniorum. sol. 3 vnc.
Marenarum. sol. 3 vnc.
Granatorum. sol. 3 vnc.
Aceti Scyllitici. sol. 4 vnc.
—— Roſati. sol. 3 vnc.
Aceti ſolutiui. sol. 8 vnc.
—— dicti Cordialis. sol. 6 vnc.
Succi Myrti. sol. 6 vnc.
Agrimoniæ sol. 6 vnc.
Bethonicæ sol. 6 vnc.
Acetoſæ depurat. sol. 2 vnc.
Fumoterræ. sol. 2 vnc.
Succorũ omniũ vſual. depur. sol. 2 vnc.

Decoctiones.

Epithymi Meſ. sol. 15 vnc.
Ioan. Baptiſtæ Montani. sol. 10 vnc.
Florum, & fructum cordial. sol. 3 vnc.
Pectoralis. sol. 3 vnc.
Carminatiuæ pro potu. sol. 4 vnc.
Eiuſdem pro Clyſter. sol. 2 vnc.
Communis pro Clyſter. sol. 12 vnc.
Hordeaceæ. sol. 4. lib.
Ptiſanæ Hordeaceæ. sol. 20 vnà.
Aquæ pectoralis long. pro potu. s. 6 lib.
Cordialis pro vna potione cum Sena, & alijs. sol. 10 vna.
Pro eadem decoctione cum aquà deſtillatà pro potione. sol. 12 vna.
Pro primà, & ſecundà decoctione de Salſa, & ligno guaiaco. sol. 60 am.
Pro tertia ebul. pro potu. sol. 24 vna.
Pro primà, & ſecundà decoctione de China. sol. 60 am.
Pro decocto Saſſafras. sol. 30 vno.
Pro decocto omniũ Sãtalorũ. sol. 30 vno.
Pro quouis alio decocto ex herbis radicibus, & eiuſmodi. sol. 24 vno.
Pro decocto Salſæ, Chinæ, & ligni guaiaci in Balneo Mariæ. sol. 80 vno.
Pro aquis ſecundis in Bal vt ſup. s. 50 vno.
Pro aqua Pulli magni facta in Alẽbico, .ſ. pro tali operatione. sol. 80 vna.
Pro expreſſione carnis. sol. 20 vna.
Pro aqua Pulli reſtaur. in B.M. pro operatione. sol. 80 vna.
Pro Galli Iuris medicati labore. s. 80 vna.
Pro Palumbi iuris, eodẽ labore. s. 62 vna.
Pro ſingulo ſuppoſ. cum ſpetiebus Hieræ, & alijs. sol. 12 vno.
Pro ſingulo ſuppoſit. ſimp. sol. 6 vno.
Pro Clyſt. communi cum oleo, & Saccaro. sol. 30 vno.
Pro quacunq; medicina in hoſtijs, & ſaccharo, & argento. sol. 6 pro dos.
Pro bolis inauratis. sol. 6 pro dos.
Seri Caprini purificati menſibus Aprilis, Maij, & Iunij. sol. 20 lib.
Alijs menſibus. sol. 24 lib.
Decoct Cicorei. sol. 4 lib.
Emulſionis communis. sol. 2 vnc.

Index Medicamentorum Hermeticorum Spagiricorum, ſiue Arte deſtillatorià paratorum.

A

AQuæ Theriacalis. sol. 50 vnc.
Cordial. Bezoard. Quer. sol. 50 vnc.
Theriacalis communis eiuſd. sol. 40 vnc.
Cordialis Saxoniæ. sol. 24 vnc.
Cordialis Salę. sol. 20 vnc.
—— dictæ ſecundæ. sol. 40 lib.
Cordialis Elixir vitæ. sol. 50 vnc.
Scorzoneræ optimæ. sol. 10 vnc.
Ex toto citro. sol. 10 vnc.
Ex cinnamomo Matthioli. sol. 30 vnc.
Ex floribus citri. sol. 6 vnc.
Ex quinque herbis Capillaribus. s. 9 vnc.
Ex Lilijs Albis in B.M. deſt. sol. 6 vnc.
Violis in B.M. deſt. sol. 6 vnc.
—— De Roſis. sol. 16 lib.
—— De Hyſſopo. sol. 16 lib.
—— De Cardo benedicto. sol. 24 lib.
—— De Cuſcuta. sol. 14 lib.
—— De Maiorana. sol. 14 lib.
—— De Abſynthio
—— De Arthemiſia.
—— De Alchachengi. } sol. 14 lib.
—— De Agrimonia.
—— De Aſparago.
—— De Pœonia. sol. 24 lib.
—— De Bethonica.
—— De Camomilla.
—— De Chelydonia.
—— De Euphragia.
—— De Fœniculo.
—— De Farfara.
—— De Gramine.
—— De Hepatica. } sol. 14 lib.
—— De Mentha.
—— De Meliſſa.
—— De Marrubio.
—— De Nenuphari.
—— De Ruta Capraria.
—— De Pentaphyllo.
—— De Pulmonaria.

Mulſa

24 a and b. Example of the medicaments listed in tariffs. Pages 15 and 16 of the *Taxa anni MDCLX seu Pretia Veneta rerum medicinalium tum simplicium tum compositarum […] anno praescripto observanda* (Venice: Typographia ducali Pinelliana, 1660).

Aqua Mulſa. sol. 4 lib.
—— Hordeacea. sol. 4 lib.
--Ex Pimpinella.
—— Ruta.
—— Saluia. } sol. 14 lib.
—— Saxifragia.
—— Scabioſa.
—— Plantagine. sol. 8 lib.
Herbarum continentium ſuccum paucum veluti, Eupatorij Auicennæ, iuę Arthetice, eorũdem aquæ, ex ſolis folijs deſt. sol. 5 vnc.
Liliorum cõuallĩũ ex floribus. sol. 8 vnc.
Geniſtæ ſeu ſparti. sol. 4 vnc.
Aquarum omnium communiũ vſualium. sol. 6 lib.
Aquarum omnium de ſuccis. sol. 4 vnc.
Aquarum ad cõminuendum calculum cum Succis radicum, foliorum, & ſeminum diuret. sol. 6 vnc.
Aceti deſtillat. sol. 3 vnc.
Aquæ Pulli, ſiue deſtillati cap. sol. 10 lib.
—— eiuſdem cum floribus, & Herbis cordialibus. sol. 18 lib.
Deſtillati Caponis in balneo Mariæ Confecti. sol. 24 lib.
Seri Caprini deſtillati. sol. 36 lib.
Aquæ a luminoſæ Fallop. sol. 6 vnc.
Antimonij Hyacinthini præp. sol. 3 gr.
—— dicti Diaphoretici. sol. 4 gr.

B

Balſami artificialis ex Gummi, & Aromatibus. sol. 26 dr.
Aquæ Balſamicę, ſiue Matris Bal. s. 20 vnc.
Balſami pro fiſtulis. sol. 30 dr.
Balſami pro vulneribus. sol. 20 dr.
Balſamicæ aquæ pro eiſdem. sol. 20 vnc.
Buttyri ſulphuris. sol. 1 gr.
Balſami ſulphuris. sol. 20 dr.

C

Croci metallorum. sol. 30 dr.
Cremoris Tartari. sol. 4 dr.
Chalybis potabiiis. sol. 16 dr.
Croci Martis. sol. 20 dr.

D

E

Extracti ex Hellebero nigro. sol. 20 dr.
Ex Rhabarbaro. sol. 80 dr.
Ex Sena. sol. 50 dr.
Ex Colocynthide. sol. 24 dr.
Ex Aloe. sol. 16 dr.
Ex Agarico. sol. 36 dr.
Ex Elaterio. sol. 4 gr.
Fx Rhapontico. sol. 120 dr.
Ex Turpetho. sol. 86 dr.
Ex panchymagogo Quer. sol. 60 dr.
Ex ſeminibus Ebuli. sol. 20 dr.
Ex Chinæ radicibus. sol. 80 dr.
Ex Radicibus Salſæ. sol. 70 dr.
Ex Ligno Guaiaco. sol. 30 dr.
Ex eiuſdem corticibus. sol. 30 dr.
Ex Santalis Rub. Albis. sol. 24 dr.
Ex Citrinis. sol. 50 dr.
Ex Xylo Aloe. sol. 100 dr.
Ex Drachena; ſiue Contrahierua Indica. sol. 24 dr.
Ex Scorzonera. sol. 12 dr.
Ex Galega. sol. 4 dr.
Ex Cardo Benedicto. sol. 8 dr.
Ex Rubia Tinctorum. sol. 8 dr.
Ex Limonibus. sol. 8 dr.
Ex Berberis. sol. 8 dr.
Ex Angelica odorata. sol. 30 dr.
Ex ligno Saſſafras. sol. 20 dr.
Extracti maioris cordialis Querc. s. 80 dr.
Extracti minoris cordialis eiuſdẽ. s. 40 dr.
Extracti ex lignis, corticibus, & radicibus arborum aromaticar. s. 40 dr
Extracti baccarum, & ſeminum. s. 24 dr
Extracti ex herbis cõmuniter vſ. s. 16 dr
Elixir vitæ maioris Querc. sol. 30 dr
—— minoris eiuſdem. sol. 12 dr.
Elixir vitæ, ſiue quintæ eſſentiæ Matthioli. sol. 16 dr
Elixir vitæ magni Ducis Hetrur. s. 30 dr
Extracti cranij humani. sol. 40 dr.
—— Pulmonis Vulpini. sol. 20 dr.
Florum antimonij ſublimati. sol. 3 gr.
—— Florum ſulphuris. sol. 6 dr.
—— Florum Benzoini. sol. 60 dr.
—— Florum liquidæ ambræ. sol. 80 dr.
—— Fæcula Bryoniæ.
—— Fæcula Scyllæ.
—— Radicum Iridis. } sol. 16 dr.
—— Aronis, & omnium radicum vſualium.
Genſæ ſerpentariæ. sol. 16 dr.

I

Iulapij Gemmarum. sol. 16 dr.

L

Laudani Nepentes Querc. præſtantiſſimi. sol. 8 gr.
Laudani Nepentes Antid. Lõd. s. 4 gr.
Laudani Nepentes Sanctorij, ſiue pilularum è citro. sol. 6 gr.
Lapis Prunellæ, ſiue Salis min. sol. 4 gr.

M

Magiſterij Ialappæ. sol. 4 gr.
Magiſterij oculorum cancrorum. sol. 124 dr.
Magiſterij Margaritarum. sol. 160 dr.
Magiſt. Mechoacan. sol. 6 gr.

Ma-

In stark contrast, in the Italian states, the granting of licenses (simple authorizations) and privileges (exclusive authorizations) for the production and commercialization of medicinal secrets was more extensively regulated and subject to the judgement of the Protomedicati and the local medical Colleges.[30] In the territories of the Venetian Republic, the production of licensed secrets involved both professional and non-professional individuals, distinguished by their knowledge of the medicinal properties of natural substances and often by the chemical manipulation of ingredients, despite the fact that the public pharmacopeias of the Italian states were almost all strictly Galenic. In this way, the authorization process helped to filter and regulate medicines that were created outside the mainstream. So extensive was the regulation that during the 1600s and then with the normative codification of the 1700s, only new pharmaceutical formulas (new as opposed to those described in local and foreign pharmaceutical codes) could be privileged as 'secrets'. The public and private pharmacopeias, which had become incredibly numerous throughout Europe, should therefore be seen merely as a basis for comparison to encourage improvement and enrichment: indeed, in Venice, if secret remedies proved effective in practice, they were always incorporated into the local pharmaceutical offer once the privilege expired.[31]

The Venetian state, besides exhibiting a massive circulation of authorized secrets, never produced an official pharmaceutical code drafted according to the criteria established by the *Capitulare of Specialibus* (*Capitular of Apothecaries*), thus granting pharmaceutical practices even greater freedom from normative theoretical dictates. Although a code had been anticipated since 1565, it was not published until the start of 1617, penned by Curzio Marinelli. In March of that year, however, Marinelli's *Pharmacopaea, sive de vera pharmaca conficiendi & praeparandi methodo, a... medicorum Venetorum Collegio comprobata* (Pharmacopeia, Or the True Method of Making & Preparing Drugs... approved by the Venetian College of Physicians) was withdrawn from sale by order of the Avogaria di Comun, to which the College of Apothecaries had appealed (fig. 25).[32] The apothecaries had found the volume detrimental to their dignity, as it was full of references to their alleged errors and malpractice. Indeed, it was based on the presumption of countless apothecary errors.[33] When asked to list the points in the Pharmacopeia that needed amending, the apothecaries chose never to respond and consigned the publication to oblivion. Consequently, a new amended edition was never produced.[34] The already-printed copies were either quietly sold off over the years or, more likely, destroyed, given that today libraries hold a minimal number of copies, despite the considerable size of the book (around 500 pages in quarto format), which should have ensured a reasonable chance of survival.[35] The deviation from the norm in the Venetian state is also confirmed by the fact that Marinelli's *Pharmacopeia* never appeared in apothecary inventories, where the books used in their shops were listed.[36] Instead, other antidotaries (both

typography. The first known advertisement on printed paper dates to 1552, indicating such a connection between printing and pharmacopeia. By 1652, the first medicinal advertisement appeared in the *Mercurius Politicus*, marking a distribution format that would triumph in eighteenth-century periodical publishing.

30. The authorization process was also applied to charlatans; see Gentilcore, *Medical Charlatanism*. Through various legislative exemptions, it could also apply to 'particular persons', including apothecaries, paint sellers, distillers, barbers, surgeons, physicians, religious figures, and those passionate about pharmaceutical research but from unrelated (musicians, shoemakers, greengrocers, etc.) or undeclared professions. See Minuzzi, *Sul filo dei segreti*.
31. There are few documented cases compared to how many likely occurred. Something similar happened to Elisabetta Amorosi Manini di Rovigo's 'Specific Antiscorbutic from Rovigo' (*Specifico antiscorbutico di Rovigo*), who was granted a privilege in 1771 and which was added to the *Pharmaceutical-Chemical Lexicon* by 1774 (p. 147). For details on the personal and professional histories of these inventors of secrets, see Minuzzi, *Sul filo dei segreti*; on the enrichment and improvement of the official pharmacopeia see Rivest's examination of the well-known Italian and European developments of the Orvietan antidote in 'Beyond the Pharmacopeia?'.
32. Two copies of the printed termination of the Avogaria di Comun (In Venice, by Antonio Pinelli, ducal printer) that mark the withdrawal of the pharmacopeia are preserved in ASVe, *Giustizia Vecchia*, b. 211, file *Speziali*.
33. The *Pharmacopeia* opens with a summary in which '*Multa errata enumerantur, quae a non paucis seplasariis in dies committuntur*' (fols 3^r–4^v). A full 168 numerated entries index the points at which Marinelli discusses the errors often committed by apothecaries.
34. More details in Minuzzi, *Sul filo dei segreti*, pp. 45–56.
35. Only three copies survive in the Italian National Library System (http://id.sbn.it/bid/UFIE001423), while typically, it's ephemeral publications, such as broadsheets or pamphlets, that tend to survive in very few copies.
36. Unlike an apothecary's personal library, the shop books were inventoried alongside the simples, compounds, and equipment found in the apothecaries' shops. So far, I have tracked down six post-1617 Venetian inventories that mention books, none of which cite Marinelli's pharmaco-

Italian and foreign) and various private Venetian pharmacopeias—especially the one created by Georg Melich and expanded by Alberto Stecchini and Antonio de Sgobbis—testify to a notable chemical bent, supported by an assortment of glassware and other appropriate tools (alembics, sublimation glasses, retort flasks, vials, cooling ducts, etc.), as well as the simple minerals and compounds inventoried in various shops.[37]

Things did not go any better with the pharmaceutical code that the Republic commissioned almost two centuries later from the professors at the Paduan Studio. After a gestation period of more than twenty years, the *Codice farmaceutico per lo stato della Serenissima Repubblica di Venezia, compilato per ordine dell'eccellentissimo magistrato della Sanità* (Pharmaceutical Code for the State of the Most Serene Republic of Venice, Compiled by Order of the Most Excellent Magistrate of Health) was published in the spring of 1790.[38] However, serious errors rendered it practically useless: it lacked scientific nomenclature, had basic gaps (absence of dosages for simple remedies and ingredients), obsolete or useless recipes, inexecutable compositions, and excessive limits in its choice of substitutes. These and other issues led health authorities to commission a detailed examination of the text, which was withdrawn from bookstores. However, the hoped-for new edition, cleansed of all highlighted defects, once again never came to fruition.[39]

It was only much later, during the eighteenth century, that in Venice a private pharmacopeia gained prominence as a reference text—*de facto* rather than *de jure*. It was not officially commissioned by physicians but was the result of research by an expert apothecary with chemical training: the *Lessico farmaceutico-chimico contenente li rimedj più usati d'oggidì di Gio. Battista Capello speziale all'insegna de' tre Monti in campo Sant'Apollinare* (Pharmaceutical-Chemical Lexicon Containing the Most Used Recipes Today of Gio. Battista Capello, Apothecary under the sign of the Three Mountains...). First published in 1728, a further ten Venetian and four Neapolitan editions had come out by the end of the eighteenth century. This was the most widely used Venetian pharmacopeia, still known to local pharmacists today, and was continually revised and enlarged first by Capello and then by his nephew Lorenzo, also a pharmacist.[40]

Venice therefore represents a unique case in the adoption of official pharmacopeia and thus in the obligation to follow pharmaceutical standards, since its apothecaries continually refused to adhere to codes drawn up by physicians and approved by the College of Physicians. However, to evaluate the impact of a pharmacological code, it is essential to examine what books were actually used in shops. The Venetian reality, with its numerous authorized secrets that enriched the pharmaceutical offerings and the many books that were consulted and used for medicinal compositions, turns out to have been particularly open to chemical practices.[41] Even the Venetian tariff reflected this: from 1660 onwards, it devoted a specific section to the *Index medicamentorum hermeticorum spagiricorum sive arte destillatoria paratorum* (*Index of Hermetic Medicaments Prepared by the Spagyric or Distilling Art*), which listed in alphabetical order the waters, balms, extracts, laudanums, magisterial compounds, oils, salts, spirits, and tinctures with an abundance of mineral substances (figs. 24a-b). It would therefore be worthwhile, should a significant number of tariffs from other Italian or European states emerge, to make a comparison with those of Venice.

peia: a Benedictine apothecary shop, 1629 (ASVe, *S. Giorgio Maggiore*, b. 26, library equipment described in http://materiamedicaintransit.eu/a/gardens/sgiorgiom-2/); the all'Abramo apothecary, 1641 (ASVe, Giudici di Petizion, f. 357, n. 58, c. 29r); a Dominican apothecary, 1682 (ASVe, SS. Giovanni e Paolo, b. 115); the apothecary at San Donato in Murano (Archivio parrocchiale, fasc. Commissaria Petronilla Chinnico, c. 1720); Gian Vincenzo Gorgazini's shop at the Cedro Imperiale, 1774 (ASVe, Giudici di Petizion, f. 463, n. 80); and Giovanni Bonamigo's apothecary at Colonna e Mezza, 1785 (ASVe, Giudici di Petizion, f. 480, n. 14).

37. For a detailed examination of the titles in post-mortem shop inventories drawn up between the sixteenth and eighteenth centuries see Minuzzi, *Sul filo dei segreti*, pp. 63-90.
38. Giormani, 'La farmacopea ufficiale della Serenissima'.
39. In Autumn of 1790, auditors produced a 256-page report against the 274-page *Code*, which left little room for corrective action. A detailed comparison between the two texts—the *Code* and the auditors' report are together in a manuscript in the Biblioteca Civica in Udine (XVII-1)—is in Caracci, 'Vicende di una farmacopea di Stato'.
40. Giovanni Battista Capello (d. 1764), *Lessico farmaceutico-chimico*. Further editions were published in Venice in 1734, 1740, 1745, 1751, 1754, 1759, 1763, 1769, 1775, 1792, and in Naples in 1761, 1769, 1775, 1780. For more on Capello, see the biographical entry in Maggioni, *Dizionario storico biografico dei farmacisti italiani*.
41. On the other hand, it is clear that—even where there was a semi-prohibitive regime for chemistry, such as in the episcopal principality of Trent—apothecaries read and made extensive use of manuals, recipe books, and collections of foreign chemical remedies. See Garbellotti, 'Libri e letture di speziali', pp. 105–06.

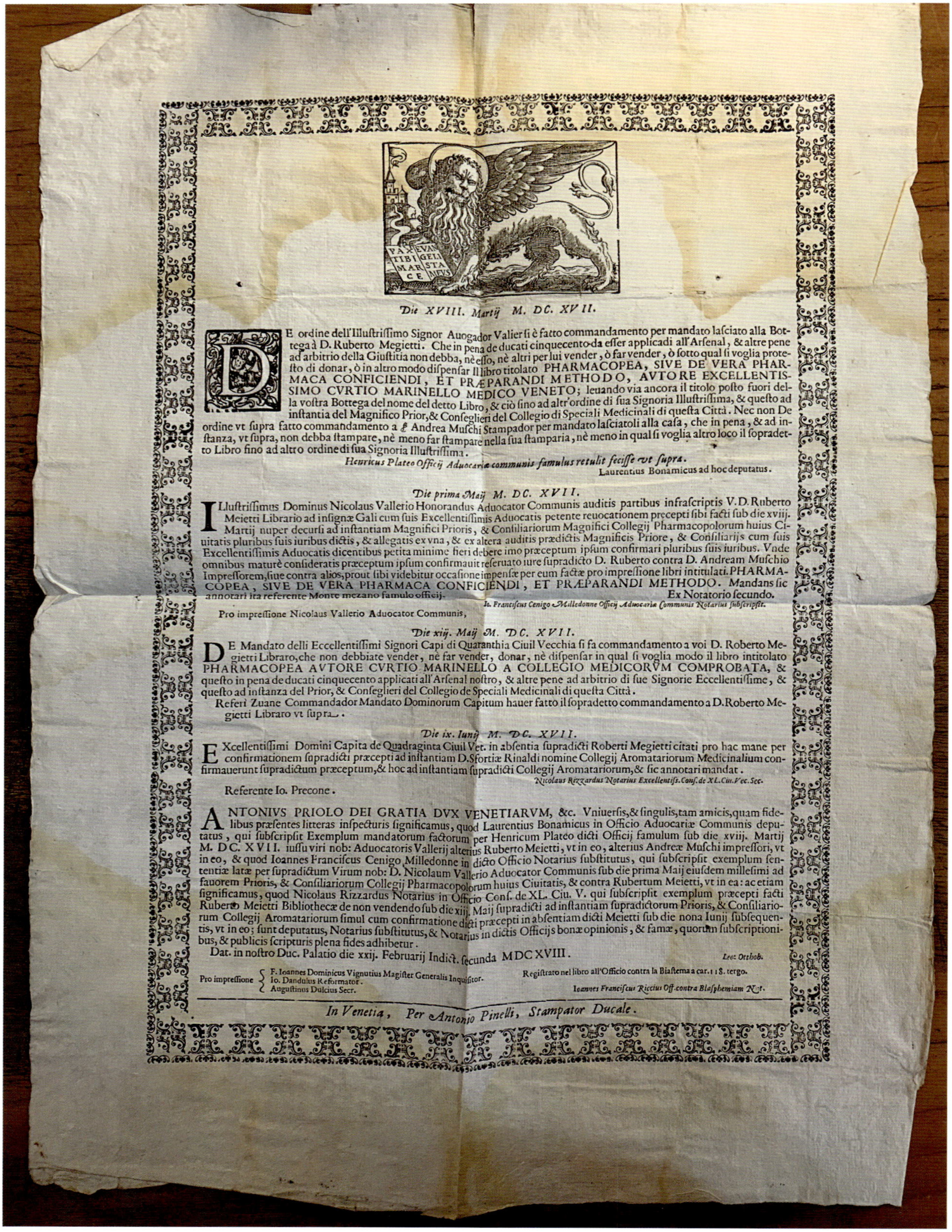

Die XVIII. Martij M. DC. XVII.

DE ordine dell'Illustrissimo Signor Auogador Valier si è fatto commandamento per mandato lasciato alla Bottega à D. Ruberto Megietti. Che in pena de ducati cinquecento da esser applicadi all'Arsenal, & altre pene ad arbitrio della Giustitia non debba, nè esso, nè altri per lui vender, ò far vender, ò sotto qual si voglia protesto di donar, ò in altro modo dispensar Il libro titolato PHARMACOPEA, SIVE DE VERA PHARMACA CONFICIENDI, ET PRÆPARANDI METHODO, AVTORE EXCELLENTISSIMO CVRTIO MARINELLO MEDICO VENETO; leuando via ancora il titolo posto fuori della vostra Bottega del nome del detto Libro, & ciò sino ad altr'ordine di sua Signoria Illustrissima, & questo ad instantia del Magnifico Prior, & Conseglieri del Collegio di Speciali Medicinali di questa Città. Nec non De ordine vt supra fatto commandamento a ℰ Andrea Muschi Stampador per mandato lasciatoli alla casa, che in pena, & ad instanza, vt supra, non debba stampare, nè meno far stampare nella sua stamparia, nè meno in qual si voglia altro loco il sopradetto Libro fino ad altro ordine di sua Signoria Illustrissima.

Henricus Plateo Officij Aduocariæ communis famulus retulit fecisse vt supra.

Laurentius Bonamicus ad hoc deputatus.

Die prima Maij M. DC. XVII.

ILlustrissimus Dominus Nicolaus Vallerio Honorandus Aduocator Communis auditis partibus infrascriptis V. D. Ruberto Meietti Librario ad insignæ Gali cum suis Excellentissimis Aduocatis petente reuocationem precepti sibi facti sub die xviij. Martij nuper decursi ad instantiam Magnifici Prioris, & Consiliariorum Magnifici Collegij Pharmacopolorum huius Ciuitatis pluribus suis iuribus dictis, & allegatis ex vna, & ex altera auditis prædictis Magnificis Priore, & Consiliarijs cum suis Excellentissimis Aduocatis dicentibus petita minime fieri debere imo præceptum ipsum confirmari pluribus suis iuribus. Vnde omnibus maturè consideratis præceptum ipsum confirmauit reseruato iure supradicto D. Ruberto contra D. Andream Muschio Impressorem, siue contra alios, prout sibi videbitur occasione impensæ per eum factæ pro impressione libri intitulati. PHARMACOPEA, SIVE DE VERA PHARMACA CONFICIENDI, ET PRÆPARANDI METHODO. Mandans sic annotari ita referente Monte mezano famulo officij.

Ex Notatorio secundo.

Io. Franciscus Cenigo Milledonne Officij Aduocariæ Communis Notarius subscripsit.

Pro impressione Nicolaus Vallerio Aduocator Communis,

Die xiij. Maij M. DC. XVII.

DE Mandato delli Eccellentissimi Signori Capi di Quaranthia Ciuil Vecchia si fa commandamento a voi D. Roberto Megietti Libraro, che non debbiate vender, nè far vender, donar, nè dispensar in qual si voglia modo il libro intitolato PHARMACOPEA AVTORE CVRTIO MARINELLO A COLLEGIO MEDICORVM COMPROBATA, & questo in pena de ducati cinquecento applicati all'Arsenal nostro, & altre pene ad arbitrio di sue Signorie Eccellentissime, & questo ad instanza del Prior, & Conseglieri del Collegio de Speciali Medicinali di questa Città.

Referì Zuane Commandador Mandato Dominorum Capitum hauer fatto il sopradetto commandamento a D. Roberto Megietti Libraro vt supra.

Die ix. Iunij M. DC. XVII.

EXcellentissimi Domini Capita de Quadraginta Ciuil Vet. in absentia supradicti Roberti Megietti citati pro hac mane per confirmationem supradicti præcepti ad instantiam D. Sfortiæ Rinaldi nomine Collegij Aromatariorum Medicinalium confirmauerunt supradictum præceptum, & hoc ad instantiam supradicti Collegij Aromatariorum, & sic annotari mandat.

Nicolaus Rizzardus Notarius Excellentiss. Cons. de XL. Ciu. Vec. Sec.

Referente Io. Precone.

ANTONIVS PRIOLO DEI GRATIA DVX VENETIARVM, &c. Vniuersis, & singulis, tam amicis, quam fidelibus præsentes litteras inspecturis significamus, quod Laurentius Bonamicus in Officio Aduocariæ Communis deputatus, qui subscripsit Exemplum mandatorum factorum per Henricum Plateo dicti Officij famulum sub die xviij. Martij M. DC. XVII. iussu viri nob: Aduocatoris Vallerij alterius Ruberto Meietti, vt in eo, alterius Andreæ Muschi impressori, vt in eo, & quod Ioannes Franciscus Cenigo Milledonne in dicto Officio Notarius substitutus, qui subscripsit exemplum sententiæ latæ per supradictum Virum nob: D. Nicolaum Vallerio Aduocator Communis sub die prima Maij eiusdem millesimi ad fauorem Prioris, & Consiliariorum Collegij Pharmacopolorum huius Ciuitatis, & contra Rubertum Meietti, vt in ea: ac etiam significamus, quod Nicolaus Rizzardus Notarius in Officio Cons. de XL. Ciu. V. qui subscripsit exemplum præcepti facti Ruberto Meietti Bibliothecæ de non vendendo sub die xiij. Maij supradicti ad instantiam supradictorum Prioris, & Consiliariorum Collegij Aromatariorum simul cum confirmatione dicti præcepti in absentiam dicti Meietti sub die nona Iunij subsequentis, vt in eo; sunt deputatus, Notarius substitutus, & Notarius in dictis Officijs bonæ opinionis, & famæ, quorum subscriptionibus, & publicis scripturis plena fides adhibetur.

Dat. in nostro Duc. Palatio die xxij. Februarij Indict. secunda MDCXVIII.

Leo: Otthob.

Pro impressione { F. Ioannes Dominicus Vignutius Magister Generalis Inquisitor. / Io. Dandulus Reformator. / Augustinus Dulcius Secr.

Registrato nel libro all'Officio contra la Biastema a car. 118. tergo.

Ioannes Franciscus Riccius Off. contra Blasphemiam Not.

In Venetia, Per Antonio Pinelli, Stampator Ducale.

25 Order by which, the Avogadori di Comun, in March 1617, withdrew the printing and sale of Curzio Marinelli's *Pharmacopoea*, with provisions confirmed in February 1618. This was done upon the request of the College of Apothecaries. The penalty for any violation of the decree was set at 500 ducats.

TARIFFS AND DISCOUNTS: PATIENTS, NURSES, AND PROXIMITY RELATIONSHIPS

Even the official annual tariffs for medicines were practically never applied. It seems that in Venice, it was common practice among apothecaries to reduce the listed prices by at least half. Other sources shed light on this, especially those concerning the management of monastic apothecaries between the mid-seventeenth and mid-eighteenth centuries. One significant eighteenth-century testimony, which also reflects on earlier decades, is the *Informazione* (Report) of two Dominicans who, along with two lay apothecaries, evaluated the state of the apothecary of the monastery of Santi Giovanni e Paolo on behalf of their confrater, Serafino Callegari.[42] After having highlighted the lack of many essential simples[43] on the shelves and the poor quality of other important items (cinchona, rhubarb, senna, cassia, manna ash), the inspectors concentrated on the lackluster recordkeeping.

Brother Serafino should have entered three price listings in the register to obtain an exhaustive balance of the shop's income and expenditure. The investigators explained how the budget should have been kept according to standard practice:

It is necessary to know that there are three ways in which drugs prices can be established. The first is the rigorous [adherence to] the *Tariff*. The second is with the discount of sixty percent, more or less, *currently in use in almost all apothecaries*. And the third is according to the actual cost and value of the medicines themselves.[44]

Brother Serafino had listed only the second price when he should have indicated at least the actual cost of ingredients and preparation, 'given all the expenses incurred in their creation and composition, the cost of their production was completely disregarded'.[45] When questioned, Serafino replied that it was difficult for him to calculate such costs because the manipulations were all done together, seamlessly, for both the religious and the secular customers. This suggests not only that external customers were numerous, even though dispensing drugs outside the monastery was forbidden, but also that the brothers did not charge for their labor. According to the Report, it was common practice for all apothecaries—religious and non—to offer large discounts on the prices fixed by the *Tariff*, sometimes exceeding 60%. Moreover, their clientele consisted of both lay and religious people without distinction.

From the rest of the report, it is clear that poor Brother Serafino, while guilty of some negligence, had been made a scapegoat for a rather unruly pattern of business management that had begun decades before him. The shop, which was opened by the Dominicans in 1674 to meet the monastery's ever-increasing medicinal needs, had almost immediately picked up the bad habit of illegally selling medicines 'a' particolari' (to laypeople). Many of these customers—including some 'companies'—were insolvent debtors against whom no legal action could be taken precisely because the sale of drugs outside the monastery was illegal.[46] If we consider these debts in conjunction with the failure to record income and expenses, it is understandable that, in 1762 (almost a century after its establishment), the Dominican apothecary was on the verge of bankruptcy.

A subsequent defense Memorandum by Brother Serafino adds important details to the picture: it provides a rather confused account of the procedures in question, suggesting that all the friars and even the prior were responsible for such irregularities. In addition, it highlights the absence of the doctor's prescriptions that should have been kept in the shop and even copied into a register. A fundamental passage of the Memorandum, signed by witnesses, recounts past and present practices:

'3rd. In spite of the directives of our fathers, the priors of all times, which stipulated that medicines should not be given out without a prescription, the fathers desired to have drugs at their own discretion; in the same way, the same father Superior did, while I had to provide the medicines even to those who went to the countryside, as I did for several fathers, namely Father Baccilieri, the

42. These expert apothecaries were Antonio Zaghetti of the Vigilanza and Francesco Orteschi of the Pomo d'Argento.
43. For the meaning of 'simple' see footnote 2.
44. ASVe, SS. Giovanni e Paolo, b. 116, file Y.XX.2°, 15, *Informazione* of 1762 of Brother Giandomenico Zorzi e Father Berardelli, in two copies. Emphasis mine: 'È necessario sapere che in tre maniere possono considerarsi li prezzi dei medicamenti. Il primo è il rigoroso a *Tariffario*. Il secondo si è col dibatimento del 60 per cento e poco più e poco meno, usato al presente da quasi tutte le speziarie. Ed il terzo considerando la pura spesa e valore che costano i medicamenti medesimi'.
45. Ibid.: 'considerandosi tutta la spesa che vi sarà andata nel farli e comporli, ma non computata per niente la fattura della loro compositione'.
46. Ibid. The four firms were 'Carminati, Feghelin, Fabro, Tavani'.

Pasoretti brothers, and Father Prudentio Rossi, who is now overseeing the new method [of running the apothecary]. And although the current Superior checks the books every three days, a lot of stuff is still dispensed without a prescription.'[47]

The bad management continued even during the internal trial involving Brother Serafino, who gave the names and surnames of the friars involved, leaving little doubt about the truthfulness of his testimony. The Memorandum continues by recounting how the brothers always requested medicines for themselves and for the temporary guests without the required prescriptions from the physician: in many cases it was Serafino himself who wrote the prescription.[48]

Confusion also reigned, according to Brother Serafino, because many friars were taking 'medicines on credit for laypersons known to them personally'—and therefore, Brother Serafino's medical prescriptions also involved customers outside the monastery. And even the two young lay assistants of the apothecary complied with all the requests of the superiors, who 'used drugs and compounds at their own liking'.[49] Serafino had tried protesting the excessive liberties taken by these youths, but they enjoyed high protection—one had been placed in the shop by the noble Pietro Giusto—as proved by the fact that among the authoritative figures he had unsuccessfully complained to was Giovanni Battista Capello, the author of the most popular private Venetian pharmacopeia.[50] The latter's involvement demonstrates how closely the religious pharmaceutical circuit was connected to the public circuit of collegiate apothecaries. It clearly illustrates the porousness of the monastic walls, in which religious figures were part of a chain that led to the external circulation of internally produced medicines. This phenomenon was not unknown in early modern Europe, but through the words of our protagonists we see just how widespread this circulation must have been, and, above all, how it occurred through intermediaries placed *within* the monastery itself. In other words, it was not just happening 'behind the counter,' but out in the open, through a network of everyday personal relationships.

Who were the people who purchased medicines from monastic pharmacies, and what kind of relationships did they have with the friars? What type of transactions did the dispensation of medicines involve?

Two further documents may help answer these questions. Both the 1762 Report and Serafino's Memorandum provide glimpses of lay customers, but a document dating to 1672 offers an intriguing perspective on the clientele of the monastic apothecary. This document contains fourteen testimonies from individuals of various backgrounds collected by the Giudici dell'Esaminador at the request of the College of Apothecaries 'for the perpetual memory of the matter'.[51] Taken between August and December, these testimonies throw light on the ways in which the monasteries of San Giobbe in the Cannaregio *sestiere* (district) and San Francesco della Vigna and San Domenico in the Castello *sestiere* dispensed their medicines to people outside their institutions.[52]

A second document sheds light on the individuals involved in the consumption of medicines from religious apothecaries: it is an *ad lites* print (print in litigation) concerning the abuses of monastery apothecaries, primarily involving the aforementioned Franciscans of S. Giobbe and S. Francesco della Vigna.[53] It reproduces various materials, including testimonies, receipts, accounting books, and notes addressed to nurses, alongside provisions from both ancient and contemporary ecclesiastical and Venetian law. These sources prompt more

47. Ibid., file Y.XX.2°, 17, *Memorandum* of Brother Serafino, undated and unbound, articulated in six points: '3° Nonostante li ordini de' padri nostri Priori, in tutti li tempi, di non dare li medicamenti senza ricetta, li padri li volevano a suo piacimento, come anco faceva il medemo superiore, dovendovi [io] anche dare il suo bisogno a quelli che andavano in campagna, come ho fatto a diversi padri, cioè padre Baccilieri, frattelli Pasoretti, e padre Prudentio Rossi hora sopraintendente del novo mettodo; ed abenché il presente superior visiti ogni terzo giorno li libri, non ostante [ciò], si dà molta robba senza ricetta'.
48. Ibid.
49. Ibid. In this case, Serafino also gives the names of one of the two youths and the superiors.
50. Ibid., point no. 6. For Capello, see footnote 41. Piero Giusto can be identified as Piero Zusto (b. 1725), son of Angelo, a senator and member of the Council of Ten who died by 1785 (the year in which his widow, Laura Valmarana, married the nobleman Piero Vettor Pisani). See CorrerVe, MS Cicogna 2504, Marco Barbaro, *Arbori de' patritii Veneti*, fols 289^{v}–290^{r}.
51. ASVe, Giudici dell'Esaminador, filza 70, 30 August 1672.
52. S. Giobbe was closed in 1806, and its friars transferred to San Francesco della Vigna.
53. ASVe, Milizia da Mar, b. 554, a printed file entitled *Spezieri medicinali* (*Medicinal Apothecaries*). The forty-four-page publication traces the legal actions brought by the College of Apothecaries against the monasteries of San Francesco della Vigna, San Giobbe, San Domenico, Santi Giovanni e Paolo, and the Servi di Maria between 1657 and 1732.

general considerations that will assist in answering the questions posed above. The documents reveal how religious apothecaries served a non-exclusive clientele and customers shopped around, visiting different religious apothecaries as well as lay ones. In times of illness, 'signor Francesco Zavori [son] of the late signor Antonio, living in Castello,' acquired medicines both from the nurse of San Francesco della Vigna and that of San Domenico.[54] A certain 'signor Z. Battista Andreolli, [son] of the late signor Gerolamo,' also from Castello, declared:

'The last time I was sick, I bought medicines partly from the monastery of San Domenico di Castello and partly from the apothecary near the San Domenico bridge, and also from the one near the Rielo bridge in Castello. But the medicines I obtained from the monastery cost me half of what I pay at the public apothecaries.'[55]

Like Andreolli, 'signor Alvise Boldù, [son] of the late signor Zuanne, living in Castello', used medicines from San Domenico and San Francesco della Vigna, as well as those from lay apothecary shops.[56] Women from the house of 'signor Z. Battista Negri, [son] of the late signor Andrea, living at San [Giobbe]', went to the friars of San Giobbe to get some 'waters, oils, and other trifles' without paying anything in exchange: 'I don't give them money, the said friars being my benefactors, and I purchase medicines from the apothecary at [the sign of] the Mermaid'.[57] Another customer of the Mermaid apothecary was 'signor Alessandro Felippi, [son] of the late signor Bortolamio, who lives [in the parish of] San Giobbe'; meanwhile, for medicated waters, he turned to the monastery of San Giobbe, which seems to have specialized in these basic remedies: 'the infirmary of San Giobbe gives waters to my house when we need them, and I give them charity when they need it, but I don't pay them anything and for the apothecary I go to the Mermaid Apothecary'.[58] In all the testimonies, many individuals went to the Mermaid (Sirena, Serena) apothecary in Castello, managed by a lay master, while also visiting monastic apothecaries.

As for the pricing, the standard practice for religious apothecaries was to dispense the simplest remedies freely or in exchange for a small donation, and to sell more elaborate compositions at half of what was on offer in lay shops, which (as we have seen above) was already heavily discounted. Religious apothecaries thus dispensed some drugs at practically cost price, as confirmed by other testimonies. A certain signor Zanmaria Tasso, a resident of Castello, says that when he needed medications, he went to San Domenico di Castello, and the nursing friar provided him with good quality items 'at cost price, that is, at half the price of what one buys from the [lay] apothecary; [and] it's good quality stuff'.[59] A fruit-seller named Alvise received a small bottle of water and some syrup for his sick child from the Observant Minor Friars of San Giobbe. They did not ask for any payment, so he left a voluntary donation as a gesture of gratitude.[60]

The practice of cutting prices to cost was not the only way in which religious apothecaries dispensed medications. Sometimes they were traded in exchange for services or bartered, and in one case were even given for a lien: a small ossicle of Saint Charles was exchanged for medicine that would be paid for later, at which point the relic would be returned to its owner.[61] The shoemaker who served the San Domenico friars paid a low price and supplemented costs with shoes for the nurses:

'I'm a shoemaker who serves the reverend Friars of San Domenico for the most part, and also the nurse friar, so in times of sickness he's given me medications and I've given

54. ASVe, Giudici dell'Esaminador, f. 70, 8 November 1672.
55. Ibid., first testimony, 30 August 1672: 'Questa ultima volta che sono stato amalato ho tolto li medicamenti al convento di San Domenico di Castello parte, et parte alla spiciaria al ponte di San Domenico et anco al ponte de Riello [o Rielo, a Castello] ma quelli che ho havuto dal convento li me costava a bon prezzo la mettà di quello che pago alle spiciarie'.
56. Ibid., same date.
57. Ibid., 28 September 1672: 'non li do danari, essendo detti padri miei benefatori, *et io mi servo di medicine dal spicier della Serena*'. Emphasis mine.
58. Ibid., 1 October 1672. Emphasis mine: 'Io sono calegher che servo li reverendi Padri di San Domenico la maggior parte, anco il padre infermier, qual in occasion di malatia mi ha datto delli medicamenti et io li ho datto delle scarpe et quanto alli medicamenti sono stati perfetti et a bon prezzo'.
59. Ibid., 30 August 1672. Emphasis mine: 'Ho ricevuto qualche bagatella de medicamenti de infermeria di San Iobbe ma non ghe le ho [pagada], ma all'incontro ghe dagho delle cere secondo mi ordinano et alle volte anco qualche soldo come ghe bisogna, perché l'infermier è mio amico e compadre'.
60. Ibid., 10 September 1672.
61. Ibid., 30 August 1672. The testimony of Alvise Boldù cited above on the cure of a priest friend, Battista di Alvise (who later died), with drugs acquired from both Dominican and lay apothecaries.

him shoes, and as for the medications, they're perfect and at a good price.'[62]

A waxmaker, Antonio Martini, did not pay for the medicines but traded for it with the wax that the friars at San Giobbe needed or by offering some money in return:

'I've received some trifling medications from the infirmary at San Giobbe but didn't [pay] for them. Instead, I gave them the wax they ordered from me, and I also offered some money, depending on their needs, because the nurse is my friend and godfather.'[63]

Smaller artisans thus repaid drugs with the products and services they already offered to the friars, while a friendship had also been established with the nursing friar.

Common denominator of all the testimonies is the emergence of various types of proximity relationships, with geographical proximity being the most prominent. Most customers lived in Castello and Cannaregio, the same districts as the monasteries. Some of them maintained work-related relationships with the friars—providing labor in various capacities—sometimes strengthened by friendship or kinship, as in the case of the shoemaker or of the aforementioned Alvise Boldù, who had 'a brother in the monastery of San Francesco della Vigna'.[64] As Lorenzo Soldà declared, 'I've gotten some remedies from the infirmary of the monastery of San Domenico, but I didn't give them anything in payment because I'm the son of a lay brother'.[65] The members of the Scuola e sovvegno di San Diego, a devotional confraternity based near the Church of San Giobbe, also regularly turned to the San Giobbe apothecary.[66] A series of receipts from the monastery's infirmary testifies to the sale of drugs to treat members of the Scuola di San Diego, often through the mediation of the charity's caretaker.[67] These receipts, issued between 1716 and 1724, were found in the confraternity's records following a search ordered during the investigations that ensued after the complaint filed by the College of Apothecaries. Typical receipts recorded as a sample in the *ad lites* print read:

'On 17 March 1718, San [Giobbe] | I received through Gio. Pietro da Venezia, nurse of San Giobbe, from signor Giacomo Zallo, caretaker of the Charity of San Diego, eighty-six *lire de piccoli*, which are for the medication given to signor Giacomo Tomasi, and [to] signor Iseppo Sagramora. Val.—L. 86.

On 20 June 1728 | I received through Giuseppe di Venezia, nurse at San Giobbe in the monastery, thirty-six-and-a-half *lire* for the medication administered to Domenico Fattori, who was a brother of the aforesaid confraternity, from the aforesaid caretaker Milesio. Val.—L. 36:50.'[68]

It is not clear whether there was consultation with medical professionals behind the sale of medicines, or simply with the friar nurse. It is likely that the two situations coexisted. The minutes of two interrogations conducted by the Avogaria di Comun in August 1730 refer to regular medical prescriptions.[69] When explicitly asked if they had purchased drugs upon presenting prescriptions, a carpenter from the Arsenal and a beadmaker ('margariter') testified that they always presented their prescriptions; both residents in the Castello district, they attested to having regularly been served by the apothecary of San Francesco della Vigna, demonstrating this with repeated prescriptions. One had done so for a year, while the other had been going for around twelve years, with open accounts at the religious apothecary.[70] The *ad lites* print also contains the transcription of a note from a Giovanni Battista Peceti, asking the nurse at San Francesco della Vigna, Giuseppe, to urgently prepare some medication prescribed by the doctor.[71]

62. Ibid., 7 November 1672: 'Io sono calegher che servo li reverendi Padri di San Domenico la maggior parte, anco il padre infermier, qual in occasion di malatia mi ha datto delli medicamenti et io li ho datto delle scarpe et quanto alli medicamenti sono stati perfetti et a bon prezzo'.
63. Ibid., 10 September 1672: 'Ho ricevuto qualche bagatella de medicamenti de infermeria di San Iobbe ma non ghe le ho [pagada], ma all'incontro ghe dagho delle cere secondo mi ordinano et alle volte anco qualche soldo come ghe bisogna, perché l'infermier è mio amico e compadre.'
64. Ibid., Alvise Boldù, 30 August 1672.
65. Ibid., 28 September 1672, declaration of Lorenzo Soldà, who lived at the Fondamenta Quintavalle in Castello. By 'lay brother' (*converso*), he meant a man who lived a monastic lifestyle but had not taken vows.
66. Vio, *Le Scuole Piccole*, pp. 474–75.
67. ASVe, Milizia da Mar, b. 554, *Spezieri medicinali*, pp. 17–19.
68. Ibid., pp. 17–18: 'Adì 17 marzo 1718, S. Giobe | Ho ricevuto io fra Gio. Pietro da Venezia infermiero di S. Giobe dal signor Giacomo Zallo custode del Sovegno di San Diego lire ottantasei de picoli, quali sono per medicamenti dati al signor Giacomo Tomasi murer, e [al] signor Iseppo Sagramora. Val L. 86. | Adì 20 giugno 1728 | Ho rcevuto io f. Giuseppe di Venezia infermiero in San Giobe nel monastero lire trentasei e meza per medicamenti sominístrati al qu. Domenico Fattori fu fratello del sudetto Sovegno, dal sudetto Milesio custode. Val L. 36:10.'
69. The Avogaria di Comun (Advocacy of the Municipality) ensured the principle of legality, namely the correctness in the application of laws.
70. ASVe, Milizia da Mar, b. 554, *Spezieri medicinali*, pp. 30–31.
71. Ibid., p. 42.

The physicians active in Venice were apparently neither annoyed nor surprised that their patients obtained the medicines they prescribed from religious apothecaries. Among the Giudici dell'Esaminador's documents, we find the testimony of Doctor Francesco Bertoldi, who declares that he is aware that some of his patients visited monastery apothecaries because they were cheaper than the lay apothecaries:

'I know that the nurse friars of San Domenico in Castello and San Francesco freely sell waters and medicaments, and this I know because I have ordered medicine for the sick many times and I know that they have gotten them at the said monasteries and that they also paid for them saying that they have a greater advantage [there] than at the [lay] apothecaries.'[72]

The Dominican friars seem to have been more organized according to the testimony of a Gian Leone Catena, who lived in Castello in 1672. They had a walled garden, outside of which was a cord attached to a bell within. Those who needed medicines would pull the cord and a friar would look out of an opening (*buso*) in the wall. After hearing their request, the Dominican would bring the drugs in exchange for a small payment. This practice was so consolidated and commonly accepted that the friars of San Domenico had a messenger of the Republic, the 'comandador' Bertocco, intervene for them in cases of insolvent debts.[73] In fact, the same Bertocco was called immediately afterward to testify about the recovery of one such debt, which he had carried out with zeal, even though it was not at all legal.[74]

The customers of the religious apothecaries were not only from the poorest social strata, or the artisans we have heard from so far. A note addressed to the nurse of San Francesco della Vigna reads:

'Master father my lord, | For the most illustrious signore Antonio Thiera my relative, who finds himself sick here, thy person [might] be pleased to provide for all the needs that shall satisfy him, & I [shall] be [thy] guarantor in all ways. | On 12 March 1700, thy most affectionate Servant Gio. Doglioni. | Reverse: To the master nurse father of San Francesco della Vigna | His hands [only].'[75]

The author of the note, who guarantees payment for any medication his relative needs, belonged to the Doglioni, a well-known and esteemed family of Venetian notaries, jurists, and physicians, and can perhaps be identified as the 'doctor of law & lawyer' to whom the Bellunese poet Ercole Rudio dedicated a sonnet in 1686.[76] The relative was perhaps Antonio Tiera, an 'eminent lawyer of Portogruaro' and dilletante poet active in the early seventeenth century.[77] Accounts consisting of several dozen—sometimes hundreds—of *lire*, paid in installments, were registered between 1725 and 1728 in the ledger books of San Francesco della Vigna. These entries include surnames of people with non-manual occupations: the 'most Illustrious signor Francesco Donà, public accountant', Zuanne Vigo (over 300 *lire*), a 'Piscopoli', an unspecified 'Reverend Mother' (fifty-three *lire*), the sacristan of San Giacomo da l'Orio (one of the oldest parochial churches in Venice), and a 'Marin in the Nunciature' (that is, an employee at the Apostolic Nunciature in Venice).[78] A carpenter named Antonio Roschin (perhaps a misspelling of Boschin) held a large open account with San Francesco della Vigna (139:14 *lire*), while around ten members of the Scuola e Sovvegno di San Diego paid smaller bills to San Giobbe, totaling approximately 200 *lire*.[79] These were indeed respectable bills, and even prestigious figures sought services from religious apothecaries, thereby showcasing the diverse clientele that religious apothecaries served, which was

72. ASVe, Giudici dell'Esaminador, f. 70, 1 September 1672: 'So che li padri infermieri di San Domenico di Castello et di San Francesco vendono liberamente aque e medicamenti, et questo lo so per haver io più volte ordinato a più persone per infermi medicine et so che le hanno tolte a detti conventi et che le hanno anche pagate dicendo che havevano più avantaggio che da spicieri'.
73. Ibid., 22 November 1672.
74. Ibid., the same date as Bertocco's deposition.
75. ASVe, Milizia da Mar, b. 554, *Spezieri medicinali*, p. 41, transcription of a handwritten note put on record: 'Padre maestro mio signore, Per l'illustriss. sig. Antonio Thiera mio congionto, che s'attrova qui amalato, V.P. si compiacia si somministrarli tutto il bisogno che lui sodisferà, & io sono pieggio in tutti li casi. Adì 12 marzo 1700, suo affetionatiss. Servitore Gio. Doglioni. Tergo: *Al Padre Maestro Infermier di S. Francesco della Vigna Sue Mani*'.
76. Rudio, *Sonetti amorosi & varii*, p. 50. Further biographical investigations should be done, but the note is certainly from a member of the Doglioni family. A Giovanni Nicolò Doglioni was a notary of the Republic between 1573 and 1610. See 'Notai di Venezia. Atti [e testamenti]', pp. 335–38, available for consultation at the ASVe.
77. Zambaldi, *Monumenti storici di Concordia*, p. 323. While not being *tout court* identifiable as our Antonio Thiera, the geographical area, profession, and poetic inclination make him very close to the author of the note, displaying a certain expressive elegance.
78. ASVe, Milizia da Mar, b. 554, *Spezieri medicinali*, p. 43.
79. Ibid., pp. 17–19.

comparable to that of any other secular apothecary. It is also highly likely that the selection of witnesses examined by the judges of the Avogaria, as well as the selection of documents to be published in the *ad lites* print, aimed to avoid implicating nobles and particularly prominent individuals—as was the tacit custom in the Republic. It is therefore probable that the nobility and the upper echelons of society are underrepresented in the sample of figures who appear in these documents.

CONCLUSIONS

By reconstructing the exceptions to and transgressions from the normative theory, we grasp certain aspects of the past that would otherwise go unnoticed. First, that new medicinal remedies were approved in derogation of the general laws prohibiting anyone from creating and selling them. The act of licensing and/or granting a privilege only to those remedies that were innovative compared to those listed in the official and private pharmacopeias in circulation is a significant indicator of the Republic's political drive towards pharmaceutical innovation, particularly in the direction of chemical medicines.

Second, the widespread practice of significant price reductions, which was also common in non-religious apothecaries, suggests that the affordability of medicines was far greater than implied by the official Tariffs, which only indicated the full cost of medicines. As one witness made clear, 'it is a well-known fact that [the religious apothecaries] sell medicines,'[80] and even medical practitioners had equal confidence in religious and secular apothecaries. Customers frequented both without prejudice, and medical professionals had no objections. Moreover, customers sometimes sought therapeutic advice from the male nurses who ran the religious apothecaries.

Religious and secular apothecaries were complementary realities, and together offered a space in which the range of transactions was extremely wide: sale at half price, sale at cost, or in exchange for donations, services, or other products. Secular apothecary shops were places of encounter and exchange of opinions and knowledge, while religious ones represented a place of 'deferred' or mediated encounters.[81] Religious apothecaries could not count on the same continuity between the inside and the outside, but had many internal intermediaries (from priors to ordinary friars) and links with the outside (of kinship, friendship, service provision, physical proximity, etc.), suggesting a similar continuous exchange of medical-pharmaceutical knowledge, albeit deferred in time and space. If a counter with scales, jars, boxes for lozenges, and long benches along the walls for waiting customers are the classic representations of the public apothecary from the late Middle Ages onwards, the bell with a cord in the monastery of San Domenico and the '*buso*' (hole) from which the nurse friar peeped out, might better represent the secluded circuits of religiously manufactured medicines.[82] These circuits were reserved but never closed, complementing the shops run by collegiate masters and appealing to a variety of customers who availed themselves of both.

WORKS CITED

Printed Primary Sources

Aldrovandi, Ulisse, *Antidotarium Bononien. a medicinae Collegio nuperrime auctum, et emendatum, et amplissimo eiusdem ciuitatis Senatui dicatum* (Bologna: apud haeredem Victorij Benacij, 1641).

Capello, Giovanni Battista, *Lessico farmaceutico-chimico contenente li rimedj più usati d'oggidì di Gio. Battista Capello speziale all'insegna de' tre Monti in campo Sant'Apollinare* (Venice: per Domenico Lovisa, 1728).

Cordus, Valerius, *Dispensatorium pharmacopolarum, ex omni genere bonorum authorum, cum veterum tum recentium collectum, & scholijs utilissimis illustratum, in quibus obiter, plurium simplicium, hactenus non cognitorum, vera noticia traditur… Item De collectione, repositione, & duratione simplicium* (Nuremberg: apud Joh. Petreium,1546).

Du Chesne, Joseph, *Pharmacopoea dogmaticorum restituta, pretiosis selectisque hermeticorum floribus abunde illustrata* (Paris: apud Claudium Morellum, 1607)

Marinelli, Curzio, *Pharmacopaea, siue De vera pharmaca conficiendi, & praeparandi methodo, a praestantiss. et excell.mo Medicorum Venetorum Collegio comprobata, libri duo, Curtio Marinello… autore…* (Venice: apud Robertum Meiettum, 1617).

Nuovo receptario composto dal famosissimo Chollegio degli eximii doctori della arte et medicina della inclita cipta di Firenze

80. ASVe, Giudici dell'Esaminador, f. 70, 22 November 1672.
81. De Vivo, 'Pharmacies as Centres of Communication'.
82. Shaw and Welch, *Making and Marketing Medicine*, pp. 53–78. See also images 3.2 and 3.3.

(Florence: per la Compagnia del Dragho, ad instantia delli signori chonsoli della Università delli spetiali, 1498).

Pharmacopœia Londinensis in qua medicamenta antiqua et nova usitatissima sedulo collecta, accuratissime examinata, quotidiana experientia confirmata describuntur, diligenter revisa, denuo recusa, emendatior, auctior. Opera medicorum Collegii Londinesis, ex serenisimi Regis mandato (London: printed [by E. Griffin] for Iohn Marriot and are to be sould at his shop in Fleetstreete in St Dunstons Churchyarde, 1618).

Renou, Jean de, *Institutionum pharmaceuticarum libri quinque. Quibus accedunt De materia medica. Libri tres. Omnibus succedit Officina pharmaceutica, siue Antidotarium ab eodem auctore commentariis illustratum* (Paris: apud viduam Gulielmi de la Noue et Dionys. de la Noue, via Iacobaea sub signo nominis Iesu, [1608]).

Rudio, Ercole, *Sonetti amorosi & varii* (Venice: appresso il Miloco, 1686).

Secondary Sources

Ait, Ivana, *Tra scienza e mercato: Gli speziali a Roma nel tardo Medioevo* (Rome: Istituto di studi romani, 1996).

Alden, John, 'Pills and Publishing: Some Notes on the English Book Trade, 1660-1715', *The Library*, 7 (1952), pp. 21–37.

Benocci, Carla, *A ciascuno il suo paradiso. I giardini dei cappuccini, dei minimi, dei gesuiti, degli oratoriani, dei camaldolesi e dei certosini in età moderna* (Rome: Istituto Storico dei cappuccini, 2020).

Brambilla, Elena, 'Dagli antidoti contro la peste alle Farmacopee per i poveri: Farmacia, alchimia e chimica a Milano, 1600-1800', in *Ricerche di storia in onore di Franco Della Peruta*, ed. by Maria Luisa Betri and Duccio Bigazzi (Milan: Franco Angeli, 1996), II, pp. 303–52.

Brockliss, Laurence and Colin Jones, *The Medical World of Early Modern France* (Oxford: Clarendon Press, 1997).

Caracci, Piercarlo, 'Vicende di una farmacopea di Stato della Serenissima Repubblica di Venezia', *Acta historiae Patavina*, 28 (1981-82), pp. 29–44.

Cargnelutti, Liliana, *Inventario dell'Archivio dell'Ospedale di Santa Maria della Misericordia* (typewritten volume, available at the Archivio Capitolare in Udine).

Corradi, Alfonso, *Le prime farmacopee italiane ed in particolare Dei Ricettari Fiorentini. Memoria* (Milan: Rechiedei, 1887).

De Vivo, Filippo, 'Pharmacies as Centres of Communication in Early Modern Venice', *Renaissance Studies*, 21: 4 (2007), pp. 505–21.

Debus, Allen G., *Chemistry, Alchemy and the New Philosophy, 1550-1700: Studies in the History of Science and Medicine* (London: Variorum Reprints, 1987).

Debus, Allen G., 'La medicina chimica nella prima età moderna', in *Storia del pensiero medico occidentale*, ed. by Mirko D. Grmek, II, *Dal Rinascimento all'inizio dell'Ottocento* (Rome-Bari: Laterza, 1996), pp. 51–92.

Drugs on the Page: Pharmacopoeias and Healing Knowledge in the Early Modern Atlantic World ed. by Matthew James Crawford and Gabriel, Joseph M. (Pittsburgh: University of Pittsburgh Press, 2019).

Furdell, Elizabeth L., *Publishing and Medicine in Early Modern England* (Rochester: University of Rochester Press, 2001).

Galluzzi, Paolo, 'Motivi paracelsiani nella Toscana di Cosimo II e di don Antonio dei Medici: Alchimia, medicina "chimica" e riforma del sapere', in *Scienze, credenze occulte, livelli di cultura* (Florence: Olschki, 1982), pp. 31–62.

Garbellotti, Marina, 'Libri e letture di speziali. Cultura farmaceutica trentina tra fine Seicento ed inizio Settecento', *Medicina & Storia*, 15 (2008), pp. 103–26.

Gentilcore, David, *Medical Charlatanism in Early Modern Italy* (Oxford: Oxford University Press, 2006).

Giormani, Virgilio, 'La farmacopea ufficiale della Serenissima nel 1790: Un libro sfortunato', *Atti e memorie dell'Acc. Patavina di scienze lettere ed arti*, 102: 2 (1989-90), pp. 95–119.

Henderson, John, *The Renaissance Hospital. Healing the body and Healing the Soul* (New Haven, London: Yale University Press, 2006).

Isaac, Peter C. G., 'Pills and Print', in *Medicine, Mortality, and the Book Trade*, ed. by Robin Myers and Michael Harris (New Castle: Oak Knoll Press, 1998), pp. 25–47.

Jepson, Michael H., 'From Secret Remedies to Prescription Medicines: A Brief History of Medicine Quality', in *Making Medicines: A Brief History of Pharmacy and Pharmaceuticals*, ed. by Stuart Anderson (London: Pharmaceutical Press, 2005), pp. 223–42.

Jones, Colin, 'The French King's Physicians in and Beyond the Royal Court in the 17th and 18th Centuries', in *Être médecin à la cour (Italie, France, Espagne, XIIIe-XVIIIe siècle)*, ed. by Elisa Andretta and Marilyn Nicoud (Florence: Sismel-Edizioni del Galluzzo, 2013), pp. 199–209.

Kolega, Alexandra, 'Speziali, spagirici, droghieri e ciarlatani. L'offerta terapeutica a Roma tra Seicento e Settecento', in *Roma moderna e contemporanea. Rivista interdisciplinare di storia*, 6:3 (1998), pp. 311–48.

Maggioni, Giuseppe, ed., *Dizionario storico biografico dei farmacisti italiani* (Padova: Accademia italiana di storia della farmacia, 1990).

Marangoni, Giuseppe, *Le associazioni di mestiere nella Repubblica Veneta (vittuaria, farmacia, medicina)* (Venice: Filippi, 1974).

Minuzzi, Sabrina, *Inventario di bottega di Antonio Bosio veneziano (1646-1694). Catalogo delle edizioni e delle incisioni* (Venice: Edizioni Ca' Foscari, 2013), also available online: http://doi.org/10.14277/978-88-97735-47-2.

Minuzzi, Sabrina, *Il secolo di carta. Antonio Bosio artigiano di testi e immagini nella Venezia del Seicento* (Milan: FrancoAngeli, 2009).

Minuzzi, Sabrina, *Sul filo dei segreti. Farmacopea, libri e pratiche terapeutiche a Venezia in età moderna* (Milan: Unicopli, 2016).

Minuzzi, Sabrina, review of Alisha Rankin, *The Poison Trials* (2021), in *Early Science and Medicine*, 27 (2022), pp. 119–22.

Monticolo, Giovanni, ed., *I capitolari delle arti veneziane sottoposte alla Giustizia e poi alla Giustizia Vecchia, dalle origini al 1330* (Rome: Forzani & C. tipografi del Senato, 1896), I, pp. 159–69, 383–92.

Moran, Bruce T., 'Courts and Academies', in *The Cambridge History of Science*, III, *Early Modern Science*, ed. by Katharine Park and Lorraine Daston (Cambridge: Cambridge University Press, 2006), pp. 251–27.

Palmer, Richard, 'Pharmacy in the Republic of Venice in the Sixteenth Century', in *The Medical Renaissance of the Sixteenth Century*, ed. by Andrew Wear, Roger K. French, and Iain M. Lonie (Cambridge: Cambridge University Press, 1985), pp. 100–17.

Patronage and Institutions: Science, Technology and Medicine at the European Court, 1500-1750, ed. by Bruce T. Moran (Rochester: Boydell Press, 1991).

Pedani, Maria Pia and Andrea Pelizza, 'Notai di Venezia. Atti [e testamenti]', typewritten document [1995-2015] available for consultation at the AAV.

Porter, Roy, *Health for Sale: Quackery in England, 1660-1850* (Manchester-New York: Manchester University Press, 1989).

Rankin, Alisha, *The Poison Trials: Wonder Drugs, Experiment, and the Battle for Authority in Renaissance Science* (Chicago: The University of Chicago Press, 2021).

Rankin, Alisha and Justin Rivest, 'Medicine, Monopoly, and the Premodern State: Early Clinical Trials', *The New England Journal of Medicine*, 375: 2 (2016), pp. 106–9.

Rivest, Justin, 'Beyond the Pharmacopoeia? Secret Remedies, Exclusive Privileges, and Trademarks in Early Modern France', in *Drugs on the Page*, pp. 81–100.

Shaw, James and Evelyn Welch, *Making and Marketing Medicine in Renaissance Florence* (Amsterdam-New York: Rodopi, 2011).

Strocchia, Sharon T., *Forgotten Healers. Women and the Pursuit of Health in Late Renaissance Italy* (Cambridge MA: Harvard University Press, 2019).

Strocchia, Sharon T., 'The nun apothecaries of Renaissance Florence: Marketing medicines in the convent', *Renaissance Studies*, 2011, 25 (5), pp. 627–47.

Urdang, George, 'Pharmacopoeias as Witnesses of World History', *Journal of the History of Medicine and Allied Sciences*, 1: 1 (1946), pp. 46–70.

Villotta, Luisa, *L'archivio storico dell'ospedale di Cividale (sezione antica)* (Udine: Società Filologica Friulana, 2013).

Vio, Gastone, *Le Scuole Piccole nella Venezia dei dogi: Note d'archivio per la storia delle confraternite veneziane*, (Costabissara, Vicenza: A. Colla, 2004).

Zambaldi, Antonio, *Monumenti storici di Concordia* (San Vito: Pascatti, 1811).

9

Assessing Treatments for Wounds and Ulcers in Eighteenth-Century Italy:

Theory, Practice, and the Value of Hospital Experience

Maria Pia Donato

In 1714, Domenico Cecchini, surgeon in Rome, published a short treatise on wounds, *La difesa dei diritti di Cesare Magati*. Cecchini's aim was, as the title stated, to uphold the superiority of the 'rare medication', to prove it 'valid by anatomical and physical-mechanical reasons' and refute the abuse of compound ointments and other techniques to induce oozing pus.[1] The rare method advocated by Cesare Magati (1579–1647) followed the idea that pus was not instrumental in healing and therefore consisted in leaving bandages in place rather than medicating several times a day. Disputes on it had been rekindled some years previously by French and Italian authors and continued intermittently throughout the eighteenth century intersecting with wider conversations on the best management of wounds and ulcers and on the merits of simple methods of dressing as opposed to overmedication, now scorned as the hallmark of rancid Galenism.

Of course, the controversy about the treatment of wounds that is the subject of this chapter was not the first one in European surgery, and not the most acrimonious either. As several historians have noted, surgeons had always been keen on using the printing press to advance their ideas or extoll their methods and skills, for their status and income were largely dependent on both reputation and the market. The flourishing early modern market for health and beauty services prompted a range of 'artisans of the body' to promote their services in multiple ways and through a variety of media.[2]

The controversy over wound treatment was also closely tied to issues of reputation and the market. One of its features were indeed the economic implications of frequent bandaging, which several surgeons rebuked as unnecessary, costly and even detrimental to the sick—patients usually paid medical practitioners on a rough per diem basis, and a significant fraction of their income came from the drugs they prescribed, and medical ethics and guild regulations condemned immoral profits made out of unduly sophisticated and long medications, with or without the conspiracy of greedy apothecaries.[3]

The scope of the dispute, however, was broader, focusing on selecting therapies that were effectual and fitted into the framework of contemporary medical theories. It thus encapsulated crucial issues of surgical knowledge and practice. By the early eighteenth century, in fact, Galenic qualitative physiology, and the Aristotelian natural philosophy that underpinned it, had been challenged by developments in anatomy and physics, leaving practitioners with the task of reframing the rationale of treatments, whose arsenal, however, had not changed equally fast. Surgery, whose theoretical and therapeutic edifice had also rested on Galenism for centuries, was no exception. This chapter analyses how such developments impacted the cure of wounds—more

1. Cecchini, *La difesa dei diritti di Cesare Magati*.
2. For an introductory overview, see Rabier, 'Medicalizing the Surgical Trade'. On the growth of vernacular print, see Fissell, 'The Marketplace of Print', and Cavallo, 'Early Vernacular Medical Advice Books'. See further, for Italy, Cavallo, *Artisans of the Body*; Gentilcore, *Medical Charlatinism*; Savoia, 'Skills, Knowledge, and Status'.
3. Park, *Doctors and Medicine;* Pomata, *Contracting a Cure;* Gentilcore ed., *The World of the Italian Apothecary*; Shaw and Welch, *Making and Marketing Medicine.* Of note, chemical medicines, after some initial resistance, were accommodated into the framework of late Galenism. See further, Wallis, 'Competition and Cooperation'.

precisely, how these developments impacted the way in which surgeons rearticulated epistemic categories such as reason, experience, and evidence in endorsing rare dressing.

In relation to the aim of this volume, which is to explore the connection between theory and practice in medicine, the controversy over wound treatment is significant in other respects as well. As we shall see, the proponents of 'simple' methods, such as Magati's or similar ones, whose work I examine, were hospital practitioners. Generally speaking, it is not surprising that these practitioners engaged in public debate. Hospitals were key institutions in urban life, and doctors working there were ipso facto part of the professional elite. Furthermore, hospitals were competitive arenas, where practitioners progressed in their career, and gained a reputation that attracted wealthy patients and fee-paying pupils. As Susan Lawrence has noted, through publishing, hospital practitioners established a professional identity among the elite and participated in 'subtle exchanges marking status, learning, and authority'.[4]

What is more interesting for the purpose of this essay is that, while mobilizing a range of justifications, theoretical as well as empirical, and using hospital experience as a paramount argument, these practitioners tried to broaden the empirical basis of their assessment and translated experience in different ways, including numerical and tabular synthesis. This relatively minor dispute in Italy thus sheds light on how novel physio-pathological ideas combined with new skills and practices that were inherent to hospital life. It shows that evidence increasingly relied on new systems of accountability that were generating a growing flow of paperwork in hospitals, which, in turn, contributed to enhance the role given to empirical arguments in the controversy, and ultimately led to innovation.[5]

In other words, this chapter attempts at reconsidering debates on wound treatment against the backdrop of intellectual, social and institutional changes. It tentatively reconnects these debates to a wider web of knowledge and practice, while exploring the ways in which surgeons collected and shaped information, how they used experience as a validating argument, and the different genres and formats they chose to recount experience and connect it to theory.

MODERN PHYSIOLOGY, REASON, EXPERIENCE AND NUMBERS

Debates on how to treat wounds using a 'simple' or 'rare' method, purportedly more effective and faithful to Hippocrates's teachings, were sparked in the late seventeenth century by Augustin Belloste, surgeon to Louis XIV's army in France and Italy, in his *Le chirurgien de l'hôpital* (1696).[6]According to Belloste, introducing probes, drains, and cloth threads in wounds, and inducing abundant suppuration to be cleansed frequently, as was common in contemporary surgery, hindered healing. Rather than replacing dressings daily and applying ointments of all sorts, he suggested, linen should be left in place for some days, not least because exposing wounds to the air could be detrimental. To support his theory, Belloste recounted the histories of wounded soldiers cured in this way in military hospitals—which, incidentally, were at that time a primary political and sanitary focus of concern in France and elsewhere. The book went through several editions, and Dionigi Andrea Sancassani, physician, surgeon and man of letters, translated it into Italian, but credited his fellow citizen Magati with devising rare dressing in his 1616 *De rara medicatione vulnerum*.[7]

Like many literati of his day, Sancassani was eager to prove the primacy of Italian science and disregarded the fact that Magati and Belloste explained their method in different terms. Whereas Magati adopted an Aristotelian-Galenic stance on the healing power of natural heat and posited that its preservation should guide the surgeon's course of action, Belloste drew upon a chemical understanding of air to plead for leaving bandages in place. Both, however, challenged common therapeutic practices,

4. Lawrence, *Charitable Knowledge*), pp. 220-21.
5. On paperwork and knowledge, see Hess and Mendelsohn, 'Case and Series'; Dinges et al. eds, *Medical Practice* (especially Hess and Schlegelmilch, 'Cornucopia Officinae Medicae'). More generally, Blair, 'The Rise of Note-Taking'.
6. Belloste, *Le Chirurgien d'hôpital*. As highlighted by Le Minor and Clair, 'Augustin Belloste (1654-1730)', Belloste was a proponent of mercurial treatment, but recommended it to be assumed orally rather than topically.
7. Sancassani, *Il lume all'occhio*, and *Chirone in campo*. Magati and Sancassani were both from Scandiano, near Reggio in Emilia. On Magati, see Loris Premuda's entry in *Complete Dictionary of Scientific Biography* https://www.encyclopedia.com/science/dictionaries-thesauruses-pictures-and-press-releases/magati-cesare (accessed January 17, 2023); *Cesare Magati medico e religioso*.

such as inducing overabundant pus, with the aim of 'digesting' unconcocted bad humors and cooling the injured part with costly composed drugs.[8] Sancassani's writings sparked further controversy, particularly among Italian practitioners, and a flurry of tracts like Cecchini's scrutinized the pros and cons of the 'rare method'.[9]

In the 1710s, Domenico Cecchini (?-1751?) was a young but well-connected surgeon. His father, Mario, was chief surgeon at the hospital of San Giacomo in Rome, surgeon to the conclave in 1692 and 1699, then to Pope Innocent XIII, and at Santo Spirito. Domenico followed in his father's footsteps. Trained at Santo Spirito under Bernardino Genga, he graduated in philosophy and medicine and embraced a career in surgery. He would later be appointed chief surgeon and lecturer at the hospital of San Salvatore and surgeon to Benedict XIII, a position that he held during the following two papacies, while moving to Santo Spirito.[10] It was actually Mario who first endorsed Magati's ideas and presumably encouraged Domenico to follow suit.[11] Domenico acknowledged his 'father and master' in promoting rare dressing at Santo Spirito, in spite of old-fashioned methods of other surgeons working there and the criticisms he faced for leaving bandages in place, which was seen as negligence.[12] Arguably, Domenico's book was part of a family strategy to enhance both men's reputation and possibly secure a more prestigious appointment in Rome's competitive arena. It was not accidental that the book was dedicated to Sinibaldo Doria, the powerful Commendator of Santo Spirito.

In his short polemical text, Domenico Cecchini demonstrates an awareness of the theoretical discrepancies between Magati's Galenic approach and later authors. His goal is to advocate Magati's method through contemporary philosophical and physiological explanations while advancing those modern doctrines in medicine in general. Mechanical medicine and the correct interpretation of Hippocrates are the unifying threads of his text, which sheds light on the incipient Enlightenment reinvention of Hippocrates the Anti-Dogmatic Observer, parallel to the demise of Galenism as a self-supported medical system.[13]

Five chapters address, respectively: the harmfulness of cloth threads in wounds; how some wounds are fatal not per se but become so due to improper management; that most compound remedies are not only ineffectual but also harmful; that any foreign body must be removed; that a wound can be considered fatal if the patient dies within seven days, but if death occurs later, it is attributed to the surgeon's errors.

The first section is the longest and most important, as it allows Cecchini to lay out his practical arguments while introducing the principles underpinning them: circulatory physiopathology and a corpuscularian appraisal of both the human body and the ingredients of medicines—which would be Cecchini's credo throughout his career, as recorded in his students' notebooks.[14] Eclectic and hardly original as these notions were, they had several implications for practice. Cecchini does not subscribe to the idea that air causes inflammation (although cold is always harmful for capillaries). His main point is that inducing abundant suppuration, either with threads or with aggressive ointments, is wrong—those who think that rot helps healing simply ignore 'the law of circulation'.[15] Magati's method is correct, but his ideas on radical humidity and vital heat in the wake of Galen are not: the true reason why rare dressing works is that it does not hinder the movements of fluids and solids.[16] Venesection is useful for controlling the mass of fluids, and foreign objects must be removed, but most canonical medicines—especially putrefactive (*ammarcianti*) and

8. For an introduction to early modern theory and practice on wound care, see Girolamo Fabrici d'Acquapendente (I have used the 1685 Padua edition of his *Opere*, pp. 56-66). For an overview, Tracy and DeVries eds, *Wounds and Wound Repair,* and, in a retrospective medical perspective, Altmeyer et al. eds, *Wound Healing and Skin Physiology.*
9. Haller, *Bibliotheca Chirurgica*, I, pp. 552–55; De Renzi (himself a late proponent of the Italian tradition of conservative surgery), *Storia della medicina,* IV, pp. 482-95.
10. Marini, *Degli Archiatri,* II, pp. XLVII-XLX.
11. Mario's involvement is mentioned by Maraviglia (alias Ruggero Calvi), *Giunta di alcune lettere,* p. 4; Sancassani, *La chirurgia svellata,* p. 100, 114, 116.
12. Cecchini, *La difesa*, pp. 112-14. Santo Spirito was organized in four main wards and services, and employed four primary physicians and two primary surgeons, each attended by a deputy (who lived on the premise), and helped (seconded) by apprentices.
13. On the numerous reinventions of Hippocrates throughout the centuries, and his different images and uses thereof in the Renaissance and the Enlightenment, see Cantor ed., *Reinventing Hippocrates;* Nutton, 'Renaissance Galenism'; Donato "Galen in an Age of Change'.
14. Donato, 'Surgeons' Training and Hospital Life'.
15. Cecchini, *La difesa,* p. 45.
16. Ibid., pp. 44-45.

digestive preparations—and frequent dressings irritate fibers that are already contracted by trauma.[17] Only light balsamic oils and gentle demulcents should be used, particularly on gunshot wounds, while baths and mineral waters are beneficial for chronic ulcers. Substances are to be understood through the properties, shape and size of their components, not through imaginary virtues. In a nutshell: simplicity and minimal medication are the real foundations of wound management according to Hippocrates's true principles and modern philosophy. He therefore established a few rules: no cloth thread or probes, no sophisticated salves (including those purportedly miraculous preparations like powder of sympathy, whose virtues are 'mere tales')[18], rare medication, and an overall simplicity in approaching any ailment and injury.

To make his points, Cecchini mobilizes arguments of reason, authority and experiment—the pillars of learned surgery.[19] His tract is in fact typical of learned medical controversy in its structure and argumentative style, and basically rests on systematic anatomical and physiological doctrines. References to observation on humans and animals, as well as repeated appeals to professional common sense, are interwoven in the text. Mentions of hospital life are also included to underscore the consequences of wrong treatments at Santo Spirito, where patients 'scream and moan, not only when their wounds are cleansed and copious excretions are dried out, but also when they are medicated and the aforementioned threads inserted in the wounds, and this for no other reason than the sheer pain they suffer, which I cannot believe only depends on the practitioners inability'.[20] In other words, arguments from practice are more experiential than factual. Domenico, however, also mentions 'calculations done to this purpose' in Roman hospitals to prove the superiority of Magati's and his father's method.[21]

The figures that are only hinted at in 1714 were published some years later under the title of *Bilancio fatto in Roma dal Sig. Mario Cecchini fra li due modi di curare le ferrite, comunale e del celebre Magati*, where sets of data drawn from hospital records are tabled down.[22]

In the early eighteenth century, numerical data and observations in the form of tables were not unknown in medical literature, as vital statistics, meteorological observations and natural histories of diseases in the wake of Sydenham gained momentum.[23] More precisely in Cecchini's work, lists of patients treated at Santo Spirito in 1696 and 1700 by his father Mario with the rare method are compared with lists of patients cured with the 'common method' by Ippolito Magnani and Pietro Cesconi, respectively.[24] The information provided in these tables matches that commonly recorded in hospital books: date of entrance, name, very short definition of the injury such as 'wound in the abdomen' or 'wound on the forehead', and the date of death or discharge. Two additional tables of the days spent in hospital show that patients treated with rare dressing spent an average of 59 days in hospital compared to 69 days for those treated with the common method, and experienced fewer fatalities. Basic as the statistics of Cecchini and his editor Sancassani were, they combined with all other arguments in documenting the superiority of simple methods for the benefit of patients, the reputation of surgeons, and, last but not least, public finances.[25]

17. Ibid., p. 50.
18. Ibid., p. 133.
19. Agrimi and Crisciani, *Edocere medicos*; McVaugh, *The Rational Surgery*.
20. Cecchini, *La difesa*, p. 22: 'gridano, e si lagnano, non solo nel pulirsi ed assorbirsi dalle loro piaghe copiosi escrementi, com'anche nel medicarsi, ed introdursi dette turande nelle loro ferrite, e ciò per non altra cagione, che pel dolore che soffrono, e pur mi dò a credere non poter procedere all'imperizia de' professori'.
21. Ibid., pp. 113–14.
22. Now in *Dilucidazioni fisico-mediche*, pp. 230–50.
23. Rusnock, *Vital Accounts*. Only in the late 18th century, though, tabling down numerical data in assessing treatments became widespread, see Tröhler, '"To Improve the Evidence of Medicine"'; Charters, *Disease, War, and the Imperial State*.
24. Magnani was active in two Roman hospitals, S. Maria della Consolazione and Santo Spirito before Mario Cecchini. BNCR, MS Sessoriano 355, a transcript of his lectures on wounds at Consolazione in 1696, documents that Magnani, drawing upon ancient, medieval and Renaissance authorities (especially Galen, Celsus, Avicenna, Guy de Chauliac, Della Croce, and Paré), maintained that wounds should be treated with cold remedies and drained with cloths or bandaged daily. Both Cecchini sr and jr might have been aware of Magnani's opinion on wound management; yet, Magnani is not explicitly targeted in the text, only in tables without further comments.
25. Sancassani, 'Il Magati redivivo per benefizio de' feriti, e per buon regolamento di chi li cura', now in *Dilucidazioni fisico-mediche*, pp. 169-232, esp. pp. 226-30. Additional layers of "reason and experiments" were woven together by the anonymous editor of the 1731 anthology featuring these

239

NUMERO

De' Feriti ricevuti, e Medicati nel Quartiere

DEL SIGNOR

MARIO CECCHINI

Chirurgo di S. SPIRITO, in tutto l'Anno M. D. CC.

ENTRATI		USCITI
li 12. Gennajo	B*onaventura Verningo* ferito nel Braccio finiftro, al num. 6. S. Giacinto.	partì li 4. Febrajo
li 14. Gennajo	*Pietro Mario* ferito nel mezzo dell'Occipite, al num. 21. Ofpidaletto.	partì li 18. Gennajo
li 14. Gennajo	*Giofeppe Braco* ferito nella Mano deftra, al num. 22. Ofpidaletto.	partì li 30. Gennajo
li 20. Gennajo	*Francefco Cecci* ferito nel Mufculo Temporale finiftro, al num. 16. Ofpidaletto.	partì li 7. Febrajo
✠ li 4. Febrajo	*Stefano Martini* ferito nell'Abdomine, al num. 25. C. Ofpidaletto.	morì li 6. Febrajo
li 5. Febrajo	Il Signor *Giufeppe Galuzzi* Computifta di Cafa, ferito d'Archibugiata nella Spalla, medicato in Camera fua.	Guarì
li 17. Febrajo	*Michel-Angelo Bettini* ferito nella Sutura Coronale, al num. 28. Ofpidaletto.	partì li 28. Febrajo
li 21. Febrajo	*Lorenzo Mozzi* ferito nel Carpo, e Metacarpo deftro, al num. 21. Ofpidaletto.	partì li 5. Marzo
li 21. Febrajo	*Giofeppe Navati* ferito nel mezzo della Fronte, al n. 19. C. Ofpidaletto.	partì li 2. Marzo
Primo Marzo	*Gio: Maria Maggi* ferito nell'Offo Coronale, al n. 20. C. Ofpidaletto.	partì li 17. Marzo
li 3. Marzo	*Giovanni Cafoli* ferito fopra la Sutura Coronale, al num. 30. Ofpidaletto.	partì li 12. Marzo
li 10. Marzo	*Gio: Battifta Caftelletti* ferito nell'Offo Coronale finiftro, al num. 18. Ofpedaletto.	partì li 17. Marzo
li 10. Marzo	*Francefco Regnicolo* ferito nel Braccio deftro, al n. 28. C. Ofpidaletto.	partì li 14. Aprile

Dome-

26. A list of patients treated by Mario Cecchini in the year 1700, recording the outcome of their cure.

SIMPLE MEDICINE AND RARE DRESSING IN MID-EIGHTEENTH-CENTURY FLORENCE

Disputes on the rare method raged in Italy for decades. It is worth noting that, like Cecchini, proponents of this and other similar 'simple' approaches neglected the core of Magati's argument (that is, vital heat), and disparaged the absurdity of producing overabundant pus, the uselessness of enlarging and bandaging wounds too frequently, and the benefits of cleansing them with lightly medicated medicaments or plain water. Some advocated the use of cold water, especially mineral waters.[26] Like Cecchini's, their rationale was no longer that of cooling pathologically hot humors, but of making the most of substances according to eclectic corpuscular philosophies. And like Cecchini, many argued that modern physics and circulatory physiology rendered Galenic notions of virtues, qualities and concocted humors obsolete. The obsolescence of old therapies, such as composing ointments of numerous ingredients each supposedly endowed with specific qualities, was explicitly pointed out by Sancassani, who vehemently criticized those 'who nowadays continue to use them, and moreover persist in defending their use, overstretching their imagination to adapt explanations to use' out of ignorance, laziness and greed.[27]

Clearly, these debates on wound management echoed broader discussions in European medicine, as Galenism waned and was not replaced by any equivalently hegemonic medical philosophy. Many Italian practitioners were keen on defending mechanical interpretations in the wake of what they considered a national lineage of modern science, extending from Galileo to Malpighi, Bellini and Borelli. But those who credited specific drugs with effects on specific pathologies, like quinine on fever, also pleaded for the use of simples.[28] Corpuscular philosophy, either chemically or mechanically oriented, provided a framework for endorsing simples—the expansion of global trade was making some of these widely available on European markets. More generally, calls for simplicity in medication and diet grew louder in all areas of medicine, as did the emphasis on the social responsibility of medical practitioners and the State in promoting the welfare of a larger number of people.[29]

Tuscany was a stronghold of such a stance. Authoritative figures like Francesco Redi and Antonio Cocchi eloquently pleaded against the abuse of medicines.[30] Famous surgeons such as Bernardino Falcinelli and Giuseppe Cignozzi claimed to follow Hippocrates's true method in treating wounds and ulcers with minimal medication.[31] This was precisely the approach defended by Angelo Nannoni (1715-1790), master surgeon at the hospital of Santa Maria Nuova in Florence

Nannoni was not academically trained, as was customary in Florence (contrary to other Italian cities). He had climbed the ladder from apprentice to master at the hospital, gained a reputation with a treatise on breast cancer, *Trattato sopra le malattie delle mammelle* (1746), and then spent some time studying in France. In 1749, in the context of a reform of health provision and surgical training at Santa Maria Nuova, he was appointed to the new lectureship of 'operations'.

A student's notebook of Nannoni's lessons on ulcers offers glimpses of his main arguments. Writers, beginning with Hippocrates 'who was the first [...] to draft some kind of system in the healing method', Nannoni explains, called ulcer any dissolution of continuity, regardless of the damaged tissue or whether the disruption was 'purulent with recent pus, or with old pus caused internally by corrupted humors'; nobody dared to think otherwise, until

materials along with old and new texts. Interestingly, the editor (possibly Virgilio Cocchi, from Perugia) also excerpted fifty 'observations', (meaning) including both patients histories and general remarks, from Magati's text, clearly aiming at reinforcing its empirical scope.

26. See, e.g., Cocchi, *Il buon'uso dell'acqua fredda*. Later historiography retrospectively fashioned Magati into the precursor of modern wound management, see, e.g., Magni, *Cesare Magati*; Münster and Romagnoli, *Cesare Magati (1579-1647)*, up to Fughelli, 'Cesare Magati'.
27. Sancassani, 'Il Magati redivivo', now in *Dilucidazioni fisico-mediche*, p. 189: 'ma ne' giorni nostri non è poca vergogna de' cerusici il continuare a praticarli, e più l'ostinarsi nel difenderne l'uso, accomodandovi le ragioni con [...] sforzo vivace d'ingegno'.
28. Jarcho, *Quinine's Predecessor*.
29. Brambilla, 'La medicina del Settecento'; Porter ed., *The Medical History of Waters*; Cavallo and Storey eds, *Conserving Health*; Kennaway and Knoeff eds, *Lifestyle and Medicine in the Enlightenment*.
30. Cocchi, 'Discorso primo di anatomia... letto pubblicamente in Firenze il dì xix settembre XDCCXLII nel teatro del grande ospedale di Santa Maria Nuova', in his *Discorsi toscani*, I, pp. 16-19, and 'Del vitto pitagorico per uso della medicina', in *Scritti scelti*, pp. 101-31.
31. Mannacio, 'Teoria e pratica della chirurgia'.

Galen restricted the term to purulent sores in the fleshy parts.[32] For his part, Nannoni includes any sores 'provided that the corrosion exudes some foul humor, commonly called rot'—which was Avicenna's definition as incorporated in medieval and early modern surgery.[33] As was customary in hospital lectures, which reproduced the academic style, albeit simplified,[34] he differentiates ulcers according to six criteria ('essence', which is in fact shape, 'causes', type of exudation, offended part, 'accidents', such as pain), then proceeds with the treatment of ulcers in general, before addressing specific types of ulcers and fistulas. Causal explanations emphasize blood and its disorders, namely acridity, as was common sense in contemporary medicine and surgery. Therapies canonically rely on a mix of lenitive and drying medications.

Nannoni also insists on the management of the non-naturals. His emphasis on hygiene is ambivalent: on the one hand, it implies a holistic understanding of the body, whose imbalance causes acridity and eventually lesions; on the other hand, this perspective supports the rejection of overmedication. Nannoni repeatedly expatiates on the uselessness of fashionable remedies. In dealing with urethral ulcers, for instance, he vehemently criticizes the use of small cylinders impregnated with corrosive ingredients, which some claim have 'the faculty of corroding excrescences, and leaving all other parts intact', but are in fact useless and harmful, for 'corrosives so selective do not exist, and in fact [...] practice proves that such cylinders excite the inflammation, corrode and ulcerate any part of the urethra they touch, and as a consequence, they always make the evil worse'.[35] To prove his point, Nannoni cites cases from printed collections of *observationes*.[36]

In his printed books, Nannoni adopts a more combative attitude, particularly in his *Trattato chirurgico... sopra la semplicità del medicare i mali d'attenenza della chirurgia*.[37] His goal is stated in the introduction: 'to demonstrate the uselessness and sometimes the manifest harm of a few manual operations and of many ad hoc remedies, taken for granted by those who ignore the nature, seat, true cause, and most probable outcome of ailments [...] with great prejudice for the sick oppressed by the disease and by medicines'.[38] The text itself begins with similar, possibly more polemical statements against false claims that there exist 'drugs capable of stopping wounds from inflaming, and to stop inflammation generate suppuration, corruption and caries', and sets out to prove the opposite through 'experiments, observations and reflections, which are the true guides leading in seeking the truth'. In a time of reform at Santa Maria Nuova, he goes on, 'the simplicity in healing progresses more and more steadily in our surgery school [...]. Such a laudable advancement [...] would be far greater if we set out with truth-seeking minds to take courage to experiment on the course of diseases, positive as well as negative, and observe what is the effect of nature, and what can be positively attributed to medicines, to most of which we credit qualities they do not really have'.[39]

Contrary to Cecchini, Nannoni refrains from quoting ancient and modern authorities, and claims to follow reason and experiment only. He does not even refer to Magati and his followers, although he defends a similar 'simple' approach to wound management. His doctrine can

32. London, Wellcome Library, MS 3659, fol. 1: 'Il primo [...] il quale tessé qualche sistema nel metodo di medicare [...] senza farvi alcuna distinzine marciosa recente o vecchia prodotta da cagione interna per via d'umori viziosi.'
33. Ibid., fol. 2: 'purché dalla corrosione della sostanza gronda un qualche umore vitioso che comunemente marcia viene addomandata'.
34. Donato, 'Surgeons' Training'.
35. Wellcome Library, MS 3659, fol. 245: 'io posso assicurare non esservi corrosivi cotanto discreti, anzi dirò confermato dalla prattica, che così fatte candelette eccitano l'infiammazione corrodono e esulcerano l'uretra in ogni sito che toccano e per conseguenza rendono sempre mai peggiore il male.'
36. Among these, Antonio Molinetti's *Dissertationes anatomicae et pathologicae* (1669) about a 'bassa turcho' - the student misspelled the word pasha, *pascià* in Italian.
37. Nannoni, *Trattato chirurgico*.
38. Ibid., p. III: 'dimostrare l'inutilità e talvolta il danno manifesto d'alcune operazioni manuali e di molti medicamenti propriamente inventanti e adottati per buoni da chi ignora la natura, sede, cagione vera, ed esito più probabile de' mali [...] con pregiudizio notabile dell'ammalato molte volte oppresso dal male e da' medicamenti'.
39. Ibid., p. 2: 'La semplicità del medicare s'avanza sempre più nella nostra scuola di chirurgia del Regio Spedale di Santa Maria Nuova di Firenze. Questo tanto lodevole avanzamento [...] sarebbe di gran lunga maggiore se con animo determinato a scuoprire la verità [...] noi c'incoraggiassimo a sperimentare e osservare nelle mutazioni tanto buone che cattive dei mali è effetto della natura, da ciò che positivamente è referibile ai medicamenti ai più dei quali noi siamo soliti attribuire certe qualità ch'ei veramente non anno (sic) [...]. Per esempio vi è chi costantemente crede che vi sieno medicamenti capaci d'impedire che le ferite non s'infiammino, e che dalle infiammazioni non nascano le suppurazioni, le corruzioni, le cancrene e le carie'.

be summarized as follows: the best treatment for wounds, and more generally for surgical pathologies, is cleansing, stitching, or bandaging to help repair by 'first intention' (that is, reuniting the wound's edges) whenever possible, dressing with clean, dry gauze, and waiting for Nature to heal. Strong caustics and irritating remedies, compound ointments, purportedly digesting and regenerative powders are ineffectual at best and more often noxious. It is likewise harmful to enlarge lesions, introduce probes, cloth and iron drains or replace bandages daily, as air can cause inflammation and infection. Invasive operations and amputation must be avoided but, if necessary, must not be delayed. Incidentally, *kairos*, the right time, was probably the single most important and unifying element in medicine and surgery from Antiquity onwards.

In some passages, Nannoni elucidates the rationale for his rebuttal of overmedication, that is, circulatory physiology. All bodily operations depend on the circulation of the blood, but there are no remedies to artificially restore it aside from time, rest, and patience, 'as human art has no other resources to help nature restore the movement of those humors that are trapped in the cells [...] and to believe otherwise goes against anatomical observations and knowledge of physiology'.[40] These ideas, however, are incorporated into histories, rather than in lengthy explanations, learned commentaries, or argumentative reasoning.

More precisely, the first section of Nannoni's book is a dissertation on wounds in which the main theme is interwoven with patients' histories, while the second is made solely of self-contained 'observations'. Stories invariably extoll simple cures as they depict opposite clinical situations to illustrate general precepts through singular instances.[41] For example, the successful cure of a girl plagued with a tumor in her knee after enduring painful and useless treatment with mercury is contrasted with the story of young nobleman who died because his doctors refused to amputate and treated inflammation with salsaparilla and topical injections.[42] Some observations relate to more than one person suffering from the same ailment, with titles stating the point of their histories (e.g., 'uselessness of blistering').[43] As a matter of fact, Nanonni does not offer detailed instructions and largely relies on tacit knowledge as he addresses a reading community of apprentices and fellow practitioners. Histories are meant to translate a general therapeutic approach into action, based on the assumption that 'simplicity in healing afflictions pertaining to surgery can be extended to other ailments'.[44]

The paramount importance of patients' histories in Nannoni's economy of proof as opposed to arguments of reasons and authority is arguably connected to his status as a non-academically trained surgeon. Of course, emphasis on experience must not be misunderstood: empirical knowledge without the study of anatomy and physiology, Nannoni states repeatedly, is fallacious, and cures are fortuitous 'unless they are based on a method acquired through the profoundest knowledge of the causes of diseases and the solid understanding of what the art [of surgery] can do and what Nature is capable to restore health.'[45]. Clearly, however, his aim is not that of advancing physiological doctrines in general (as was Cecchini's) but a *methodus medendi*, while asserting his own status of elite surgeon mastering reason and experience and serving the main city hospital—his narratives are carefully crafted to convey all these ideas at once. In an effort to strengthen his arguments, Nannoni also repeatedly recalls what he observed in French hospitals, and criticizes invasive surgeries performed by renowned surgeons in Paris, as opposed to 'simple methods' practised at Santa Maria Nuova.[46]

The hospital does indeed provide the intellectual and material framework for Nannoni's *Trattato chirurgico*. As countless authors of surgical *curationes* and *observationes*,[47] Nannoni is eager to discuss patients from distinguished families from his private practice to promote his personal prestige inside and outside the hospital microcosm. Yet the vast majority of his stories deal with men and women

40. Ibid., pp. 30-31: 'non avendo l'arte umana altri capitali che questi per mettere la natura in stato di far ripigliare moto a quegli umori che essendo trattenuti nelle cellule [...] il credere diversamente è contro le osservazioni anatomiche e repugna alle migliori cognignizioni fisiologiche'.
41. Siraisi, 'How to Write a Latin Book on Surgery'; Donato, 'Practical Knowledge'.
42. Nannoni, *Trattato*, pp. 46-59.
43. Ibid., p. 370.
44. Ibid., p. 296 'questo trattato della semplicità del medicare i mali appartenenti alla chirurgia estender si può anco ad altri mali'.
45. Ibid., p. 429, 'senza ragione di metodo acquistato colla più perfetta cognizione della cagione dei mali e colle notizie sicure di quel che può l'arte, e di quel tanto che è capace la natura in vantaggio del recuperamento della salute'.
46. Ibid., p. 178, 'l'abbiamo osservato tante volte che possiamo fare autorità irrefragabile'.
47. Pomata, 'Sharing Cases'; Nutton, 'Pieter Van Foreest'; Donato, 'Practical Knowledge'.

treated at Santa Maria Nuova. We do not know from what source precisely Nannoni drew his material—possibly a personal casebook or hospital registers. What we do know is that by the mid-eighteenth century, the writing tasks assigned to surgical senior and junior staff to manage patients and treatments expanded notably.[48] Furthermore, apprentices were now supposed to explain cases assigned to them by lecturers in practical surgery to familiarize themselves with the exposition of patients' histories.[49] Notably, Nannoni's book reproduces the structure and style of *Dissertazioni... aggiuntevi quaranta osservazioni... di chirurgia* published in 1747 by his master Antonio Benevoli, possibly the first anthology of this kind by a master surgeon at Santa Maria Nuova, at a time when this and other hospitals were under revision by the newly established government of Habsburg-Lorraine.[50]

As a matter of fact, like Benevoli's, one of the underlying themes of Nannoni's writings is the good care provided in Florence. In 1774 and 1776, Nannoni published two further volumes on *semplicità del medicare* that are, in fact, anthologies of case narratives.[51] Dozens of additional histories, mostly drawn from his hospital activity, tout the same principles: the high quality of health provision in Florence and the superiority of the Tuscan, and his own, 'simple surgery'.

COLLECTING FACTS 'IN THE STYLE OF GEOMETERS'

Nannoni's writings stirred further controversy, in a period when the management of wounds through deep manual debridement (that is, the removal of fibrous connective tissue and pus), especially endorsed by French authors, was gaining traction.[52] Meanwhile, another surgeon in Florence set himself the task of assessing best practices in curing surgical ailments through 'reason and experiment' and resumed the conversation on Magati's method as part of this broader intellectual enterprise.

Giuseppe Cavallini (?-1791) was born in Cevoli, near Pisa. Like Nannoni, he was not academically trained, but raised through the ranks as an apprentice, then aide, and finally master at Santa Maria Nuova, although he presumably received a more solid education than his predecessor, or at least he showed it off more overtly.[53] His *Collezione istorica di casi chirurgici metodicamente disposti e con note illustrate*, three volumes in six tomes published between 1762 and 1779, claimed to be no less than a 'historical collection of surgical cases, methodically arranged and illustrated with notes', all from Santa Maria Nuova. The work progressed from easier to more difficult cases in 'the style of geometers', elucidating their differences and what 'moderns and ancients thought about them.'[54]

Adopting a bold Enlightenment posture, Cavallini introduces his treatise by stating that all knowledge must be based on facts, the 'sole guide that makes it possible to discover truth' that transformed science from a 'conglomerate of chimeric inventions [...] into an orderly series of ideas based only on experience.'[55] To this end, Cavallini provided hundreds of patients' histories, which he presumably drew from hospital records and his own notes—in 1767 he was officially appointed *istoriografo dei casi chirurgici*, a task that he was probably already performing. Either way, the large number and the arrangement of cases is in keeping with Cavallini's stated goal: assembling facts about surgical ailments according to their essence, treatment, and outcome.[56] Observations are clustered by types of afflictions, interspersed with 58 *riflessioni*, and complemented with annual synopses of illnesses treated in the hospital.

As I have argued elsewhere, Cavallini's *Collezione* is a good instance of Enlightenment Hippocratism, as it

48. *Regolamento dei regi ospedali di Santa Maria Nuova*, esp. for junior staff and apprentices, pp. 20-21, 41, 44, 59-64, 77-78, 103, 138, 175, 212.
49. *Ordini di medicheria*, p. 15; 'Regolamento delle scuole di chirurgia del Regio Spedale di Santa Maria Nuova', in Cocchi, *Relazione dello spedale di Santa Maria Nuova*, p. 217.
50. See Pasta, 'L'ospedale e la città'.
51. Nannoni, *Memorie di chirurgia*, and *Memorie... sopra alcuni casi rari*. It should be noted, however, that in the third volume, which is a sort of late life review, Nannoni explicitly relates conflicts among senior practitioners who followed different methods within Santa Maria Nuova.
52. Castellani and Coturri, 'Una polemica'; Reichert, 'The Historical Development'; Dos, *French Surgery*, pp. 384-86 and passim.
53. See the entry by Ugo Baldini in *Dizionario biografico degli italiani*, vol. 22 (Rome: Istituto dell'Enciclopedia Italiana, 1979), s.v.
54. Cavallini, *Collezione istorica di casi chirurgici*, I/1, pp. 3-4: 'passando dai semplici casi a più complicati, avvertendone inoltre le differenze, e ciò che dagli antichi e moderni sopra di essi è stato pensato.'
55. Ibid.: 'un aggregato di invenzioni chimeriche, si vide in breve ridotto a un'ordinata serie di riflessioni fondate solo sopra l'esperienza'.
56. Daston, 'Perché i fatti'.

attempts a synthesis of collected qualitative information.[57] Florence's local tradition of conservative surgery resonates with faith in Nature's healing power that had been rekindled in Enlightenment medicine and culture at large. The general thread of the volume on wounds, published in 1767 and dedicated to none other than Grand-Duke Peter Leopold for improving health care and restoring science in Tuscany, is the excellency of the Tuscan tradition of simple medicine. Cavallini, however, also heralds confidence in progress, as further improvements are still to be achieved by those who follow reasons and experiments. He therefore sets out to review a great number of patients' records, '[so that] we will hopefully be able to assess the different methods of cure'.[58]

In a short introductory dissertation on scar formation, Cavallini summarizes canonical notions on the essence and differences of wounds in light of blood circulation. Scars are produced by what he sees as 'inorganic substance' carried by blood, gluten. Indeed, circulation is the sole physiological phenomenon responsible for the growth of tissues. Cavallini's medical philosophy, however, is not purely mechanical as is the case with earlier authors like Cecchini. Drawing eclectically upon van Swieten, Haller, Priestley, Caldani and other contemporary authors, he posits the irritability of tissues and the existence of an 'elastic fluid' (which he at times calls elasticity or flexibility) inherent to fibres and indispensable for healing.

Consequently, conditions for wound repair are 'unobstructed communication of the extremities of arterial vessels from the wound to the heart; the vitality of [the heart] movement; the flexibility of the parts; their shape and contact; the absence of internal and external causes that hinder [the parts'] extension'.[59] More practically stated, healing implies 'a certain diameter of the arterial vessels; rest; rare medication; the proximity of the edges, and the absence of certain secretions hindering coagulation' that are necessary for gluten to build up scar tissue.[60] This is where the praise of rare dressing enters the picture. Cavallini attributes the primitive idea to Asclepiades and Galen, followed by Magati; these, however, explained it on ground of 'reasons no longer intelligible in our century', and must be reframed according to modern medicine in order to be put it into practice correctly.[61] A dozen *riflessioni* address points of theoretical or practical interest and learnedly review a large and diverse body of ancient and modern literature, expatiating on surgical matters as much as natural philosophy—especially on air and the atmosphere, its alterations and effects on the human body, the salubriousness of hospitals and how to assess it.[62]

The bulk of the book, however, is composed of brief case histories. A total of 118 occurrences of wounds are assembled, beginning with a 4-inch cut in the lower left calf of a 50-year old woman, Caterina Orsolini, cured in five days by bandaging alone to the surprise of her family, and ending with the attempted suicide of Giovan Gualberto Santini, 22 years old, who slashed his throat with a razor in a 'fit of melancholic delirium'. Although the cartilage was damaged, and notwithstanding inflammation, burning fever, very sore swelling, aphonia, and difficulties in swallowing, he was eventually cured thanks to live stitches to the integuments, emollients, light diet, and some silver nitrate on the scar.[63]

In the selection and arrangement of patients' histories, Cavallini clearly intends to document the superiority of a plain approach to wounds, and to surgery in general, as practiced in Florence. Like his senior colleague Nannoni, Cavallini is keen on praising the care provided at Santa Maria Nuova and the ability and charity of the surgeons working there. There are reports of failed cures, but successful ones are more numerous, many of which only involve suturing the cut with stiches or bandages.[64] The rhetoric of fact and experiment permeates every part of Cavallini's work. Contrary to Nannoni's, his case reports are generally short and penned in an impersonal, matter-of-fact style reminiscent of Hippocrates's *Epidemics*, that is, recorded by an attentive but detached observer.[65] Furthermore, such a format is consistent with Cavallini's

57. Donato, 'Practical Knowledge'. On Enlightenment systematics, see, in a vast body of literature, *The Quantifying* Spirit; Rusnock, *Vital Accounts*.
58. Cavallini, *Collezione*, II/1, p. II: 'onde sperar si possa di valutare de' varj metodi nella cura di simili malattie'.
59. Ibid., p. XII-XIV: 'la libera comunicazione dell'estremità de' vasi arteriosi dalla ferita al cuore; la vivacità del suo movimento; la flessibilità delle parti; la direzione; la figura [...]; l'assenza di forze interne, ed esterne, che renitano al prolungamento'.
60. Ibid.: 'un certo diametro ne vasi arteriosi; la quiete; la rara medicatura; la vicinanza delle parti; l'assenza di certe secrezioni opposte al coagulo'.
61. Ibid, pp. XXIII-XXV.
62. Ibid, pp. 100-04.
63. Ibid., pp. 1 and 150-151.
64. See, e.g., cases of wound in the abdomen, ibid. pp. 110-13.
65. Rey, 'Anamorphoses d'Hippocrate'.

role as hospital *istoriografo* drawing on hospital registers as much as his own *libretto* or notebook. By that time, in fact, medical and surgical students were expressly required to note daily observations on all patients.[66]

Cavallini also relates experiments on animals and in vitro observations he conducted at Santa Maria Nuova. More precisely, tables summarize observations on human blood, fat and bile; blood serum from healthy subjects compared with blood serum of acutely ill patients; shaken blood serum of acutely ill patients with healthy blood; fat diluted in water compared with fat diluted with blood serum, and their alterations during several days and in relation to weather and atmospheric pressure. Still, the purpose of such experiments was purely practical, aiming to 'encourage clinicians to use similar observations in uncertain cases, so that they may not be misled by appearances in prognosis as much as in treatment', and ultimately to improve surgery.[67]

A TENTATIVE CONCLUSION: PAPERWORK AND HOSPITALS AS (UNINTENDED?) SITES OF INNOVATION

All the surgeons taking part in the controversy on rare dressing, whose work has been examined in this chapter, appeal to arguments of reason, authority and experiment to demonstrate the superiority of their approach to wound care, namely minimal intervention. Thus, a century-old expectant attitude to health and disease that was deeply rooted in the Hippocratic and (albeit concealed) Galenic tradition was rehabilitated on the basis of new arguments.

It is actually tempting to argue that these authors simply reframed old practices in modern terms. Canonical procedures such as bloodletting could even be better explained within a mechanical framework.[68] But this would not be entirely accurate. The waning of Galenism as a free-standing medical philosophy did not imply the rise of a similar comprehensive medical system; nonetheless, it did imply discrediting numerous remedies, procedures and overmedication typically associated with qualitative humoral medicine (including in its chemical version). Practices such as inducing overabundant suppuration to digest corrupted humors had no place within circulatory physiopathology, whereas other techniques such as rare medication or debridement appeared consistent with it. In a nutshell, adherence to novel theories could produce therapeutic styles and preferences.

No doubt, the actual pace and extent of such shifts in ordinary surgical practice largely remain to be investigated. More bluntly stated, did surgeons like Cecchini, Nannoni, and Cavallini actually treat their patients in the way they recommended in their texts?

Clues on the consumption of drugs in the treatment of wounds are difficult to glean from hospital records. Although internal rules required prescriptions to be recorded and double-checked in multiple ways, such as on single sheets, ward registers, and pharmacy master books, few have survived later selection by archivists, and it is hard to track down prescriptions for individual patients.[69] However, I suggest, pitting manuscript against printed sources, as if only the former captured real cures, is probably not the most productive way of questioning the relation of theory and practice in early modern medicine and surgery. Scrutinizing what intellectual and material resources combined that allowed practices to be theoretically formulated and (more or less extensively) introduced, and in what context, seems more rewarding.

Hospitals should be revisited in this context. As mentioned, Cecchini, Nannoni, and Cavallini were hospital practitioners. Their over-representation in debates is linked to the growing importance of hospitals, including for the practice of, and training in surgery, and, consequently, the rising status of surgeons working and teaching there. The opportunity of treating numerous patients was an experiential resource in and of itself, and by extension a source of legitimation. Therefore, unsurprisingly, all assign a central place to expertise gained there to defend the superiority of simple dressing. The hospital, however, does not only yield generic experiential topoi. As authors strive to strengthen their evidentiary claims by widening the observational basis of their argument, they draw from individual and collective activity in the wards in multiple ways, although they

66. Decree dated 7 August 1788 in *Regolamento dei regi ospedali*, p. LXXII, and in this same *Regolamento*, see also pp. 38-39 and 41-42.
67. Cavallini, *Collezione*, p. 164: 'per incoraggiare i clinici a mettere in uso nei casi dubbiosi queste osservazioni, onde non restino ingannati dall'apparenze nei prognostici, come anche nelle cure'.
68. Müller, *Blutegeltherapie*; Ruisinger, 'The Circulation of the Blood'.
69. *Regole*, pp. 30-32, 56.

translate it in different forms—tables and figures, detailed individual case histories, collected case reports.

The impact of the hospital in shaping debates on wound treatment was indeed fundamental on both an epistemic and material level. From the late seventeenth century onwards, against the backdrop of economic and demographic crisis, political, ecclesiastical, and medical authorities alike put renewed pressure on hospitals to enhance their accountability—a trend that intensified during the following century up to the reforms of the 1770s and 1780s. Increased scrutiny of their activities and expenditures aimed at improving the medical, religious, and especially financial management to deal with falling revenues and expanding demand.[70] More precisely, it aimed at curbing maladministration and selecting welfare recipients to secure the financial viability of these complex organisms, while at the same time augmenting their capacity and maintaining standards of care consistent with public expectations, as many of these *luoghi pii* passed under direct State control. Hospitals were renowned for offering inmates and outpatients costly drugs they could not afford otherwise. Santo Spirito in Rome was particularly famous for its richly endowed *spezieria*, which was central to Catholic and papal propaganda, but constantly posed a problem for hospital finances.[71] Likewise, the number, workload, and behavior of medical, surgical, and other staff raised recurrent complaints and concerns, while the improvement of medical, and especially surgical, training became a central issue.

The importance of paperwork rose accordingly. Needless to say, hospitals had always been multifaceted establishments that combined landownership with financial and charitable activities, and therefore required sophisticated accountancy systems. Books of the inmates had always been kept.[72] Nonetheless, from the late seventeenth century onwards, all types of registers, including weekly, monthly and yearly tables, reports, and all sorts of books and records—both produced internally and by external commissioners, both secular and ecclesiastical—multiplied to cope with these conflicting imperatives. At Santo Spirito, for instance, comparative tables of patients' turnover in different wards, similar to those used by Cecchini, appeared in the late seventeenth century. Regardless of their original scope (i.e., controlling attendance by medical staff and to repress negligence), these tables became standard thereafter and available for different uses.[73] Tabular overviews of sick persons treated, orphans assisted, and food and medicines provided were first introduced as tools for internal reviews and were later printed and released to the public.[74] As noted, the role of medical and surgical staff in producing paperwork, both medical and administrative, also grew under eighteenth-century regulations.[75]

Set against such a backdrop, this minor dispute on wounds acquires more complex nuances. Hospital practitioners writing on rare dressing clearly aimed at advancing their personal excellency and distinguishing themselves in the professional arena by responding to what they perceived to be the primary goal of authorities: rationalising health provision. By endorsing a method they credited with advantages in terms of attendance and expenditure for drugs, they were 'epistemological imitators', to borrow Susan Lawrence's definition, as different regimes of evidence continued to coexist.[76] Still, over time empirical evidence shifted from an experiential to a more factual understanding, as practitioners relied on information that presupposed the paperwork generated by reforms in hospital management and daily routine. These, along with novel theories, created the institutional circumstances for empirical evidence to gain a more prominent place in assessing treatments, and ultimately for new practices to be introduced.

70. *Health Care and Poor Relief*; Jones *The Charitable Imperative*; Cavallo, *Charity and Power.*
71. De Angelis, *La spezieria dell'arcispedale di Santo Spirito;* Colapinto, 'La speziera dell'Ospedale di S. Spirito'; De Renzi, 'A Fountain for the Thirsty'.
72. Savoia, 'The book of the sick'. More generally, in a very vast body of scholarship, see *L'uso del denaro.*
73. Early instances of numerical tables of patients and turnovers can be found in AAV, MS Chigi H II 50; Spada, *Stato della casa dell'Archispedale di Santo Spirito*, and *Stato materiale formale et economico della casa di S. Spirito*; BAV, Congregazione della S. Visita apostolica, *Acta*, 12. Of note, at the end of the seventeenth century, other Roman hospitals introduced additional books of the sick to double-check prescriptions, turnover and expenditure, e.g., S. Salvatore (1671), S. Giacomo (1697).
74. See, for ASRo, Ospedale Santo Spirito, b. 1414. See also Piccialuti, *La carità come metodo di governo,* esp. pp. 127-29; Dominici, 'Il governo dell'ospedale di Santo Spirito'. Alike tables were of course introduced in hospitals throughout Europe and were even used for international comparisons, e.g., by the French Royal Commission for the reform of hospitals in the 1770s, see Foucault et al., *Les machines à guérir*, pp. 151-52.
75. See above, and for comparison, Thalamy, 'La médicalisation de l'hôpital'; Hess, 'Das Material einer guten Geschichte'; Hess and Schlegelmilch, 'Cornucopia'. More generally, *The Impact of Hospitals*; *Accounting for Health.*
76. Lawrence, *Charitable Knowledge*, p. 217.

To conclude, Christopher Lawrence has shown that the history of surgery has been shaped by the concerns of practitioners from its origins and is often told as a story of courage and antidogmatism.[77] Classic disciplinary histories usually focus on major operations, rather than on day-to-day practice, and highlight innovation in manual techniques, rather than shifts in the medical theories underpinning treatments and consequent shifts in the treatments themselves. Moreover, they rarely question how such shifts happened. As a consequence, pre-modern surgery is commonly viewed as an indistinct age of traditionalism and inertia.

Much of all this is probably not to be disputed. Still, this chapter has tentatively argued that to conceptualize change in early modern surgery, innovation should be understood as slight mutual adjustments of theory and practice rather than major breakthroughs. More generally, by pointing at the link between surgical theory and practice and hospital management, this chapter has suggested that understanding medical practice in a broader sense than a set of therapeutic actions in opposition to a set of notions and beliefs might contribute to reframing the question of theory and practice in pre-modern medicine that is at the core of this volume.

WORKS CITED

Printed Primary Sources

Belloste, Augustin, *Le Chirurgien d'hôpital, enseignant une manière douce et facile de guérir promptement toutes sortes de playes, avec un moyen d'éviter l'exfoliation des os, et une plaque nouvellement inventée pour le pansement des trépans* (Paris: L. d'Houry, 1696).

Cavallini, Giuseppe, *Collezione istorica di casi chirurgici metodicamente disposti e con note illustrati* (Florence: stamperia Bonducciana, 1764-1779).

Cecchini, Domenico, *La difesa dei diritti di Cesare Magati, discorso ...nel quale mostrasi la sussistenza del metodo Magatino con ragioni anatomiche e fisico-meccaniche* (Rome: Domenico Antonio Ercole, 1714).

Fabrici d'Acquapendente, Girolamo, *Opere* (Padua: per Giacomo Cadorino, 1685).

Cocchi, Antonio, *Discorsi toscani* (Florence: Doncuddi, 1761).

Cocchi, Antonio, *Scritti scelti* (Florence: Giunti 2000).

Cocchi, Antonio, *Relazione dello spedale di Santa Maria Nuova di Firenze*, ed. by Anna Mannelli Goggioli (Florence, Le Lettere, 2000).

Cocchi, Virgilio, *Il buon uso dell'acqua fredda nelle malattie tanto interne, quanto esterne* (Perugia: Costantini, 1735).

Dilucidazioni fisico-mediche tendenti a richiamare la medicina pratica alla preziosa purità in cui ce la lascio il grande Ippocrate (Rome: Giorgio Plancho, 1731).

Haller, Albecht von, *Bibliotheca Chirurgica* (Bern-Basel: Schwighauser, 1773–74)

Maraviglia, Pandolfo (alias Ruggero Calvi), *Giunta di alcune lettere...* (Ravenna: stamperia camerale, 1713).

Marini, Gaetano, *Degli Archiatri pontifici* (Rome: Pagliarini, 1784).

Nannoni, Angelo, *Trattato chirurgico... sopra la semplicità del medicare i mali d'attenenza della chirurgia* (Florence: Francesco Moücke, 1761).

Nannoni, Angelo, *Memorie di chirurgia... per servire alla formazione del secondo tomo del Trattato sopra la semplicità del medicare i mali curabili coll'ajuto della mano* (Siena: Bindi, 1774).

Nannoni, Angelo, *Memorie... sopra alcuni casi rari di chirurgia* (Florence: nella stamperia già Albizziniana, 1776).

Ordini di medicheria da osservarsi nell'esercizio e nello studio della chirurgia da i maestri e dalli studenti di essa nel Regio Spedale di Santa Maria Nuova di Firenze (Florence: Bernardo Paperini, 1747).

Regolamento dei regi ospedali di Santa Maria Nuova e di Bonifazio (Florence: Cambiagi, 1789).

Regole da osservarsi nel sacro, ed apostolico Archiospedale di Santo Spirito (Rome: Pagliarini, 1751).

Sancassani, Dionisio Andrea, *Il lume all'occhio* (Forlì: Dandi, 1707).

Sancassani, Dionisio Andrea, *Chirone in campo* (Venice: Girolamo Albrizzi, 1708).

Sancassani, Dionisio Andrea, *La chirurgia svellata, o sia continuazione dello Chirone in campo* (Venice: Giambattista Albrizzi, 1716).

Stato materiale formale et economico della casa di S. Spirito di Roma, avanti, e nel governo di Monsignor Arcivescovo Febei, con diversi fogli, nè quali apparisce (Rome: Reverenda Camera Apostolica, 1677).

Secondary Sources

Accounting for Health: Calculation, Paperwork, and Medicine 1500-2000, ed. by Axel C. Hüntelmann and Eliver Falk (Manchester: Manchester University Press, 2021).

Agrimi, Jole and Chiara Crisciani, *Edocere medicos. Medicina scolastica nei secoli XIII-XV* (Milan: Giuffré, 1988).

Altmeyer, Peter et al., *Wound Healing and Skin Physiology* (Berlin-Heidelberg: Springer, 1995).

77. Lawrence, 'Democratic, Divine and Heroic'.

Blair, Ann, 'The Rise of Note-Taking in Early Modern Europe', *Intellectual History Review*, 20 (2010), 303–16.

Brambilla, Elena, 'La medicina del Settecento: dal monopolio dogmatico alla professione scientifica', in *Storia d'Italia, Annali 7, Malattia e medicina*, ed. by Franco Della Perruta (Turin: Einaudi, 1984), pp. 3–147.

Cantor, David, ed., *Reinventing Hippocrates* (New York–London: Routledge, 2001).

Castellani, Carlo and Enrico Coturri, 'Una polemica tra Gianalessandro Brambilla ed Angelo Nannoni a proposito della "medicazione semplice" delle ferrite', *Castalia*, 15 (1959), 65–78.

Cavallo, Sandra, *Charity and Power in Early Modern Italy: Benefactors and Their Motives in Turin, 1541-1789* (Cambridge: Cambridge University Press, 1995).

Cavallo, Sandra, *Artisans of the Body in Early Modern Italy. Identities, Families and Masculinities* (Manchester: Manchester University Press, 2007).

Cavallo Sandra and Tessa Storey (eds), *Conserving Health in Early Modern Culture: Bodies and Environments in Italy and England*, (Manchester: Manchester University Press, 2017).

Cavallo, Sandra, 'Early Vernacular Medical Advice Books and their Popular Appeal in Early Modern Italy', *Nuncius. Journal of the Material and Visual History of Science*, 36 (2021), 264–303.

Cesare Magati medico e religioso. Atti del Convegno di Studi (Rome: l'Italia Francescana Editrice, 1978).

Charters, Erica, *Disease, War, and the Imperial State: The Welfare of the British Armed Forces During the Seven Years' War* (Chicago: The University of Chicago Press, 2014).

Colapinto, Luigi, 'La speziera dell'Ospedale di S. Spirito in Saxia a Roma', *Atti e memorie della accademia italiana di storia della farmacia*, 12 (1995), 217–20.

Daston, Lorraine, 'Perché i fatti sono brevi?', *Quaderni Storici*, 36 (2001), 745–70.

De Angelis, Roberto, *La spezieria dell'arcispedale di Santo Spirito in Saxia e la lotta contro la malaria* (Rome: Coluzza, 1954).

De Renzi, Salvatore, *Storia della medicina in Italia* (Naples: nella tipografia del Filiatre Sebezio, 1846).

De Renzi, Silvia, 'A Fountain for the Thirsty and a Bank for the Pope: Charity, Conflicts, and Medical Careers at the Hospital of Santo Spirito in Seventeenth-century Rome', in *Health Care and Poor Relief in Counter-Reformation Europe (1620-1720)*, ed. by Ole P. Grell, Andrew Cunningham, and Jon Arrizabalaga (London: Routledge, 1999), pp. 102–131.

Dominici, Silvia, 'Il governo dell'ospedale di Santo Spirito e dei suoi annessi nel secolo XVII. Coninuità e riforme', in *L'antico ospedale di Santo Spirito. Dall'istituzione papale alla sanità del terzo millennio*, ed. by Luigi Cardilli (Rome: il Veltro, 2001), pp. 239–51.

Donato, Maria Pia, 'Galen in an Age of Change (1650–1820)', in *Brill's Companion to the Reception of Galen* ed. by Petros Bouras-Vallianatos and Barbara Zipser (Leiden: Brill 2019), pp. 487–507.

Donato, Maria Pia, 'Surgeons' Training and Hospital Life in Seventeenth- and Eighteenth-century Rome', in *Transforming Medical Education*, ed. by Delia Gavrus and Susan Lamb (Montreal, ON–Kingston, ON: McGill University Press, 2022), pp. 136–60.

Donato, Maria Pia, 'Practical Knowledge and the Rhetoric of Experience: Three Italian Surgeons and Their Observations', *Early Science and Medicine*, 27 (2022) 235–56.

Dos, Serge J., *French Surgery of the Eighteenth Surgery. The Royal Academy of Surgery (1731-1793)* (Xlibris US, 2021).

Fissell, Mary, 'The Marketplace of Print', in *Medicine and the Market in England and its Colonies, ca 1450-1850,* ed. by Mark Jenner and Patrick Wallis (Basingstoke: Palgrave MacMillan, 2007), pp. 108–32.

Foucault, Michel et al., *Les machines à guérir (aux origines de l'hôpital moderne)* (Paris: Institut de l'environnement, 1976).

Fughelli, Patrizia, 'Cesare Magati. Spanning over Centuries', *Medicina Historica*, 1 (2017), 7–12.

Gentilcore, David, *Medical Charlatinism in Early Modern Italy* (Oxford: Oxford University Press, 2006).

Health Care and Poor Relief in 18th and 19th- Century Southern Europe, ed. by Ole P. Grell, Andrew Cunningham, and Bernd Roeck (Aldershot: Ashgate, 2005).

Hess, Volker and Andrew J. Mendelsohn, 'Case and Series: Medical Knowledge and Paper Technologies, 1600–1900', *History of Science*, 48 (2010), 287–314.

Hess, Volker, 'Das Material einer guten Geschichte. Register, Reglemente und Formulare', in *Fakta, und kein moralisches Geschwätz. Zu den Fallgeschichten im 'Magazin zur Erfahrungsseelenkunde' (1783-1793)*, ed. by Sheila Dickson, Stefan Goldmann, and Christof Wingertszahn (Gottingen: Wallstein, 2011), pp. 115–39.

Hess, Volker and Sabine Schlegelmilch, 'Cornucopia Officinae Medicae: Medical Practice Records and Their Origin', in *Medical Practice. Physicians and Their Patients*, ed. by Martin Dinges et al. (Leiden-Boston, Brill & Rodopi, 2016) pp. 11–38.

The Impact of Hospitals 300-2000, ed. by John Henderson, Peregrine Horden, and Alessandro Pastore (Bern: Peter Lang, 2007).

Jarcho, Saul, *Quinine's Predecessor: Francesco Torti and the Early History of Cinchona* (Baltimore: Johns Hopkins University Press, 1993).

Jones, Colin, *The Charitable Imperative; Hospitals and Nursing in Ancien Regime and Revolutionary France* (London: Routledge, 1989).

Lawrence, Christopher, 'Democratic, Divine and Heroic: The History and Historiography of Surgery', in *Medical Theory, Surgical Practice. Studies in the History of Surgery*, ed. by Christopher Lawrence (London: Routledge, 1992), pp. 1–47.

Lawrence, Susan, *Charitable Knowledge: Hospital Pupils and Practitioners in Eighteenth-Century London* (Cambridge: Cambridge University Press, 1996).

Le Minor, Jean-Marie and Paul Clair, 'Augustin Belloste (1654-1730), de la chirurgie militaire à la thérapeutique mercurielle', *Revue d'histoire de la pharmacie*, 89 (2001), 369–80.

Lifestyle and Medicine in the Enlightenment. The Six Non-Naturals in the Long Eighteenth Century, ed. by James Kennaway and Rina Knoeff (Abingdon: Routledge, 2020).

Magni, Egisto, *Cesare Magati e la sua riforma nella chirurgia* (Bologna: Gamberini e Parmeggiani, 1919).

Mannacio, Anna Teresa, 'Teoria e pratica della chirurgia nella Scuola dello Spedale fiorentino di Santa Maria Nuova tra XVII e XVIII secolo', *Atti e Memorie dell'Accademia di scienze e lettere La Colombaria* 54 (2003), 189–206.

McVaugh, Michael, *The Rational Surgery of the Middle Ages* (Florence: Sismel, Ed. del Galluzzo, 2006).

The Medical History of Waters and Spas, ed. by Roy Porter (London: Wellcome Institute for the History of Medicine, 1990).

Müller, Ingo Wilhelm, *Blutegeltherapie im 17. und 18. Jahrhundert*, Wolfenbüttel, s.e., 1985.

Münster, Ladislao and Giovanni Romagnoli, *Cesare Magati (1579-1647) lettore di chirurgia nello studio ferrarese, primo chirurgo dell'Arcispedale di S. Anna e il suo geniale e razionale metodo per la cura delle ferite* (Ferrara: Università di Ferrara, 1968).

Nutton, Vivian, 'Pieter Van Foreest: The Physician as Writer in Surgery', *Journal of the History of Medicine and Allied Science*, 72 (2017), 87–97.

Nutton, Vivian, 'Renaissance Galenism, 1540–1640: Flexibility or an Increasing Irrelevance?', in *Brill's Companion to the Reception of Galen*, ed. by Petros Bouras-Vallianatos and Barbara Zipser (Leiden: Brill, 2019), pp. 472–486

Park, Katharine, *Doctors and Medicine in Early Renaissance Florence* (Princeton: Princeton University Press, 1985).

Pasta, Renato, 'L'ospedale e la città. Riforme settecentesche a Santa Maria Nuova', in *La bellezza come terapia. Arte e assistenza nell'ospedale di Santa Maria Nuova a Firenze*, ed. by Enrico Ghidetti and Esther Diana (Florence: Le Lettere, 2005), pp. 271–91.

Piccialuti, Maura, *La carità come metodo di governo. Istituzioni caritative a Roma dal pontificato di Innocenzo XII a quello di Benedetto XIV* (Turin: Giappichelli, 1991).

Pomata, Gianna, *Contracting a Cure: Patients, Healers, and the Law in Early Modern Bologna* (Baltimore: Johns Hopkins University Press, 1998).

Pomata, Gianna, 'Sharing Cases: The Observationes in Early Modern Medicine', *Early Science and Medicine*, 15 (2010), 193–236.

The Quantifying Spirit of the Eighteenth Century, ed. by Tore Frängsmyr, J.L. Heilbron and Robin E. Rider (Berkeley: University of California Press, 1990).

Rabier, Christelle, 'Medicalizing the Surgical Trade, 1650–1820: Workers, Knowledge, Markets and Politics', in *The Palgrave Handbook of the History of Surgery*, ed. by Thomas Schlick (London: Palgrave, 2018), pp. 71–94.

Reichert, Frederick L., 'The Historical Development of the Procedure Termed Débridement: Pierre Joseph Desault', *Bulletin of the Johns Hopkins Hospital*, 42 (1928), 93–104.

Rey, Rosalyn, 'Anamorphoses d'Hippocrate au XVIIIe siècle', in *Maladie et maladies: Histoire et conceptualisation. Mélanges en l'honneur de Mirko Grmek*, ed. by Danielle Gourevitch (Geneva: Droz, 1992), pp. 257–276.

Ruisinger, Marion Maria, 'The Circulation of the Blood and Venesection: On the Relation between Medical Theory and Practice in the Early 18th Century', in *Medical Therapy and Therapeutic Practice in the Eigteenth Century*, ed. by Jürgen Helm and Renate Wilson (Stuttgart: Franz Steiner, 2008), pp. 37–60.

Rusnock, Andrea, *Vital Accounts: Quantifying Health and Population in Eighteenth-Century England and France* (Cambridge: Cambridge University Press, 2009).

Savoia, Paolo, 'The Book of the Sick of Santa Maria della Morte in Bologna and the Medical Organization of a Hospital in the Sixteenth-Century', *Nuncius*, 31 (2016), 163–235.

Savoia, Paolo, 'Skills, Knowledge, and Status: The Career of an Early Modern Italian Surgeon', *Bulletin of the History of Medicine*, 93 (2019), 27–54.

Shaw, James and Evelyn Welch, *Making and Marketing Medicine in Renaissance Florence* (Amsterdam: Rodopi, 2011).

Siraisi, Nancy G., 'How to Write a Latin Book on Surgery: Organizing Principles and Authorial Devices in Guglielmo da Saliceto and Dino del Garbo", in *Practical Medicine from Salerno to the Black Death*, ed. by Luis Garcia Ballester and others (Cambridge: Cambridge University Press, 1994), pp. 88–109.

Thalamy, Anne, 'La médicalisation de l'hôpital', in *Les machines à guérir (aux origines de l'hôpital moderne)* (Paris: Institut de l'environnement, 1976), pp. 43–53.

Tröhler, Ulrich. '"To Improve the Evidence of Medicine": Arithmetic Observation in Clinical Medicine in the Eighteenth and Early Nineteenth Centuries', *History and Philosophy of the Life Sciences*, 10 (1988), 31–40.

L'uso del denaro. Patrimoni e amministrazione nei luoghi pii e negli enti ecclesiastici in Italia (secoli XV-XVIII), ed. by Alessandro Pastore and Marina Garbellotti (Bologna: il Mulino, 2001).

Wallis, Patrick. 'Competition and Cooperation in the Early Modern Medical Economy', in *Medicine and the Market*, ed. by Jenner and Wallis, pp. 47–68.

The World of the Italian Apothecary, ed. by David Gentilcore, *Pharmacy in History* 45 (2003).

Wounds and Wound Repair in Medieval Culture, ed. by Larissa Tracy and Kelly DeVries (Leiden: Brill, 2015).

10

'Malignità che s'infonde': *Rice Fields, Space, and Medicine in Counter-Reformation Milan*[1]

Lavinia Maddaluno

In 1584, in the countryside of Novara, an unknown individual requested that the local health deputies, physicians, the bishop, and the representative of the Magistrato Ordinario gather at the home of a Mr. de Campoz. This mysterious organizer subsequently compiled a chronicle detailing the most salient moments of the meeting and its participants. He described how those present began to observe a drawing (*disegno*) by a local engineer, Giovanni Battista Clarici. Although the author did not reveal the drawing's content, it is inferred that it depicted a city in the Duchy of Milan and its rural surroundings. The report, in fact, concerned the rice fields around Novara.

The report highlighted how state institutions established the distance between the stagnant waters of paddy fields and urban areas. It was accompanied by a series of documents expressing the opinions of clergy and landowners on the medical, moral, political, and economic arguments for and against rice cultivation near Novara. The issues at stake were both medical and technical. On the one hand, rice fields were considered a threat to public health because their stagnant waters were believed to produce miasmas. On the other hand, many rice fields were plots of land unsuitable for other crops due to their wet and humid environment. Edicts and proclamations issued since the sixteenth century mandated that paddy fields be situated at least four miles from the center of any city.[2] However, measurements were often questioned, and some landowners accused Clarici of miscalculating the distance between their rice fields and Novara. According to these accusations, Clarici had used a different unit of measurement, making the canonical four-mile distance equivalent to three and a half miles. This led to discontent among landowners who found their activities suddenly outlawed.

Engineers such as Clarici were frequently involved with various magistracies in the Duchy, including the *Magistrato Ordinario* and *Straordinario*, the *Vicario di Provvisione*, and the *Magistrato di Sanità*, offices responsible for settling conflicts and controversies concerning the management of lands, marshes, stagnant waters, and paddy fields.[3] More specifically, while land surveyors, who held a lower status than engineers, took measurements on contested sites, engineers used those measurements to make drawings and sketches, which were then used as evidence in legal proceedings. The key magistracy for the preservation of public health in the Duchy of Milan was the *Magistrato di Sanità*. It had an internal court, the *Tribunale di Sanità* or Health Board Court, which was called into session each time there was a controversy between two or more parties

1. This article is part of the 'Water-Cultures–The Water Cultures of Italy, 1500–1900' project, which has received funding from the European Research Council (ERC) under the European Union's Horizon 2020 research and innovation program (grant agreement no. 833834). The information and views set out in this article reflect only the authors' views and the Agency (ERCEA) is not responsible for any use that may be made of the information it contains. I would like to thank the two volume editors, Sandra Cavallo and John Henderson, as well as Elisa Andretta, Lucia Dacome and Craig Martin for reading the text and providing feedback.

2. ASMi, Atti di Governo, Agricoltura Parte Antica 64, page unnumbered. These distances kept varying in the legislation throughout the early modern period.

3. To be precise, the *Magistrato Ordinario* dealt with the state budget, duties, taxes, and fortifications, while the *Magistrato Straordinario* managed the prince's possessions and addressed questions concerning the grain trade, fines, and confiscations. The *Vicario di Provvisione* managed grain prices and the *annona* and controlled the maintenance of roads, water channels, and bridges.

concerning matters of public health, be it a cesspit emanating foul air, a rice field situated too close to inhabited areas, or a stagnant pond. Most importantly, even though the *Magistrato di Sanità* was established in response to a plague epidemic, it did not deal exclusively with epidemic containment measures. In general, its role was preventative and proactive, identifying environmental threats and reducing their impact on the health of the community.[4]

The goal of this essay is to offer a multifaceted perspective on strategies of healthscaping in a rural and peri-urban milieu in the sixteenth- and seventeenth-century Spanish Duchy of Milan. It also aims to show the complex interconnections between medical theories and the management and control of natural resources and spaces. Scholarship on early modern practices of public health and cultures of prevention has tended to focus on the urban dimension, shedding light on the multiplicity of actors who shaped material public health infrastructures such as systems of water provision and organic waste collection and disposal, as well as domestic practices such as dietary regimens in aristocratic households.[5] This essay will instead focus on the rural and mobile dimension, exploring medical practices resulting from human engagement with transitional spaces such as rice fields and, more broadly, stagnant waters. More generally, the essay aims to reinstate the importance of spatial awareness as key in unpacking public health practices and medical concepts and revealing their social, cultural, and political imbrications.[6] Rice fields were particularly contested spaces where various jurisdictions clashed, and negotiations between different forms of knowledge and expertise took place. They were trading zones, imbued with multiple meanings, and sites of exchange between tenant farmers, migrant workers, and institutions such as the offices of the *Magistrato Ordinario*, *Magistrato Straordinario*, and *Magistrato di Sanità*, whose ramifications were represented by engineers sent to take measurements, civil servants ensuring the local application of edicts, and physicians assessing the noxiousness of water and air.[7]

Indeed, the Lombard plains of the Cinquecento were characterized by diverse forms of migration, ranging from *famuli*—salaried workers who lived on the farms of their employers and had a somewhat stable occupation, lasting from a few months to a few years—day laborers, who came from both the surrounding hills and mountains and the contiguous plains.[8] Day laborers worked side by side with salaried workers, even though the former did not live on the farms but rather in the so-called *cassine*, small and temporary dwellings built seasonally, following the harvesting of hay and rice.[9] Rice played an important role in the economy of late sixteenth- and seventeenth-century Milan. However, rice fields also represented a pervasive environmental threat. Despite their increasing importance in the Duchy of Milan, rice fields were also seen as places of transit, material, spiritual corruption, and vulnerability. Their purpose was constantly reconsidered and projected upon.[10] Contemporary manuscripts indicate that the same piece of land could be viewed as either barren unless cultivated with rice, or potentially capable of producing alternative crops such as wheat and rye. While landowners favored the latter view, representatives of Spanish institutions often held the former, and opposed paddy fields. As we will see, visions of stagnant waters and rice fields were fluid, embodying constantly evolving medical as well as political and moral cultures of knowledge.

The present essay consists of three sections. The first section focuses on the report and set of documents introduced earlier, using them to explore the intersecting cultural and medical–intellectual dimensions of rice fields management. The section reveals that some of these rice field controversies not only concerned public health but also exposed visions of the political and jurisdictional conflicts, whose main protagonists were Cardinal Carlo Borromeo (1538–84) and the Governor of the Duchy of Milan, the Spanish Marquis d'Ayamonte. To examine the

4. See Maddaluno, 'Public Health in Milan'.
5. In particular, see Cavallo and Storey, *Healthy Living in Late Renaissance Italy*. On plague prevention practices in the Renaissance, see Henderson, *Florence under Siege*, pp. 51–84. On cultures of cleanness, see Rawcliffe and Weeda, *Policing the Urban Environment*. For a discussion of current trends in the history of public health, see Geltner and Coomans, 'The Healthscaping Approach', pp.18–33.
6. Baker, Nijdam, and van 't Land eds., *Medicine and Space*, pp. 1–3. On geographical awareness and disease, see Dobson, *Contours of Death and Disease*. For a more recent take on the spatial dimension, see Crawshaw, *Cleaning up Renaissance*.
7. Long, 'Trading Zones', pp. 840–47.
8. See di Tullio, 'Domestici e agricoltura capitalista', pp. 87–97.
9. See di Tullio, 'Rese agricole', pp. 293–318.
10. See the work on the imaginary surrounding stagnation in Bachelard, *L'eau et les rêves*; Durand, *Le strutture antropologiche*.

link between the political domain and the sphere of territorial and environmental control, we will draw on the works of Giovanni Botero (1544-1617), particularly his *Della Ragion di Stato* (1589).

The second section analyzes the medical dimension, focusing on Ludovico Settala's writings on Hippocrates and his considerations on reason of state and public health. Specifically, this section engages with Settala's five commentaries on Hippocrates's *Airs, Waters, and Places*, the *Librum Hippocratis Coi de aeribus, aquis, locis, Commentarii V* (1590), particularly passages addressing the physician's role in identifying environmental threats and those concerning water use and stagnant waters. Settala acted as *Protofisico* in 1628, during the plague epidemic cycle that struck Milan between 1627 and 1630. At that time, he also authored a less well-known political text about reason of state, *Della Ragion di Stato Libri Sette* (1627), where he elaborated on the contemporary concept of reason of state in connection with medical practice and the knowledge and control of state territories. Botero's and Settala's texts offer a broad insight into the intellectual and medical debates taking place at the time of our rice field controversies, highlighting the intersection of medical theories with contemporary political stances and public health practices in the Spanish Duchy of Milan. The final, shorter section explores the contribution of engineers to medical theory, through their involvement in assessing the distances between rice fields and inhabited areas.

Even though most of the documents considered date from the end of the sixteenth century, as a whole, they cover a fairly broad chronology, from 1584 to the 1660s. The reason for this chronological breadth is that most of these conflicts first emerged in the sixteenth century but ended only in the late seventeenth, with the majority sealed by a medical ruling issued by the physicians under the *Magistrato di Sanità*. Finally, the essay will also shed light on some non-medical actors involved in these conflicts, particularly engineers. Overall, it seeks to nuance our understanding of the way public health and medical knowledge were practiced in sixteenth- and seventeenth-century Milan and emphasize the spatial and mobile dimension of healthscaping practices.

RICE, CORPOREAL DEATH, AND THE DEATH OF THE SOUL IN COUNTER-REFORMATION MILAN

Rice cultivation was a divisive practice in early modern Lombardy. Land reclamation interventions on the vast marshes that characterized part of the Lombard landscape in medieval and early modern times had facilitated the cultivation of wheat, combined with hay, since the mid-sixteenth century. However, the increase in rice production, which represented an important crop not only for local and rural communities but also for the provision of larger urban centers, created environmental anxieties. Novara, the city at the center of one of the nine provinces into which the Duchy of Milan was divided, enjoyed the perfect geography for rice cultivation, lying in a plain rich in water springs. Moreover, rice was key to feeding the Spanish army, which often settled in Lombardy for months at a time for military training or used the region as a stopover on its way to Flanders from the time of the Dutch revolt from 1567 onwards.[11] The author of the report on rice fields in Novara highlighted that the main reasons for central institutions to loosen the prohibition of sowing rice around the city were precisely the presence of 'continuous army quartering', along with the need for tenant farmers to pay tax levies.[12] Rice was the answer to the social instability resulting from a potential dearth of wheat and a means to counteract the constant increase in taxation due to the decades of warfare that had plagued the Duchy since the Quattrocento. Another anonymous commentator, who provided a memoire giving the reasons in favor of rice cultivation in Novara, claimed that even the traditional reason for the prohibition of rice cultivation close to urban centers, that is, the *pubblica salute*, did not hold: in fact, he argued, water did not stagnate in the countryside around Novara but rather had a 'libero decorso', that is, it kept flowing freely, thus not representing a health threat.[13] However, this was not a universal view. Yet another author who wrote about rice in Novara expressed his opinion against cultivating this crop. According to him, the stagnating water of rice fields filtered underneath the lands devoted to other forms of cultivation, damaging not only crops such as wheat and hay but also wine production:

11. d'Amico, 'Spanish Milan', pp. 46–68.
12. ASMi, Atti di Governo, Agricoltura Parte Antica 53, page unnumbered.
13. Ibid.

> The malignant and rotten water of rice fields broadly percolates underground causing worms, *zuchette* (as they are called), and other animals that damage wheat, vineyards, forests, hay, and other produce, as can be seen based on past and present experience.[14]

This excerpt formed part of the same set of documents with which we opened this essay. The author, likely a member of the local clergy, presented a narrative of the countryside of Novara as a wasteland, a space that was once inhabited by a 'great quantity of people, robust, of good color, and red-blooded' but that, after being cultivated with rice, was affected by significant depopulation and a lack of *industria*. In his view, rice triggered a negative transformation of lands and spaces, which went from being fruitful and generative of 'everything' to being corrupt and affected by uncontrolled growth of organic matter.[15]

Rice cultivation embodied the fear of ungodly chaos, of the possibility that living creatures could be generated spontaneously from putrefying matter, a notion that brought into question the tenet that the origin of life and living creatures could be explained only by recourse to God's intelligent intervention.[16] Ideas regarding such spontaneous generation were circulating in the Renaissance, based on the reading of Aristotle's *De generatione animalium,* which relied in turn on the fourth book of the Hippocratic treatise *Diseases* (Chapter 54).[17] For example, the Milanese Girolamo Cardano (1501–76) in his *De subtilitate* (Nuremberg, 1550) appropriated the Aristotelian passage where the Greek philosopher explained that living beings were generated in earth and water due to the presence of water in the earth and *pneuma* and animating heat in water. As Hiro Hirai has recently highlighted, Cardano used this passage to justify his panvitalism and claim that the Aristotelian animating heat formed the foundation for the generation of all creatures, including animals and minerals.[18] That inanimate matter could generate living beings was a notion articulated in various ways in the Cinquecento, from Pietro Pomponazzi (1462–1525) and Bernardino Telesio (1509–88) to Giordano Bruno (1548–1600) and Ulisse Aldrovandi (1522–1605) to name just a few. However, this notion often clashed with the theological agenda of the Counter-Reformation because it cast doubt on the role of God as the first cause.[19]

From the available archival material, we know that the hoped-for destruction of rice fields and instigation of projects of land reclamation would serve the purpose of reinstating the original purity of lands, their 'pristina bontà', thereby reclaiming a lost moral order.[20] Observations on the general bodily appearance of those living and working close to rice fields, particularly their skin color, recalled the contemporary Galenic medical framework, in which skin could reflect humoral balance or imbalance and thus the presence of disease.[21] Of course, as we will see in the next section, such observations are also revealing of the impact of Hippocratic medicine and, more generally, of the six non-naturals, the control of which was a condition for a healthy life.[22] More broadly, the emphasis on geography, population, and *industria* had considerable cultural and intellectual significance at the end of the

14. 'Nelli terreni vicini alli risati per rispetto della refrigeratione che ricevono dall'acqua maligna et putrefatta de detti risati la quale penetrando sotto terra si sparge nelli terreni circonvicini in grande spatio si causano vermi, zuchette (come si dice) et altri animali che danno notabile danno a li grani, alle viti, alli boschi, alli fieni, et altri frutti come si vede per l'esperientia che se n'è fatto e che si può fare.' On rice-related food provisioning, see di Tullio, 'Rese agricole', pp. 293–318.
15. Even though the term of *industria* does not feature in the manuscript source analyzed, it appeared in the writings of contemporary authors such as Giovanni Botero, standing for all those activities involving a manipulation of raw materials and an increase in land productivity. See Botero, *Della Ragion di Stato*, pp. 210–14.
16. On how the concept of spontaneous generation emerged in 'popular' cultures and was seen as an unsettling form of 'naturalism' by the Inquisition, see Ginzburg, *Il formaggio e i vermi*, pp. 211–12. For a criticism of Ginzburg's view, see Zambelli, 'From Menocchio to Piero Della Francesca', pp. 983–99.
17. Manning and Wilberding, 'Reflection II', pp.177–85. On Aristotle's spontaneous generation, see Kress, 'Aristotle on Spontaneous Generation'. For Hippocrates, see the critical edition of *Diseases* IV in Lonie, *The Hippocratic Treatises*, pp. 350–51.
18. Hirai, 'Cosmic Heat in Telesio', pp. 71–83. See also Hirai, 'Prisca Theologia and Neoplatonic Reading of Hippocrates', pp. 95–96.
19. The question of spontaneous generation in the Cinquecento merits a more in-depth analysis than is within the scope of the present essay. For more on the topic, see Hirai, *Medical Humanism and Natural Philosophy*, pp. 1–19. On Pomponazzi, see Perrone Compagni, 'Un'ipotesi non impossibile', pp. 99–111. On Bruno, see Knox, 'Giordano Bruno'.
20. ASMi, Atti di Governo, Agricoltura Parte Antica 53, unnumbered page. On Cardano's celestial heat, see Giglioni, 'Girolamo Cardano e Giulio Cesare Scaligero', pp. 313–39.
21. Murphy, 'Skin and Disease', pp.179–214.
22. Cavallo and Storey, *Healthy Living in Late Renaissance Italy*, p. 3.

Cinquecento, when modern European states, especially the Duchy of Milan under Spanish rule, were developing strategies for political and economic consolidation to remain competitive on the international market.[23] Overseas exploration and the encounters of Europeans with new climates, diseases, and people brought to the fore how important knowledge, improvement, and control of local circumstances and environments were for social and political organization and policymaking.[24] The case of Novara took place at around the time when reason of state theorist Giovanni Botero was counselor and secretary to two of the key figures of Counter-Reformation Milan, Cardinal Carlo Borromeo and his cousin, Federico Borromeo (1564–1631).[25] Botero is particularly relevant in the context of the archival documents we are considering in that he reflected on how statecraft practices and economic growth depended on princes and counsellors having access to knowledge of geography, population, medicine, and, more generally, nature. Botero articulated a novel approach to reason of state, rethinking the dimension of the political and integrating, as highlighted by Harald Braun, a concern for the protection of Christendom with a concern for the new forms of statehood that arose in the context of religious conflicts and global expansion.[26]

In *Delle cause della grandezza delle città* (1588), Botero underlined the centrality of population and industry in reinforcing the state's economy, claiming that true wealth did not lie in mines filled with precious metals but in how humans worked the soil and transformed and traded raw materials. He argued that 'the duties on Milanese goods bring more money into the King of Spain's coffers than the mines of Zacateca and Jalisco'.[27] Even though Botero mostly referred to manufactured goods, his concept of *industria* linked true wealth to the human transformation and amelioration of nature, claiming that '*industria* advances nature'. In the eighth book of his *Della Ragion di Stato* (1589), dedicated to the 'ways to increase population and force', Botero extolled the importance of princely intervention in improvement projects, such as 'drying marshes, deforesting and cultivating useless woods, [and] supporting and aiding those who would like to invest in these enterprises'.[28] He praised the creation of water channels for commercial purposes in the earlier Duchy of Milan through the diversion of larger rivers such as the Ticino and Adda, as well as the (ultimately unsuccessful) land reclamation interventions enacted on the Pontine marshes in Latium by Pope Leon X.[29] In *Della Ragion di Stato* and *Delle cause della grandezza delle città*, Botero mostly focused on rivers as key to what he called *commodità della condotta*, that is, the ease of connecting communities and transporting raw and manufactured materials within the state or abroad.[30] However, in his later *Discorso intorno allo Stato della Chiesa* (1599), Botero also dedicated space to river floods and stagnant waters.

Although Botero mostly addressed the projects aiming to divert the Aniene River toward Rome to improve the city's air quality, he also reflected on a broader aspect that shed light on the documents concerning Novara. Botero emphasized the structural and orderly aspect of rivers and dikes, contrasting them with the pervasive, uncontrollable, and shapeless nature of floods and the stagnant waters they produced. He insisted that reclaimed lands, whose rivers and waters ran freely, were characterized by active and industrious communities, while marshlands were instead places of transit and marginality: 'Peasants fall sick, hit by malignant air and soil, by the heat of the sun during the day, and by the cold of the Moon during the night'.[31] The documents concerning rice fields in Novara partook in what was not only Botero's but a broader early modern trope, evident in other geographical contexts such as France, in the work of another reason of state theorist, Jean Bodin. Bodin interpreted marshes and stagnant waters as symbols of backwardness and weak state policies, contrasting them

23. See Miglietti and Morgan, eds., *Governing the Environment*, pp. 1–21.
24. For an example of environmental governance in the early modern period, see Appuhn, *A Forest on the Sea*. On improvement, see Slack, *The Invention of Improvement*. For an example of land reclamation intervention, see Morera, 'Mise en valeur des zones humides'.
25. See Continisio, 'Giovanni Botero'.
26. Braun, 'Knowledge and Counsel', pp. 270–89.
27. Giovanni Botero's *Delle cause della grandezza delle città* (1588) is incorporated in his *Della Ragion di Stato*, p. 41. On Botero and *industria*, see Miglietti, 'Debating greatness', pp. 239–57.
28. Botero, *Della Ragion di Stato*, p. 207.
29. Ibid., pp. 208–10.
30. For Botero's view on rivers, see Andretta, 'Il filo dell'acqua', pp. 363–400.
31. Botero, 'Discorso sullo Stato della Chiesa' (1599) in Botero, *Relatione della repubblica venetiana*, p. 114.

with drained and cultivable lands, which he saw as the epitome of power and state control.[32]

The stagnant waters surrounding Novara were not marshes but rice fields. They were productive and generative. Nonetheless, in the anonymous Novara report, they were still portrayed as transitional spaces, inhabited by migrants rather than by sedentary communities, whose bodies were permanently diseased. Another aspect of rice cultivation is that one would not only cultivate but also eat rice. Indeed, the author of the report noted that the significant introduction of rice into the countryside provoked changes in the diet of local communities, unsettling their bodily economies. This remark is not surprising, as rice only started to be used as a food staple at the end of the sixteenth century, having previously been known mostly as a remedy, as we know from a contemporary source, Castore Durante's *Herbario Novo* (1585).[33] Durante extolled the virtues of rice as a medicament for infertility (cooked with cinnamon, sugar, and milk) and dysentery (in the form of a decoction). A contemporary of Durante, Girolamo Cardano, in his *De methodo medendi lectiones quatuor* (1565), discussed the use of rice in a medical context, criticizing the widely held view that its whiteness could be particularly appropriate for feeding the sick.[34] Rice also appeared in dietary regimens in sixteenth-century Milan, being sold by local retailers to charities and parishes together with rye during the 1576 plague epidemic.[35]

However, even though contemporary evidence shows that rice could be used as a remedy and represented an important food staple, it was still seen as a deadly danger. The author of the Novara document argued that the presence of rice paddies was incompatible with life and especially with the presence of children. The young could not be raised too close to rice fields, not only because stagnant water corrupted the air and created a permanent fog (*nebbia*) but also because the water from rice paddies penetrated (*malignità che s'infonde*) wells and fountains, making it undrinkable.[36] The author made a connection to the plague, stating that 'this infection of air caused by rice fields has the same effect as the plague, as we have seen in some lands'.[37] This last comment is telling because it highlights the vividness of the cultural memory of plague epidemics and the connection between the impact of environmental factors such as water and air on the presence of disease, on the one hand, and the relatively recent plague outbreak that struck the Duchy of Milan in 1576, on the other.[38] The corruption of the body caused by environmental factors was also coupled with a corruption of the soul:

> Sowing rice does not only provoke the corporeal death of human beings but also that of their soul, in that many poor foreigners are encouraged to come to clean rice, and because of that, they get sick and die without confessing; also, since harvesting rice takes a long time, very few people come to mass on festive days, and they never cease to fight and quarrel.[39]

According to the author of the report, clergymen refused to serve God in places where rice was cultivated, thus abandoning entire areas, and leaving them to their inescapable and sinful fate. Even non-human animals such as livestock despised rice, refusing to eat the hay that grew close to rice fields. Unlike other crops meant for the internal market, rice was mostly produced for export, which the author saw as a dissipation of the state's internal wealth. Moreover, even when the rice produced remained in the Duchy of Milan, the author of the report remarked, it mostly brought benefit to a few people rather than the community at large, serving individuals and not society. The evocation of seasonal migration and the circulation of rice produce suggests that rice fields were seen not only as an environmental threat to public health, comparable to

32. Bodin, *Six Books*, p. 547. On Bodin's view, see Morera, 'Marshes as Microclimates', pp. 56–75.
33. Durante, *Herbario Novo*, pp. 393–94.
34. Cardano, *De methodo medendi*, p. 132; quoted in Siraisi, *The Clock and the Mirror*, p. 74. On Cardano and diet, see Gentilcore, *Food and Health*, pp. 65, 106.
35. BTMi, *Materie 349*, document dated 18 October 1576.
36. On practices regarding drinking water, see Gentilcore, 'From "Vilest Beverage" to "Universal Medicine"', pp.683–703.
37. '[Q]uesta infettione d'aria causata da' risati fa il medesimo effetto all'interno de' detti risati, come suol fare la peste, come si è visto in alcune terre.'
38. Cohn, *Cultures of Plague*. On shared plague memory, see also Carmichael, 'The Last Past Plague', pp.132–60.
39. '[N]on solo noce il seminerio delli risi alla morte corporale delli uomini, ma anche a quella dell'anima, percioché molti poveri forastieri si lasciano indurre a venir a mondar li risi e stando nell'acqua per tal effetto s'infermano e moiono di necessità, per le cascine, strade, et sopra li istessi argini senza confessione oltre di che durando il racoglier delli risi poca giente vengono à messa il giorno delle feste, et mai cessano tra loro discordie, liti, risse et morti.'

the plague in their effects, but also as the cause of potential upheaval and disruption of social and economic order, a geographical space that rendered fragile the dynamics between social groups and modes of agricultural production.[40] The Counter-Reformation imperative of controlling souls entailed the policing of bodily economies and the knowledge and improvement of specific territories.[41]

On this note, Carlo Borromeo also tried to extend his control by breaking the old Sforza and Spanish legislation on the distance to be maintained between rice fields and inhabited areas. As mentioned earlier, such legislation required a four-mile distance to be maintained between rice fields and the center of any given town, measured from the navel of the city, the metropolitan church, or, sometimes, the city walls. Around 1576, the Cardinal issued an edict regarding rice cultivation to help his tenant farmers, even threatening to excommunicate anyone who opposed his measures. The year 1576 was, of course, one of crisis in the Duchy since it coincided with one of the worst plagues, which affected population and workforce in the countryside as well as agricultural productivity, unsettling and changing social and economic structures. The governor of the Duchy of Milan, the Spanish Marquis d'Ayamonte, wrote a critical letter to Borromeo, arguing for the primacy of 'public utility and public health,' which ought to supersede individual needs and even economic imperatives. Ayamonte asked Borromeo to consider not only the 'evident air corruption and infection' as causes of high mortality but also 'the frequent news concerning the progress of the plague around the borders of the Duchy'.[42] Cardinal Borromeo's edicts represented a threat not only to public health but also, perhaps mostly, to the sovereignty of the state. Governor Ayamonte reported that the Cardinal,

> had an edict published in his name that was similar in substance to the edict of S. E. Velasco but differed from it for it reclaimed the faculty and autonomy to determine whether lands are fit to produce rice or not and it imposes other specific and arbitrary punishments, even excommunication, independently of whether those under his jurisdictions were members of the clergy or laymen.[43]

The representatives of state institutions, in this specific case the *Magistrato Straordinario*, tried to convince the Cardinal 'through well-founded reasoning' ('con li veri fondamenti di ragione') of why he lacked the authority to issue edicts that conflicted with state legislation and posed a threat not only to state sovereignty but also to the preservation and government ('governo') of public health ('pubblica sanità'). The case of Borromeo evokes the contemporary Counter-Reformation tensions and complexities between different jurisdictions and the connection between public health and politics. At the same time, it sheds light on forms of environmental governance, particularly the governance of water and air, in a rural context and, more specifically, in lands dedicated to rice production. However, Borromeo tried to turn rice paddies into the site of his political, social, and spiritual control by capitalizing on the presence of separate jurisdictions and bypassing the required four-mile distance established by Duchy institutions. The presence of rice paddies and the policing of these spaces engendered fears of contamination and prompted contemporary intellectual debates about marginal territories and land improvement. Embedded within a neo-Hippocratic medical framework, these forms of environmental governance naturally revealed ways of applying medical knowledge. This knowledge was far from monolithic, being constantly negotiated and re-produced by the actors involved, the spaces where those conflicts took place, and the symbolic and religious dimensions mobilized at the time of the Counter-Reformation. This section has highlighted how medical knowledge was embedded in the material, political, spiritual, and social government of rice cultivation. We might wonder, however, if a political stance was also present in printed medical texts of the time, particularly in commentaries on the Hippocratic *Airs, Waters, and Places*.

40. di Tullio, 'Tra ecologia ed economia', pp. 283–99.
41. de Boer, *The Conquest of the Soul*, pp. 43–45. See also Prosperi, *Tribunali della Coscienza*, pp. 243 ff. On social and environmental regulation, see again Crawshaw, *Cleaning up Renaissance*, p.22.
42. 'Manifesta corrutione et infetione d'aere e per conseguente mortalità grande et aggiungendosi a questo gli avvisi frequenti del progresso che la peste andava facendo intorno ai confini.' ASMi, Atti di Governo, Agricoltura Parte Antica 53 (*c.*1576), unnumbered page.
43. 'Fece pubblicare un editto in suo nome, simile in sostanza alla grida di S.E. (Velasco) ma differente in questo, che riserva a sé [...] la facoltà di conoscere e dichiarare se i terreni siano o non siano atti a produrre altro che riso et impone certe altre pene precise, et arbitrarie, anche della scomunica, che siano ecclesiastici o laici e non sottoposti alla sua giurisdizione.' In ibid.

MEDICAL KNOWLEDGE

Even though the documents concerning Novara did not refer explicitly to medical theories, their emphasis on the negative effects of stagnant waters resonates with the broader cultural legacy of the humanistic readings of the Hippocratic corpus, especially *Airs, Waters, and Places* (henceforth *AWP*). This Hippocratic text had inspired two commentaries connected to Milan and its territories by the end of the sixteenth century: the first, published in Basel in 1570, by Milanese physician Girolamo Cardano (1501–76), who praised Hippocrates for his appeal to experience as foundational to medical practice; and the second, published in Cologne in 1590, by the physician and later *Protomedico* of plague-ravaged Milan, Ludovico Settala (1552–1633).[44] We will focus here on Settala's commentary.[45]

As a medical deputy during the Milanese plague of 1576–77, Settala combined his humanist training with medical practice on the ground and later, in the 1620s, with political discourse.[46] As Craig Martin argues, in Settala's 1632 discussion of Aristotle's *Problemata*, a key text on contagion, Settala advocated for integrating natural philosophy and medicine. He wanted to legitimize and strengthen the status of medical knowledge, and he did so by showing that the *Problemata* drew on the Hippocratic *AWP*.[47] Settala placed noxious vapors at the center of his explanation of plague and disease transmission, thus distancing himself from 'seeds' and corpuscular theories.[48] He explained that there was no need to resort to the theory of seeds to account for the causes of diseases, as in the tradition of Girolamo Fracastoro's *De contagione* (1546), arguing that disease was caused by a corruption of mixture communicated from one body to another through heat and humid vapors. Settala's interest in disease transmission was consistent with his active engagement in the preservation of public health.

In his later text, *Della Ragion di Stato* (1627), Settala compared practices aimed at protecting the community, such as politics, and those concerned with the preservation of public health, such as medicine. He claimed that reason of state, the theme at the core of his book, had a descriptive goal and involved the study of various forms of government, including both virtuous and tyrannical ones. In a similar fashion, he argued, physicians studied venoms not to prepare them but to identify remedies and antidotes.[49] Settala began writing *Della Ragion di Stato* when he was appointed *Protofisico*, an authoritative position in matters of public health that he held during the plague epidemic cycle in Milan between 1627 and 1630 (he would die soon afterward, in 1633). However, the physician had already developed his views on reason of state while teaching moral philosophy at the Canobian Schools in Milan.[50] Settala's interest in reason of state combined his political Tacitism, which harmonized reason of state theories with the moral stances of the Counter-Reformation, with his material engagement in public health.[51] His earlier (1590) and significant work on Hippocrates, however, unveils a different aspect of the intersection between political control and medicine: the centrality of knowledge of specific geographies in medical discourse and practice. Experiential knowledge is one of the key themes of Settala's commentary on Hippocrates. In this four-hundred-page treatise, the physician presented Greek passages from the Hippocratic *AWP*, followed by a Latin commentary, portraying Hippocrates as someone who 'used to take note of everything he observed, either by demonstration or by his everyday experience of the sick'.[52] However, Settala further emphasized how physicians' experience ('experientia') of sick bodies was coupled, in Hippocrates' work, with a knowledge ('cognitio') of the air ('aeris ambientis'), the winds, and, more generally, the sites ('locorum') where medical healing took place ('in quibus mederi velis medicus'). Settala also

44. Cardano, *Commentarii in Hippocratis de aere, aquis, et locis opus*. See further Siraisi, 'Girolamo Cardano and the Art of Medical Narrative', p. 591. See also Nutton, 'Hippocrates in the Renaissance'. On medical commentaries in the sixteenth century, see again Siraisi, *The Clock and the Mirror*, pp. 123 ff.
45. Settala, *Librum Hippocratis* (Cologne: Ciotti, 1590).
46. Cohn, *Cultures of Plague*, p. 262.
47. Martin, 'Lodovico Settala's Aristotelian *Problemata* Commentary', pp.19–42.
48. Ibid., p. 41. On seeds theory, see Nutton, 'The Seeds of Disease', pp. 418–39. On the long history of seed theory, see Hirai, *Le concept de semence*.
49. Botero, *Della Ragion di Stato Libri Sette*, p. 8.
50. Mellerio, 'Ludovico Settala'. The Canobian schools were founded by Paolo Canobio (XVI century) and dedicated to the teaching of philosophy and dialectics. See Caselli, *Nuovo ritratto di Milano*, p. 100.
51. On Tacitism in the medical profession, see d'Alessio, 'Usi politici della medicina', pp. 269–82.
52. Settala, *Librum Hippocratis*, p. 2.

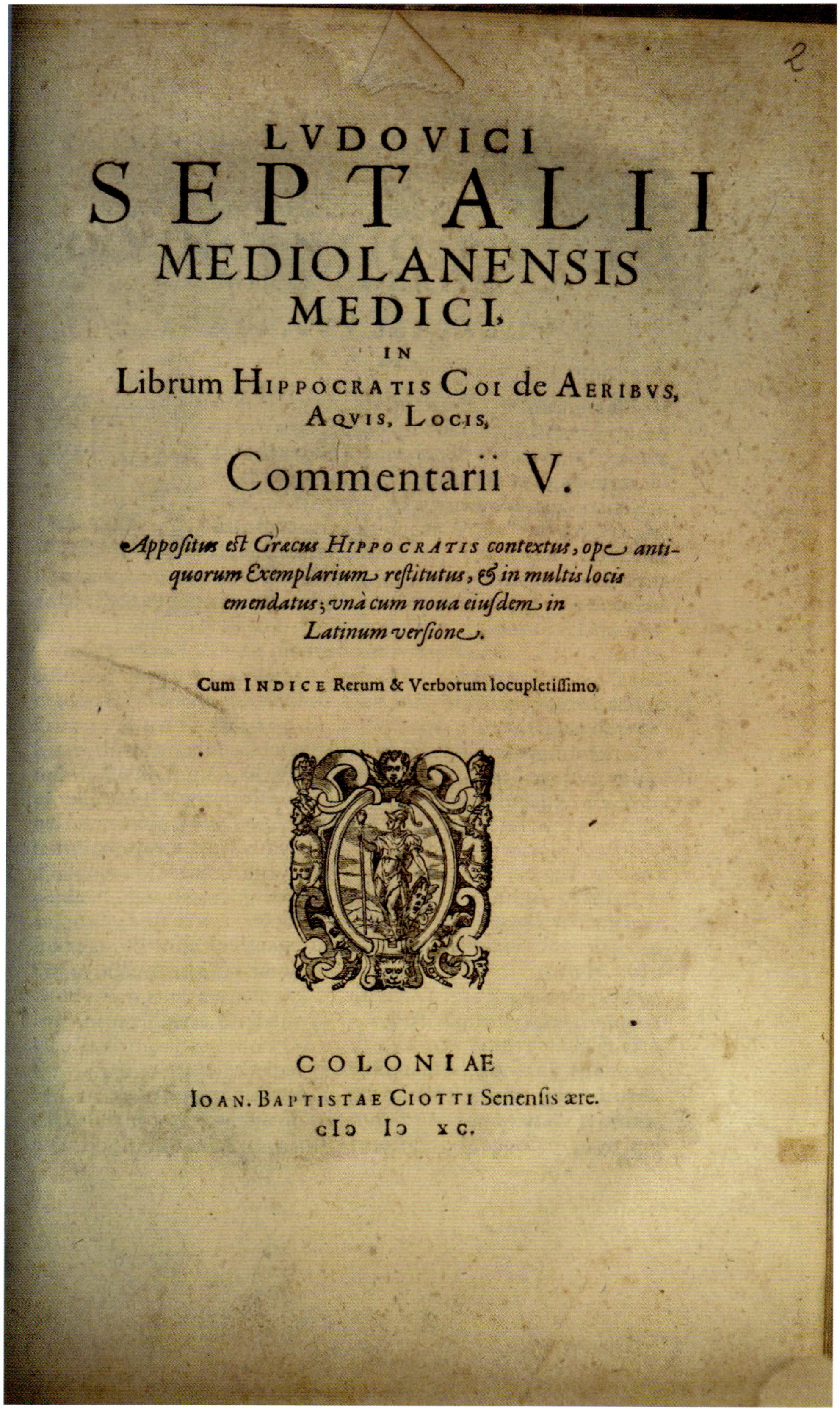

LVDOVICI
SEPTALII
MEDIOLANENSIS
MEDICI,
IN
Librum HIPPOCRATIS COI de AERIBVS,
AQVIS, LOCIS,
Commentarii V.

Appositus est Græcus HIPPOCRATIS contextus, ope antiquorum Exemplarium restitutus, & in multis locis emendatus; unà cum noua eiusdem in Latinum versione.

Cum INDICE Rerum & Verborum locupletissimo.

COLONIAE
IOAN. BAPTISTAE CIOTTI Senensis ære.
cIↃ IↃ XC.

27. Frontispiece of Lodovico Settala, *Ludovici Septalii Mediolanensis medici in librum Hippocratis Coi De aeribus, aquis, locis commentarii V* (Cologne: Ciotti, 1590).

commented on Hippocrates' passages on waters, arguing for their examination in good and bad state ('earunde perfectione et malitia'):

> The physician must know, through his art, the nature of waters ('natura aquarum'), as well as their good and evil state, for their change is usually very troublesome, and their use is often of the greatest importance, for they provoke great changes in the body.[53]

Settala dedicated various sections of his commentary to waters, pointing out that *AWP* did not address water universally ('universaliter') but rather focused on their specificities. Hippocrates's *AWP*, he argued, distinguished between geographical knowledge of waters,—such as the locations of torrents, rivers, and lakes—and a material understanding of the waters used by the inhabitants of specific sites. He claimed that whenever they ventured into uncharted territories, physicians needed to secure both forms of knowledge to make predictions and prescribe treatments.

After highlighting ancient views on water as the principle of all things, as seen in Hesiod and Pindar, Settala focused on sections of the Hippocratic *AWP* that elaborated on stagnant and marshy waters. He claimed that stagnant waters caused various diseases and were recognizable because of their unpleasant ('ingratus') and slimy ('limosus') taste, putrid odor ('putrido odore'), and dark color ('colore atro').[54] If ingested in the summer, stagnant waters affected the stomach, while in the winter, descending slowly in the bladder, they provoked pleurisy. However, Settala also addressed ambiguities in the Hippocratic *AWP*, claiming that Hippocrates did not clarify how waters with unhealthy properties, such as aluminous water ('aqua aluminosa') or salty water ('aqua salsa'), could be beneficial to bodily health, as occurred, for example, in the case of thermal baths. Thermal waters, rich in metallic properties, were noxious for drinking but beneficial for bathing. Settala dedicated an extensive commentary to analyzing the nature of marshes and stagnant and lacustrine waters, placing the first two at the peak of noxiousness. However, he discussed stagnant waters not only as a type of 'site' but also as a metaphor for everything unwelcoming and infertile. In another passage, he drew a comparison between the womb and stagnant waters, arguing that just as humidity in the maternal womb could hinder generation, stagnant waters prevented cereal seeds from taking root.[55]

The projection of a specific agricultural landscape, characterized by stagnant waters, onto the human and, more specifically, female body, connects Settala's neo-Hippocratic medical knowledge with contemporary discourses on population and depopulation processes, as previously mentioned in relation to Botero's work. In fact, in the same section in which the analogy between the female body and the desolate landscape takes shape, Settala also referred to Hippocrates's *De natura muliebri* (*On the Nature of Woman*) and *De sterilibus* (*On Barrenness*). More specifically, he noted that while there are many causes of sterility, 'an important place has been attributed to excessive humidity.' A wet environment dilated the pores of the skin, and humidity would reach the uterus, dry and cold by nature, through the head and 'superior bodily parts'.[56] The claim in the Novara report concerning the depopulation of the local countryside due to the stagnant waters of rice fields thus had a medical foundation. More generally, in the tradition of neo-Hippocratic medical thought, knowledge of places and sites was central to the training of physicians. Knowing places also meant being useful to the community and serving *salute commune*. Physicians were key in producing the final Health Board reports on the salubrity (or lack thereof) of specific sites. Their medical discourse intersected with the political and institutional drive toward territorial control and the policing of marginal and transitional spaces. In the tradition of Vitruvius's *Ten Books on Architecture*, the location and layout of homes should be chosen according to the orientation of the Sun and winds, with a preference accorded to winds coming from the north, and avoiding the geographical proximity of any other building or landscape feature which might block the airflow.[57] Vitruvius's *Ten Books* had been translated in Latin for the first time in 1486, quickly becoming a key reference in humanist architectural culture, especially in Leon Battista Alberti's *De re aedificatoria* (1485), Giuseppe Viola Zanini's *Della*

53. Ibid., p. 4.
54. Ibid., p. 30.
55. Ibid., p. 72.
56. Ibid.
57. See Vitruvius, *Ten Books on Architecture* 1. 1.

architettura (1627), and Vincenzo Scamozzi's *L'idea dell'architettura universal* (1615).[58]

ENGINEERING PRACTICE

Physicians were thus not the only actors involved in applying medical knowledge concerning the impact of the environment on the health of individuals and communities. Spaces and geographies were hybrid domains, where medical knowledge intersected with architecture and engineering. Although engineering knowledge was obviously not medical, its application went hand in hand with medical ideas and practices. Engineers and land surveyors were hired by various institutions in early modern Milan, one of those being the Health Board. The Duchy of Milan had a long-standing tradition of engineering, rooted in its strategic position in the Italian Wars of the Quattro-Cinquecento, epitomized by Leonardo da Vinci's multiple roles under Ludovico Sforza, a tradition that persisted in Milan under the French and Spanish rule in the sixteenth and seventeenth centuries. Documents such as petitions to become engineers highlight the mechanism by which authority and status were established in the discipline. These petitions, structured around set questions and answers, shed light on the essential skills required of engineers and the importance of measuring distances in the countryside. When the son of Health Board engineer Giuseppe Maria Robecco sought admission to the College of Engineers, it was another engineer who answered the questions posed by the College about the boy's abilities. This fellow engineer focused on the young Rebecco's observational competence:

> Every time that I have had occasion to deal with Mr. Giuseppe Maria Robecco, I have always seen his son, Mr. Bernardo, in his study, at a table, writing and copying texts and images of his profession with attention and diligence.[59]

Despite originating in a non-medical context, these forms of expertise acquired medical relevance, as they played a critical role in resolving public health conflicts. Although engineers' training before performing 'fieldwork' and entering the College was still typically humanistic, as the image of Bernardo in his study tells us, engineers were also highly mobile actors. They moved from one place to another, from cities to the countryside, from indoors to outdoors, from supposedly noxious sites such as marshes or rice paddies to small urban centers, where they assessed the distances between manholes, ponds, and humans. Late in the seventeenth century, when engineer Giovanni Maria Robecco asked the *Magistrato Straordinario* to make him Cameral Engineer, in the tradition of the Robecco family, he listed some of the key tasks of his predecessors, such as mastering water channels and controlling 'water and sown rice fields'.[60] Engineers turned transitional spaces, such as rice fields, into controllable places with clear boundaries, ensuring that their noxious air could not reach inhabited areas and their stagnant waters would not contaminate drinkable waters. Engineers like Clarici played a key role in visualizing contested spaces, where negotiations among various social actors centered on the harmfulness of water and air. Engineering drawings became essential tools for constructing evidence. Clarici's drawing, with which we opened this essay, supposedly represented a rural space in relation to an urban center, catalyzing the senses of various actors. This underscores the growing importance of visual experience in the making of medical and, more broadly, scientific knowledge at the end of the sixteenth century and how the concern of 'image makers' with imitation was coupled with a drive for truth in legal settings.[61] When decisions regarding whether or not to cultivate rice fields around urban centers had to be made, state institutions relied on the measurements, drawings, and maps of engineers. These objects were used to make choices that would have legal repercussions on public health practices. The concept of *disegnare* (to draw) carried significant implications, intersecting with ideas of planning, projecting, organizing, and policing territories

58. See Cavallo and Storey, *Healthy Living in Late Renaissance Italy*, p. 81.
59. 'Tutte le volte che ho avuto occasione di trattare con il Sig. Giuseppe Maria Robecco, ho sempre veduto il Sig. Bernardo suo figlio, nel di lui studio, sedendo ad un tavolino a scrivere, copiar scritture, e disegni della sua professione, con tutta attenzione e diligenza.' BTMi, Famiglie, Robecco 1312, unnumbered page. Even though this source is from the eighteenth century, procedures to enter the Collegio did not change until the 1770s.
60. 'delas aguas, y sementeras de el aroz'. ASMi, Famiglie 157 (Robecchi). Plea from Giovanni Maria Robecchi to the *Magistrato Straordinario*, 18 October 1684. See Zanetti, *Janelo Torriano*; Repishti, 'Architetti e ingegneri' and Brambilla, 'Le professioni scientifico-tecniche', pp. 345–446.
61. On this shift, see Pereda, *Crime and Illusion*, on the Spanish Golden Age. On the concept of experience in the early modern period, see Dear, 'The Meanings of Experience', pp. 106–31.

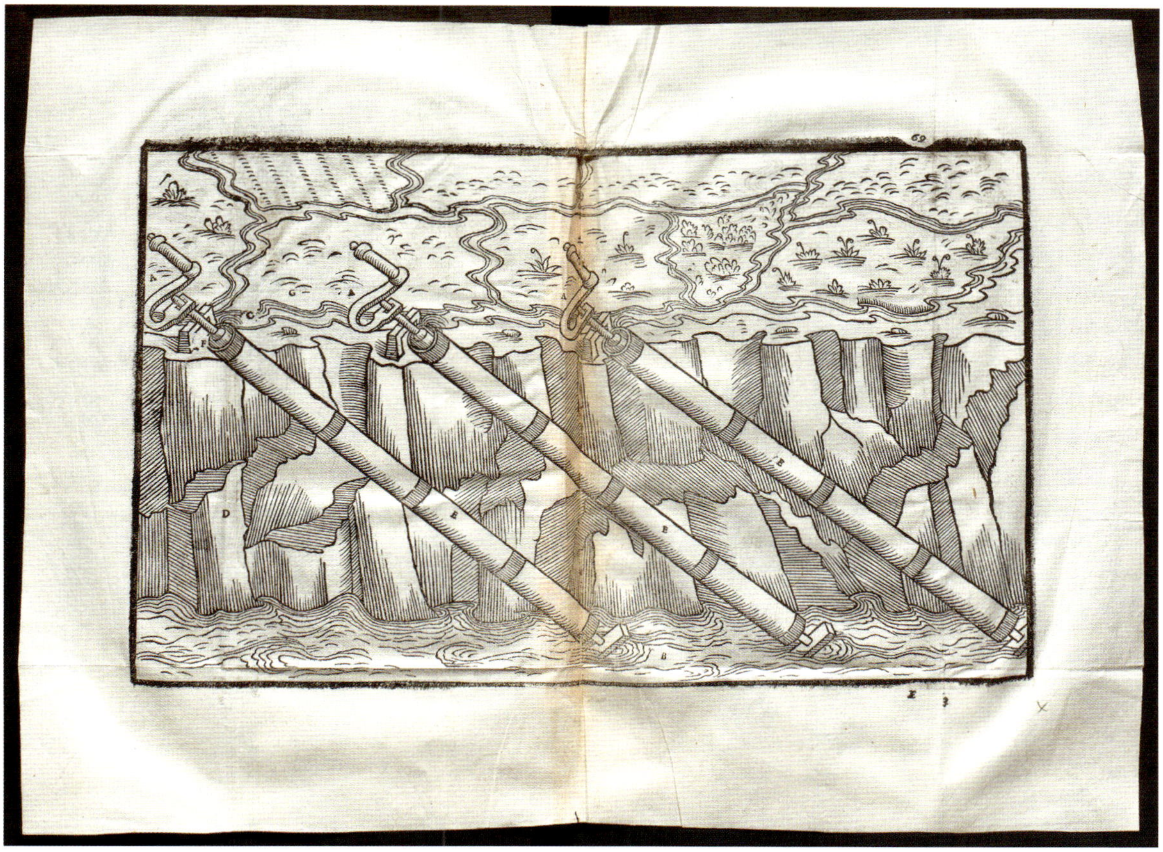

28. The image, from Giuseppe Ceredi, *Tre discorsi sul modo d'alzare l'acque da' luoghi bassi* (Parma: Seth Viotti, 1567), shows the application of Ceredi's screw on a riverbank.

and reminding us of the key role of intellectual endeavors in the process of visualizing spaces.[62]

At the same time, engineering knowledge, particularly concerning the diversion of water channels, land reclamation, and marsh drainage, garnered the interest of physicians. One notable example is that of a *fisico* from Piacenza, Giuseppe Ceredi, who in 1565 asked the Milanese magistracies to sponsor his machine—a special Archimedean screw intended to pump water from channels and streams, facilitating field irrigation.[63]

Ceredi's project faced strong opposition from the *Magistrato Straordinario* and the *Vicario di Provvisione* in Milan, Alessandro Archinto, who refused to invest public finances in the machine, seeing it as a danger to the economy of the Duchy. Archinto believed that Ceredi's machine would turn fields dedicated to wheat cultivation into pastures, posing a potential threat to urban provisioning.[64] The machine was eventually sponsored by the institutions of the Duchy on the grounds that it was useful to the cultivation of 'millet, fava, and beans', key staples in the diet of the poor.[65] However, Ceredi himself warned against the indiscriminate use of the machine for the irrigation of rice fields. He thus merged his knowledge of ancient Archimedean mechanics, which inspired the screw, with a knowledge of ancient medical texts and a neo-Hippocratic approach to the knowledge of places. Places could be transformed and tamed thanks to technological and engineering interventions, and water could be moved from one site to another to serve the needs of local economies; however, landowners, as well as

62. On this, I remind to the recent work of Murphy, *Waters and Welfare*, p. 124, n. 18.
63. ASMi, Acque Parte Antica 6. Document dated September 1565. See Maffioli, *La via delle acque*, pp. 25–30.
64. Ceredi, *Tre discorsi*, p. 94.
65. Ibid., p. 95. On fava beans in bread making, see Gentilcore, 'Il pane nell'Europa moderna', pp. 459–78.

state institutions, should still ensure that these ways of controlling nature did not violate key tenets of neo-Hippocratic medical practice.[66] Such balance could be achieved only through a proper knowledge of sites, which Ceredi clearly advocated when he claimed that the use of the machine for the cultivation of rice would be acceptable as long as 'rice fields [were] exposed to northern winds,' which would dissipate humidity and 'protect neighbors from universal infirmities'.[67]

CONCLUSION

As discussed in this chapter, stagnant waters, particularly those in rice fields, catalyzed contrasting preoccupations. They were spaces of transition, imbued with various meanings. Rice fields, in particular, became symbolic sites over which state institutions and magistracies—especially the Health Board and the Church—struggled to establish comprehensive control at a time when healthscaping practices and territorial knowledge were becoming essential to the state's existence. From a religious point of view, the migrant workforce, often eluding the practice and ritual of confession, turned rice fields into a threat to the Counter-Reformation's agenda. Furthermore, rice fields became sites where different cultures of knowledge, such as medicine and engineering, intersected. As we saw in the case of Settala's commentary to the Hippocratic *AWP*, discourses on stagnant waters were present in contemporary humanistic medical accounts. The interest in the Hippocratic corpus was not simply the expression of an erudite humanism but was intertwined with the broader imperative for physicians to understand the health threats associated with specific sites. This essay has also shown that rice fields were not only interesting from the point of view of medical practice but could be known through the drawings and measurements of engineers, who attempted to contain their murkiness and established their distance from inhabited areas. These practices of quantification and measurement reveal the relationship between the preservation of public health and the economic needs of urban centers such as Milan and Novara. The drawing by Clarici, observed by various actors trying to make sense of the dangers posed by the Novara paddy fields, visualized spaces of conflict, yet it also mirrored cultures of medical and engineering knowledge.

Debates concerning rice fields around Novara lasted until late in the seventeenth century, specifically 1661, when the Health Board prompted the Milanese College of Physicians to issue a printed report on rice cultivation in the region.[68] The author of the report, physician Paolo Maria Terzago (1625–95), claimed that the presence of paddy fields could be tolerated if their borders managed to contain their thick exhalations. He concluded that that was not the case because of winds blowing from the south. He grounded his argument on medical authorities, not only Hippocrates but also Democritus, Ibn-Sina's (Avicenna's) *De febribus* (1560), published as a commentary by Giovanni Arcolani, and the contemporary Lazarus Rivière's *Istitutiones medicae* (1656). The report was followed by a later *Consulta* (1680) from the Health Board, focusing on the corruption of the stagnant waters of rice fields in Novara. The *Consulta*, printed but unsigned, argued that stagnant waters affected the 'constitution' of air, corrupting its purity at the risk of provoking 'endless evils', which were easily 'transformable into an epidemic', disrupting ('sconcertando') the 'good symmetry of human bodies'.[69] Though the *Consulta* focused on Novara, it drew more general conclusions, which could be applied elsewhere in the Duchy. In particular, the document highlighted the 'situation' (*situazione*) of the city of Milan, located in a plain, surrounded by mountains, valleys, and bodies of water that blocked wind and air circulation. The underlying assumption of the report was that controlling the influence of stagnant waters and their noxious vapors was not only a medical imperative but also a social and economic one: 'One pestilential infection in the territory of Novara would have represented a damage and a danger to the entire body of the state, to public health, and to commerce with nearby countries'.[70] The application of neo-Hippocratic ideas merged with the goals of keeping the body politic intact and protecting the commercial potential of the Duchy. More broadly, practices of heathscaping—such as the spatial control and measurement of paddy fields by the Health Boards and engineers—intersected with theoretical discourses about the preservation of state sovereignty.

66. On practices of 'nature control' and for the specific case of air, see Cavallo, 'Health, Air and Material Culture', pp. 695–716.
67. Ceredi, *Tre discorsi*, p. 92.
68. *Parere del Collegio dei Medici della Città di Milano, Eccitato dal Magistrato di Sanità*, c. 1661.
69. *Consulta del Magistrato di Sanità fatta a S. M. à 5 ottobre 1680, toccante a provvedere agli incovenienti per lo seminerio de' risi*, pp. 3–4.
70. *Consulta del Magistrato di Sanità fatta a S. M. à 5 ottobre 1680*, p. 11.

According to the 'local' Milanese tradition of Boterian reason of state, the *grandezza* of the state was based on its population, as commercial strength relied more on human *industria* than on material wealth, be that agricultural or mineralogical. Without people, wealth could not be extracted from the soil, and the soil could not become truly productive. Discourses on rice fields thus reflected not only ideas of healthscaping, grounded on neo-Hippocratic medical theories and practices, but also models and theories of social and political order.

WORKS CITED

Printed Primary Sources

Bodin, Jean, *Six Books of the Commonwealth* (London: G. Bishop, 1606).

Botero, Giovanni, *Della Ragion di Stato Libri Tre* (Venice, appresso i Gioliti, 1598; 1st edn 1589).

Botero, Giovanni, *Relatione della repubblica venetiana* (Venice, Giovanni Varisco, 1605).

Cardano, Girolamo, *De methodo medendi sectiones quatuor* (Paris: in aedibus Rouillij [i.e. Philippe Gaultier], via Iacobaea, sub signo Concordiae, 1565).

Cardano, Girolamo, *Commentarii in Hippocratis de aere, aquis, et locis opus* (Basel: Ex Officina Henric Petrina, 1570).

Ceredi, Giuseppe, *Tre discorsi sul modo d'alzare l'acque da' luoghi bassi* (Parma: Seth Viotti, 1567).

Consulta del Magistrato di Sanità fatta a S. M. à 5 ottobre 1680, toccante a provvedere agli inconvenienti per lo seminerio de' risi, 1680, found in ASMi, Atti di Governo, Agricoltura Parte Antica 53.

Durante, Castore, *Herbario Novo* (Rome, Bartholomeo Bonfadino e Tito Diani, 1585).

Parere del Collegio dei Medici della Città di Milano, Eccitato dal Magistrato di Sanità, *c.* 1661, found in ASMi, Atti di Governo, Agricoltura Parte Antica 53.

Settala, Lodovico, *Della Ragion di Stato Libri Sette* (Milan, Giovanni Battista Bidelli, 1627).

Settala, Lodovico, *Librum Hippocratis Coi de aeribus, aquis, locis, Commentarii V* (Cologne: Ciotti, 1590).

Vitruvius, *Ten Books on Architecture*, trans. by Ingrid D. Rowland (Cambridge: Cambridge University Press, 1999).

Secondary Sources

Andretta, Elisa, 'Il filo dell'acqua: fiumi e saperi nel mondo di Giovanni Botero', in *Un mondo di Relazioni: Giovanni Botero e i saperi nella Roma del Cinquecento*, ed. by Elisa Andretta, Romain Descendre, and Antonella Romano (Rome: Viella, 2002), pp. 363–400.

Appuhn, Karl, *A Forest on the Sea: Environmental Expertise in Renaissance Venice* (Baltimore, MD: John Hopkins University Press, 2009).

Bachelard, Gaston, *L'eau et les rêves* (Paris : José Corti, 1942).

Brambilla, Elena, 'Le professioni scientifico-tecniche a Milano e la riforma dei collegi privilegiati (Sec. XVII–1770),' in *Ideologia e scienza nell'opera di Paolo Frisi*, ed. Gennaro Barbarisi, 2 vols (Milan; Franco Angeli, 1987), vol.2, pp. 345–446.

Braun, Harald, 'Knowledge and Counsel in Giovanni Botero's *Ragion di stato*', *Journal of Jesuit Studies*, 4 (2017), 270–89.

Carmichael, Ann, 'The Last Past Plague: The Uses of Memory in Renaissance Epidemics', *Journal of the History of Medicine*, 53 (1998), 132–60.

Caselli, Giuseppe, *Nuovo Ritratto di Milano in riguardo alle Belle Arti* (Milan: Francesco Sonzogno, 1827).

Cavallo Sandra and Tessa Storey, *Healthy Living in Late Renaissance Italy* (Oxford: Oxford University Press, 2013).

Cavallo, Sandra, 'Health, Air and Material Culture in the Early Modern Italian Domestic Environment', *Social History of Medicine*, 29.4 (2016), 695–716.

Cohn, Samuel, *Cultures of Plague: Medical Thinking at the End of the Renaissance* (Oxford: Oxford University Press, 2010).

Continisio, Chiara, 'Giovanni Botero', in *Il Contributo italiano alla storia del Pensiero: Diritto* (2012).

d'Alessio, Silvana, 'Usi politici della medicina nella prima età moderna', in *Interpretare e curare nel Rinascimento*, ed. by Andrea Carlino, Maria Conforti, and Antonio Clericuzio (Rome: Carocci, 2013), 269–282.

d'Amico, Stefano, 'Spanish Milan: 1535–1706', in *A Companion to Late Medieval and Early Modern Milan*, ed. by Andrea Gamberini (Leiden: Brill, 2015), 46–68.

de Boer, Wietse, *The Conquest of the Soul: Confession, Discipline, and Public Order in Counter-Reformation Milan* (Leiden: Brill, 2000).

Dear, Peter, 'The Meanings of Experience', in *The Cambridge History of Science*, ed. by Katharine Park and Lorraine Daston (Cambridge University Press, 2006), 106–31.

di Tullio, Matteo, 'Tra ecologia ed economia: uomo e acqua nella pianura lombarda d'età moderna', in *Storia economica e ambiente italiano (ca. 1400–1850)*, ed. by G. Alfani, M. di Tullio, and L. Mocarelli (Milan: Franco Angeli, 2012), 283–99.

di Tullio, Matteo, 'Rese agricole, scorte alimentari, strutture famigliari: le campagne dello stato di Milano a metà Cinquecento', in *Ricchezza, valore, proprietà in età preindustriale (1400–1850)*, ed. by Guido Alfani and Michela Barbot (Venice: Marsilio, 2009), 293–318.

di Tullio, Matteo, 'Domestici e agricoltura capitalista. Relazioni di lavoro e di potere nelle campagne lombarde della prima età moderna', *Mélanges de l'École française de Rome - Italie et Méditerranée modernes et contemporaines*, 131-1 (2019), 87–97.

Dobson, Mary, *Contours of Death and Disease in Early Modern England* (Cambridge: Cambridge University Press, 1997).

Durand, Gilbert, *Le strutture antropologiche dell'immaginario* (Bari, 1991; 1st ed. Paris, 1963).

Geltner, Guy, and Janna Coomans, 'The Healthscaping Approach: Towards a Global History of Early Public Health', *Historical Methods: A Journal of Quantitative and Interdisciplinary History* (2022), 18–33.

Gentilcore, David, *Food and Health in Early Modern Europe: Diet, Medicine and Society. 1450–1800* (Bloomsbury, 2016).

Gentilcore, David, 'From "Vilest Beverage" to "Universal Medicine": Drinking Water in Printed Regimens and Health Guides, 1450–1750", *Social History of Medicine*, 33 (2020), 683–703.

Gentilcore, David, 'Il pane nell'Europa moderna tra dietetica e alimentazione', in *La civiltà del pane: storia, tecniche e simboli dal Mediterraneo all'Atlantico*, ed. by Gabriele Archetti (Brescia: Cisam, 2015), 459–478.

Giglioni, Guido, 'Girolamo Cardano e Giulio Cesare Scaligero: il dibattito sul ruolo dell'anima vegetativa', in *Girolamo Cardano: le opere, le fonti, la vita*, ed. by Marialuisa Baldi and Guido Canziani (Milan: FrancoAngeli, 1999), 313–39.

Ginzburg, Carlo, *Il formaggio e i vermi: il cosmo di un mugnaio del '500* (Turin: Einaudi, 1976).

Governing the Environment in the Early Modern World: Theory and Practice, ed. by Sara Miglietti and John Morgan (London: Routledge, 2017).

Henderson, John, *Florence under Siege: Surviving Plague in an Early Modern City* (New Haven: Yale University Press, 2019).

Hirai, Hiro, *Le concept de semence dans les théories de la matière à la Renaissance: De Marsile Ficin à Pierre Gassendi* (Turnhout: Brepols, 2005).

Hirai, Hiro, 'Cosmic Heat in Telesio between Aristotle's "De generatione animalium" and Hippocrates' "De carnibus"', in *Bernardino Telesio tra filosofia naturale e scienza moderna*, ed. by Giuliana Mocchi (Rome: Serra, 2012), 71–83.

Hirai, Hiro, *Medical Humanism and Natural Philosophy: Renaissance Debates on Matter, Life and the Soul* (Leiden: Brill, 2011).

Hirai, Hiro, 'Prisca Theologia and Neoplatonic Reading of Hippocrates in Fernel, Cardano and Gemma', in *Cornelius Gemma: Cosmology, Medicine and Natural Philosophy in Renaissance Louvain*, ed. by Hiro Hirai (Rome: Serra, 2008), 91–104.

Knox, Dilwyn, 'Giordano Bruno', in *The Stanford Encyclopedia of Philosophy*, ed. by Edward N. Zalta (Summer 2019 ed.).

Kress, Emily, 'Aristotle on Spontaneous Generation, Spontaneity, and Natural Processes', in *Oxford Studies in Ancient Philosophy*, lviii, ed. by Victor Caston (Oxford: Oxford Studies in Ancient Philosophy, 2021).

Long, Pamela O., 'Trading Zones: Arenas of Exchange during the Late-Medieval/Early Modern Transition to the New Empirical Sciences', in *History of Technology*, xxxi, ed. by Ian Inkster (2012), 840–47.

Lonie, Iain M., *The Hippocratic Treatises: 'On Generation', 'On the Nature of the Child', 'Diseases IV'* (Berlin: Walter de Gruyter, 1981).

Maddaluno, Lavinia, 'Public Health in Milan', in *Routledge Encyclopedia for the Italian Renaissance* (Routledge, 2023).

Maffioli, Cesare, *La via delle acque (1500–1700): appropriazione delle arti e trasformazione delle matematiche* (Florence: Olschki, 2010).

Manning, Gideon, and James Wilberding, 'Reflection II: The World Soul and Spontaneous Generation', in *World Soul: A History*, ed. by James Wilberding (New York, 2021), 177–85.

Martin, Craig, 'Lodovico Settala's Aristotelian *Problemata* Commentary and Late-Renaissance Hippocratic Medicine', in *Early Modern Medicine and Natural Philosophy: History, Philosophy and Theory of the Life Sciences*, xiv, ed. by Peter Distelzweig, Benjamin Goldberg, and Evan Ragland (Dordrecht: Springer, 2016), 19–42.

Medicine and Space: Body, Surroundings and Borders in Antiquity and the Middle Ages, ed. by Patricia Baker, Han Nijdam, and Karine van 't Land (Leiden: Brill, 2012).

Mellerio, Giorgio Giacomo, 'Ludovico Settala', *Dizionario Biografico degli Italiani*, 92 (2018).

Miglietti, Sara, 'Debating Greatness from Machiavelli to Botero', in *Early Modern Philosophers and the Renaissance Legacy*, ed. by Cecilia Muratori and Gianni Paganini, *International Archives of the History of Ideas/Archives internationales d'histoire des idées*, 220 (Cham: Springer, 2016), 239–57.

Morera, Raphaël, 'Marshes as Microclimates: Governing with the Environment in Early Modern France', in *Governing the Environment*, ed. by Miglietti and Morgan, 56–75.

Morera, Raphaël, 'Mise en valeur des zones humides et associations de gestion: naissance et affirmation de nouveaux pouvoirs territoriaux (France, XVIe-XVIIIe siècles)', *Siècles* 42 (2015). URL :http://journals.openedition.org/siecles /2946; DOI :https://doi.org/10.4000/siecles.2946 [accessed 17 September 2024]

Murphy, Caroline, 'Waters and Welfare: Rivers, Infrastructure and the Territorial Imagination in Grand Ducal Tuscany, 1549–1609' (unpublished doctoral dissertation, MIT, 2023).

Murphy, Hannah, 'Skin and Disease in Early Modern Medicine: Jan Jessen's *De cute, et cutaneis affectibus* (1601)', *Bulletin of the History of Medicine*, 94.2 (2020), 179–214.

Nutton, Vivian, 'Hippocrates in the Renaissance', in *Die hippokratischen Epidemien*, ed. by Gerhard Baader and Rolf Winau (Stuttgart, 1989), 418–39.

Nutton, Vivian, 'The Seeds of Disease: An Explanation of Contagion and Infection from the Greeks to the Renaissance', *Medical History*, 27 (1983), 1–34.

Pereda, Felipe, *Crime and Illusion: The Art of Trust in the Spanish Golden Age* (Turnhout: Brepols, 2019).

Perrone Compagni, Vittoria, 'Un'ipotesi non impossibile: Pomponazzi sulla generazione spontanea dell'uomo (1518)', *Bruniana & Campanelliana* 13 (2007), 99–111.

Prosperi, Adriano, *Tribunali della coscienza: inquisitori, confessori, missionari* (Turin: Einaudi, 1996).

Rawcliffe, Carole and Claire Weeda, *Policing the Urban Environment in Premodern Europe* (Amsterdam: Amsterdam University Press, 2019).

Repishti, Francesco, 'Architetti e ingegneri comunali, ducali, e camerali nella Milano sforzesca e spagnola,' in Ingegneri ducali e camerali nel Ducato e nello Stato di Milano (1450–1706): dizionario biobibliografico, ed. by Paolo Bossi (Florence: EdiFir, 2007), pp. 23–30.

Siraisi, Nancy, *The Clock and the Mirror: Girolamo Cardano and Renaissance Medicine* (Princeton University Press, 1997).

Siraisi, Nancy, 'Girolamo Cardano and the Art of Medical Narrative', *Journal of the History of Ideas*, 52 (1991), 581–602.

Slack, Paul, *The Invention of Improvement: Information & Material Progress in Seventeenth-Century England* (Oxford: Oxford University Press, 2015).

Stevens Crawshaw, Jane, *Cleaning Up Renaissance Italy. Environmental Ideas and Urban Practice in Genoa and Venice* (Oxford: Oxford University Press, 2023).

Zambelli, Paola, 'From Menocchio to Piero Della Francesca: The Work of Carlo Ginzburg', *The Historical Journal*, 28.4 (1985), 983–99.

Zanetti, Cristiano, Janello Torriano and the Spanish Empire (Leiden: Brill, 2017).

Authors' Biographies

ELISA ANDRETTA is Directrice de recherche at the CNRS (LARHRA, Lyon, France). She is the author of *Roma Medica. Anatomie d'un système médical au XVIe siècle* (Rome, EFR, 2011) and *Le Monde sous l'œil des médecins. Nature et politique à l'Escorial et au Vatican (XVIe siècle)* (Paris, Classique Garnier, 2024), as well as of numerous works on the social and cultural history of medicine and natural history in early modern Italy and Spain. Together with Romain Descendre (ENS-Lyon) and Antonella Romano (EHESS), she is co-responsible for the project "Le monde dans une péninsule: espaces urbains, présences étrangères, économies des savoirs dans l'Italie du Cinquecento" ([MONDO500)], École française de Rome, LARHRA, Centre A. Koyré, Labex CoMod.

GASTON J. BASILE is currently senior researcher and series editor for MAP's publications, as well as professor in the Department of Classics and the postgraduate school at the University of Buenos Aires. His latest research explores the translation of scientific texts during the Italian Renaissance. He is currently leading a large-scale project on previously unstudied recipe collections from Medici Florence. His postdoctoral work has been supported by fellowships from the National Endowment for the Humanities (2022-2023), the Harvard Center for Italian Renaissance Studies (2021-2022), The Warburg Institute (2019), the Deutscher Akademischer Austauschdienst (2018), the University of Buenos Aires (2015-2017), and the University of Siena (2016, 2011). His most recent research has been published in journals such as the *Journal of the Warburg and Courtauld Institutes*, *Arts et Savoirs*, *Medievalia et Humanistica*, the *Bulletin of the Institute of Classical Studies*, *Dialogues d'Histoire Ancienne*, and *Renaissance Quarterly* (William Nelson Prize for the best research article of 2023). His forthcoming monograph investigates the role of Greek-to-Latin translation in the development of scientific knowledge in fifteenth-century Italy.

SANDRA CAVALLO is Professor Emerita of Early Modern History at Royal Holloway, University of London. She has written extensively on various aspects of the history of medicine in early modern Italy, as well as on gender, material culture and domestic space, and their relationship with health management. Her publications include the monographs *Charity and Power in Early Modern Italy* (1995), *Artisans of the Body in Early Modern Italy. Identities, Families, Masculinities* (2007, p/b 2010), and *Healthy Living in Late Renaissance Italy* (2013, co-authored with Tessa Storey), winner of the Roland Bainton prize for History 2014. Among her co-edited volumes: *Widowhood in Medieval and Early Modern Europe* (1999), *Spaces, objects and identities in early modern Italian medicine* (2008), *Domestic Institutional Interiors in Early Modern Europe* (2009), *A Cultural History of Childhood and the Family* vol. 3, *The Early Modern Age* (2010) and *Conserving Health in Early Modern European Culture* (2017). She is currently working at a monograph tentatively titled: Medicine at Home in Early Modern Europe.

LUCIA DACOME is Associate Professor and Pauline M.H. Mazumdar Chair in the History of Medicine at the Institute for the History and Philosophy of Science and Technology, University of Toronto, and cross-appointed to the History Department. Her research focuses on themes at the intersection of the social, cultural, and material history of health and medicine, the history of the body, the histories of women and gender, and the histories of slavery and race in early modern Europe and the Mediterranean world. She is the author of *Malleable Anatomies: Models, Makers, and Material Culture in Eighteenth-Century Italy* (2017) and co-editor of *Unruly Objects: Material Entanglements in the Arts and Sciences* (2020). Her research has also appeared in the *Bulletin of the History of Medicine*, *Eighteenth-Century Studies*, the *Journal of the History of Ideas*, *History of Science*, *History of Psychiatry*, *Past & Present*, *Renaissance Studies*, and *Studies in History and Philosophy of Biological and Biomedical Sciences*. She is currently at work on a book-length project on slavery, medicine, and natural inquiry in early modern Italy, focusing on Tuscany and the port city of Livorno.

MARIA PIA DONATO is CNRS Research Professor at the Institut d'Histoire Moderne et Contemporaine in Paris, and teaches History of Science and Medicine at the École Normale Supérieure in Paris. She is a historian of early modern culture and the history of science and medicine, especially in a Catholic context. Her recent publications include the monographs *Sudden Death. Medicine and Religion in 18th-Century Rome* (2014, originally published in Italian in 2010) and *L'archivio del mondo—Quando Napoleone confiscò la storia* (2019), and the edited book *Medicine and the Inquisition in the Early Modern World* (2019). She is now working on the history of surgery and surgeons, has published several works on the subject, and is currently co-editing a volume on surgical training in early modern Europe.

JOHN HENDERSON is Emeritus Professor of Italian Renaissance History, Birkbeck, University of London, and Emeritus Fellow of Wolfson College, University of Cambridge. He has published a wide range of books and articles on the history of Italy from the Renaissance to the early modern period, with a special interest in history of religion, charity, medicine and public health. Major monographs include: *Piety and Charity in Late Medieval Florence* (1994 and Chicago, 1997); *The Great Pox. The French Disease in Renaissance Europe*, with John Arrizabalaga and Roger French (1997), and *The Renaissance Hospital. Healing the Body and Healing the Soul* (2006). His most recent books include *Florence Under Siege: Surviving Plague in an Early Modern City* (2019); *Plague and the City*, edited with Lukas Englemann and Christos Lynteris (2018); and *Representing Infirmity. Diseased Bodies in Renaissance Italy*, edited with Fredrika Jacobs and Jonathan K. Nelson (2021). His latest book, *The French Disease in Renaissance Italy: Representation and Experience*, was published by Cambridge University Press in late 2024. He is co-editor with Jonathan K. Nelson of the Cambridge University Press book series 'Renaissance Elements'.

LAVINIA MADDALUNO (PhD, Cantab.) is an early modern historian working at Ca' Foscari University (Venice). Her expertise crosses the history of science and intellectual history, with a focus on early modern Europe. She has written on political economy in the Italian Enlightenment, on water management in seventeenth-century France and on public health in sixteenth-century Milan, among other themes. Her research received support from the EUI, the Warburg Institute and Villa I Tatti, the FMSH (Paris) and the Fondazione Einaudi. She is the author of *Science and* Political Economy *in Enlightenment Milan, 1760-1805*, for Oxford University Studies in the Enlightenment (Liverpool, 2024). More recently, Lavinia has been working and writing on the history of rice in the early modern Mediterranean and Europe, adopting a history of knowledge and environmental history perspective, and has been the 2024 visiting scholar at the Instituto de História Contemporanêa (Universidade Nova de Lisboa).

SABRINA MINUZZI is a historian of the book and a researcher specializing in the Social History of Medicine at the Department of Humanities and Cultural Heritage, University of Udine. She is the author of numerous essays and the monographs *Il secolo di carta: Antonio Bosio artigiano di testi e immagini nella Venezia del Seicento* (2009) and *Sul filo dei segreti: Farmacopea, libri e pratiche terapeutiche a Venezia in età moderna* (2016). She has also edited the special issue of *Nuncius: Journal of the Material and Visual History of Science* 2 (2021), titled *Printing Medical Knowledge: Vernacular Genres, Reception, and Dissemination*, which focuses on the incunabula and early modern production of medical-scientific texts. Her article 'Quick to say quack. Medicinal secrets from the household to the apothecary's shop in early eighteenth-century Venice', *Social History of Medicine* 1 (2019) has been awarded the Worth Estes Prize 2020 for the best paper published in the history of pharmacology in the previous two years.

ALESSANDRA QUARANTA is a historian specializing in social history of medicine in the early modern period. Since 2023, she has been a post-doctoral researcher at the University of Liège, Department of Historical Sciences. She is also currently collaborating with the Museum of Sciences of Trento. In April 2024 she lectured on the history of the early modern medical professions at the Department of Economics and Management of the University of Brescia, Historical Studies Unit. She was awarded postdoctoral research fellowships at the Universities of Vienna (2020–2022) and of Trento (2016–2018), and collaborated with the Friedrich-Meinecke-Institut of the Freie Universität Berlin (2020). Her main publications include: *Medici-physici trentini nella seconda metà del Cinquecento* (2019); *Medici italiani eretici nella seconda metà del Cinquecento* (2019); 'Italian Physicians at the Habsburg Courts (1550–1620)', *European History Quarterly*, 53/4 (2023),

549–578; 'Gender and the Doctor-Patient Relationship. The Casebook of Doctor Francesco Partini (1500–1569)', *Genesis. Rivista della Società Italiana delle Storiche*, 22/1 (2023), 201–227; 'The *Consilia* by Learned Physicians Pietro Andrea Mattioli and Francesco Partini. Dialectic Relations between Doctrine, Empirical Knowledge and Use of the Senses in the Sixteenth-Century Europe', *Social History of Medicine*, 35/1 (2022), 20–48.

SHARON STROCCHIA is Professor of History at Emory University (USA). A social and cultural historian, she has published widely on women, religion, health, and society in Renaissance Italy and has contributed to several ongoing digital projects. Among her major publications are *Death and Ritual in Renaissance Florence* (1992); *Nuns and Nunneries in Renaissance Florence* (2009), which received the Marraro Prize from the American Catholic Historical Association; the edited volume *Women and Healthcare in Early Modern Europe (special issue of Renaissance Studies, 2014);* the co-edited volume (with Sara Ritchey)*, Gender, Health, and Healing, 1250-1550* (2020), which won the Collaborative Project Award from the Society for the Study of Early Modern Women and Gender; and the multi-award winning book, *Forgotten Healers: Women and the Pursuit of Health in Late Renaissance Italy* (2019). Her current book project examines the commercialization of medical remedies in Italy between 1550 and 1650.

MICHAEL STOLBERG was trained as a physician but also holds a PhD in history and philosophy. After two years as a research fellow in Tuscany, he spent six years as an assistant professor at the Institute for the History of Medicine and Medical Sociology in Munich. Various research grants then took him to Venice, Cambridge (England) and Munich until 2004, when he took up the chair in the History of Medicine in Würzburg, Germany, which he held for 20 years. Since the spring of 2024, he is senior professor at the University of Würzburg. He has published widely on learned medical theory and practice, the patient experience and body history in early modern Europe. His major publications include the books *Experiencing Illness and the Sick Body in Early Modern Europe* (2011), *Uroscopy in Early Modern Europe, 1500-1800* (2015), *A History of Palliative Care, 1500-1970. Concepts, Practices, and Ethical Problems* (2017), *Learned Physicians and Everyday Medical Practice in the Renaissance* (2022) and, most recently, *Gabrielle Falloppia (1522/23-1562). The Life and Works of a Renaissance Anatomist* (2023).

Index